Fine-Needle Biopsy of Superficial and Deep Masses

G. Gherardi

Fine-Needle Biopsy of Superficial and Deep Masses

Interventional Approach and Interpretation Methodology by Pattern Recognition

Forewords by
David B. Kaminsky
Sergio Fiaccavento

Springer

Giorgio Gherardi, MD
Head, Institute of Anatomic Pathology and Cytopathology
Fatebenefratelli Hospital, Milan, Italy
Professor, Postgraduate School of Anatomic Pathology
University of Milan, Italy
giorgio.gherardi@fbf.milano.it

Chapter 7 has been written in collaboration with:
Stefania Rossi, MD
Division of Pathology, Department of Medicine,
Surgery, and Dentistry, University of Milan,
AO San Paolo and Fondazione IRCCS Ospedale Maggiore Policlinico
Regina Elena e Mangiagalli
Milan, Italy

ISBN 978-88-470-1432-9 e-ISBN 978-88-470-1433-6

DOI 10.1007/978-88-470-1433-6

Springer Dordrecht Heidelberg London Milan New York

Library of Congress Control Number: 2009931758

Cover design: Simona Colombo, Milan, Italy

Typesetting: Compostudio, Cernusco s/N (Milan), Italy
Printing and binding: Printer Trento S.r.l., Trento, Italy
Printed in Italy

Springer-Verlag Italia S.r.l, Via Decembrio 28, I-20137 Milan, Italy
Springer is part of Springer Science+Business Media (www.springer.com)

To my sons Sergio, Andrea, and Dario
and to Stefania, for her encouragement and support

Foreword

This innovative monograph by Dr. Giorgio Gherardi deconstructs the box that has, for too long, confined the safe, conventional perspective on aspiration biopsy, releasing a turbo-mechanism for its modernization. In an evolving world of targeted therapies, nanotechnologies, high definition digital imaging, genetic engineering and minimally invasive interventional procedures, aspiration biopsy prevails as an instrument of change and stability. Its efficacy has been justified scientifically, economically and socially, but its capacity has yet to be fully exposed and celebrated.

The twenty-first century demands that the pathologist who is integral to mysteries of disease transitions to the clinical interface as consultant, care provider and gatekeeper of the diminutive specimen and the triage processes which maximize extraction of its scientific information. Aspiration biopsy facilitates the cellular microcosmic panorama of deviation, targeted therapy and cure while uniting subspecialty disciplines in a process of collaborative care-giving. Dr. Gherardi promotes evolution of the niche pathologist to the interventionalist, inspiring within him or her emergence of the complete physician by encouraging pre-analytical evaluation of the patient, re-describing a customized approach to biopsy technique and sample triage for ancillary studies as prelude to interpretation.

Pathologists are becoming competent in ultrasonography for image-guided sampling and familiar with CT and MRI for tracing the needle through a trajectory to the target lesion. Radiologists and pathologists are fusing specialties mediated by acquisition, interpretation and archiving of digital images. Moreover, pathologists are interfacing with patients regarding their disease processes and take an active role in communication, education and therapy decisions. The book re-energizes the intellectual assessment of aspirated samples by redirecting critical thought processes to pattern profiling as the core of criteria-based decisions taking pattern recognition to new cognitive heights. Pattern profiling is central to each chapter and carries the intention of promoting reproducibility and limiting inter-observer variance. Trusted criteria and evidence-based information are re-formatted to achieve a visual thrust, a new awakening, a reaffirmation of vows in a technique that has revolutionized medicine worldwide. Aspiration biopsy, like cinema, is driven by its images as a common language that breaks international barriers and cultural differences.

Palm Springs, July 2009

David B. Kaminsky, *MD, FIAC*
Past President, American Society of Cytopathology
and Papanicolaou Awardee
Palm Springs Pathology Services
Palm Springs, CA, USA

Foreword

It has been my great pleasure to read Dr. Gherardi's monograph, first of all because the information conveyed in the text and images is in great concordance with my own personal experience, acquired over many years, in the practice of cytopathology. In particular, I appreciated the prominence given by the author to the issues of sampling and specimen triage, and to the importance of the active involvement of the pathologist in the diagnostic process. Although the latter is crucial to the success of the procedure, pathologists too often neglect the role they are expected to play in this aspect of patient management. In addition, as Dr. Gherardi stresses in the book, in order to continue to favorably compare with other, more invasive diagnostic procedures in daily clinical practice, fine-needle aspiration biopsy must be based upon a rigorous abidance of well-defined diagnostic algorithms. The accuracy of the text and accompanying images shows that the author has acquired his knowledge on the job, i.e., practically and not only theoretically, including extensive experience in correlating biopsy findings with the related histological ones. This is evident in each chapter.

I truly hope that this wealth of information–which is not restricted to the field of diagnostic cytopathology–is taken advantage of not only by pathologists in training but also by other specialists, thus promoting better awareness of the need for a multidisciplinary approach to improve the clinical impact of cytological diagnosis. There is no doubt that this multidisciplinary approach should begin as early as possible, i.e., from the moment of sampling the lesion, and continue until the diagnosis is reached and the therapeutic strategy decided upon.

Brescia, July 2009

***Sergio Fiaccavento**, MD*
Cytopathology Unit,
Istituto Clinico Città di Brescia,
Brescia, Italy

Preface

By definition, fine-needle biopsy (FNB) is a diagnostic procedure employing needles of small caliber that are inserted into superficial and deep-seated masses to collect, at each pass, a minimal amount of cellular sample from the lesion under investigation. The harvest is acquired with or without aspiration, and it is smeared onto a glass slide or processed for histological examination. In some cases, the use of larger-caliber and cutting needles may be required to provide a core of tissue whose histological evaluation can assist in the diagnostic process. Direct smears, cell blocks, and cores represent the diagnostic yield of FNB and they provide the pathologist with a potentially enormous amount of diagnostic information that in most cases is expected to lead, in experienced hands and in the proper context, to a reliable and tissue-equivalent diagnosis.

The field of application of FNB is the diagnosis of malignant tumors and their simulants. Nowadays, oncological treatment is becoming decreasingly destructive in surgical terms and increasingly aimed at pharmacological and patient-tailored therapies. Remarkable advances in our understanding of neoplastic progression at the cellular and molecular levels have also spurred the discovery of molecularly targeted drugs. Genomic profiling is increasingly able to allow the re-classification of cancers into new molecularly and prognostically homogeneous subgroups. In future scenarios–which already exist for some types of malignancies–the determination of molecular predictors of response will play a decisive role in defining the first line of therapy administered to the patient, with the goal of improving efficacy and maximizing the possibility of long-term control. Moreover, the discovery of molecularly targeted drugs has recently encouraged their use in patients with advanced stages of disease, with promising results.

What role for pathological diagnosis can be expected in these future scenarios? Obviously, the diagnosis of malignancy will continue to be the essential requisite for treatment and, at least for many years to come, it will be based on the consideration and proper evaluation of morphological findings. The major difference from the past, however, will be that the higher number of solid tumors amenable to first-line pharmacological therapy will result in a smaller number of tumor specimens available for pathological diagnosis, because surgical excision of the tumor will no longer represent the first event in the management of a patient with an early-stage tumor. In addition, in order to verify their possible candidacy for targeted therapies, patients presenting with advanced and inoperable disease will require a more precise and detailed tissue diagnosis than previously deemed necessary. In summary, pathologists will be faced with an ever decreasing amount of cellular material collected for tumor diagnosis and for the determination of selected biomarkers that indicate the most appropriate therapeutic regimen.

Based on these considerations, FNB is likely to experience a renaissance in its utilization in the near future. FNB gained a considerable popularity in the 1980s in the USA and in Europe, as a consequence of a significant tumor burden in those populations and the correlative escalating financial costs for disease management. Despite the initial skepticism of the medical community, the recognition of the practical advantages of FNB and its cost effectiveness led to the development of a generation of pathologists who were confident in the interpretation of such minimal cellular samples and, no less importantly, in the sampling procedure. This was a short-lived event, as problems of different kinds eventually discouraged pathologist-performed FNB. Instead, the trend reverted to the preference for incisional or excisional surgical biopsy for the diagnosis of many types of tumors. As a consequence, expertise in cytological sample interpretation and recruitment declined. Indeed, in several diverse clinical settings, pathologists eventually ignored their duty to provide the patient with the most reliable diagnosis, with the least patient discomfort, and at the lowest cost. Times are changing, however, and the need for reliable tissue-equivalent diagnosis as the first step in any decision regarding oncological treatment in patients presenting with early- or late-stage disease will soon become increasingly compelling in daily practice. Accordingly, pathologists must be prepared for these new developments.

The aim of this monograph is to testify to the applicability of FNB in these clinical settings, with the wider ambition of suggesting a relatively novel approach to tumor diagnosis. In fact, the conventional approach of many textbooks published so far concerning the practice of FNB has been to describe the cytopathological picture starting from the end, i.e., the lesion as it appears in histological preparations. This book offers the alternate approach of starting from the very beginning of the diagnostic work-up, i.e., a morphological evaluation of the specimen in the given case, and provides criteria to classify all observations according to a reliable and reproducible pattern-profiling approach. Pattern recognition is central to diagnostic reasoning in this field of pathology and assists the observer in identifying the list of possible diagnoses matching the detected profile. Once the major pattern has been identified, the diagnostic possibilities are dramatically reduced. In some cases, there will be an unequivocal correspondence between a given pattern and a disease entity, while in others multiple pathological entities can match the observed pattern profile. In the former situation, the predictive value of the morphological pattern per se is very high and a definite diagnosis can be released. In the latter situation, detecting the correct pattern helps one to identify a list of possible diagnostic alternatives, each expressed in probabilistic terms. In this context, the predictive value of the morphological pattern for a specific disease entity can be enhanced by properly considering pre-analytical data and/or by including additional findings obtained from ancillary techniques, thus reaching a sufficiently high predictive value. The addition of new data to pattern profiling brings order to a group of lesions whose least common denominator is a specific cytomorphological pattern. In summary, one can vastly simplify the cytopathological investigation and more critically express the real possibility that the given sample matches a specific diagnosis.

In the book, the classical cytology of breast carcinoma and its simulants, of thyroid nodular lesions, and of malignant lymphomas have been revisited under a pattern-profiling approach, with the aim of introducing reproducibility as much as possible in this field of pathology, which is still dominated by subjectivity. Moreover, a common pattern-recognition approach is described for most tumors and pseudotumors encountered in abdominal and intrathoracic sites, with the hope that it represents a useful key to interpret all possible morphological findings. A decision tree is subsequently described such that, when possible, a conclusive diagnosis can be reached. Last but not least in importance is an initial chapter in which some of the basic modalities of what I call "interventional cytology" and the most useful procedures for sample triage are reviewed. Central to the book is the belief that the pathologist, who is not a niche expert but rather a complete physician with distinguished wide-ranging abilities, should be involved not only in interpreting the cellular harvest but to an equal extent also in the sampling procedure and in the pre-analytical evaluation of the patient.

I am unusually indebted to several gifted teachers and friends who have inspired and guided me in more than 20 years of practice of FNB sampling and interpretation. I would like to thank Torsten Lowhagen, MD, FIAC (1929-1999) for introducing me to the "language" of fine needle aspiration cytology and David B. Kaminsky, MD, FIAC for hosting me several times in his Department. I am grateful to the numerous cytotechnologists who have supported me with their patience, professionalism, and assistance (in alphabetical order, D. Battarino, G. Cirillo, A. Jannacci, M. Tirabasso) and to the histotechnology staff, headed by Ms. O. Senesi, for their competent support. My special thanks go also to C. Marveggio, BD, F. Bianchi, MD, A. Croce, MD, for their suggestions and advice, to S. Perrone, MD, and F. Silva, MD, for their enthusiastic cooperation and incredible radiological talent, and to all the Oncologists and Surgeons in my Institution who strongly believe in the advantages of the FNB procedure for their patients. Finally, I am immensely grateful to Stefania Rossi, MD, who coauthored Chapter 7, for her invaluable suggestions and advice, as well as for her helpful and understanding support.

Milan, July 2009 ***Giorgio Gherardi***

Contents

1 Methods

1.1 Sampling

1.1.1 The Interventional Pathologist

An interventional approach by the pathologist is essential for the success of fine-needle biopsy (FNB) [1-14]. FNB is a reliable, inexpensive, minimally invasive diagnostic procedure that is immediately repeatable and very well-tolerated by the patient. However, its success depends totally upon the capacity of the physician performing the procedure to reach the target, collect a representative sample, and, finally, optimally exploit the cellular sample for proper ancillary investigations. In other words, FNB is extremely operator-dependent, which represents a great limitation that has thus far negatively impacted potential diffusion of the procedure in many clinical contexts. In addition, inadequate or poor-quality samples have prevented pathologists from developing sufficient experience in the interpretation of cytological findings, thereby further undermining the popularity of FNB.

In any clinical scenario, FNB has no chance of implementation and widespread acceptance if the task of sampling is assigned to physicians who are not well-aware of all the critical issues concerning adequacy, representativity, and processing of cytological specimens. In fact, it is well-known that, with few exceptions, surgeons, endocrinologists, radiologists, and clinicians without specialized education and training are not able to provide FNB samples of the same high quality as obtained by experienced pathologists. Ljung et al., 2001 [1], clearly demonstrated that physicians with formal training in the techniques of FNB sampling are able to achieve much more accurate diagnostic results than physicians without such training, and, not surprisingly, differences in the tumor detection rate are greatly due to errors in sampling the lesion. Pathologists are likely to obtain even better results than clinicians well-trained in FNB sampling [2,7–9,11,13,14]. This is not related to presumed superior manual skills but rather to two additional key factors. First, the pathologist's interaction with the patient, the radiologist, and/or the clinicians in charge, and his or her access to all available clinical data elicit a relevant history and allow for more precise focusing of the specific clinical question. Second, a better knowledge of the intrinsic submacroscopic and microscopic features of solid tumors, which derives from training in surgical pathology, allows the pathologist to select the most appropriate modality for sampling the lesion in order to provide the best and most reliable answer to the clinical question. The close interaction of pathologists with clinicians has a highly positive impact on patient outcome [2,8,12–14]. A further consequence of collaboration and shared responsibilities is that the attending staff intervenes in a more prudent and conservative fashion, which, in turn, promotes cost containment. In addition, pathologists are better able to provide a patient-oriented report that facilitates the decision-making process.

1.1.2 Preanalyitical Evaluation and Requirements

To carry out the procedure of FNB, complete knowledge of the clinical features of the lesion to be investigated and of the results of imaging and laboratory investigations is required. This is essential to focus on the clinical problem, plan additional ancillary and complementary tests, and decide on the most appropriate type of samples to be obtained (smears, or

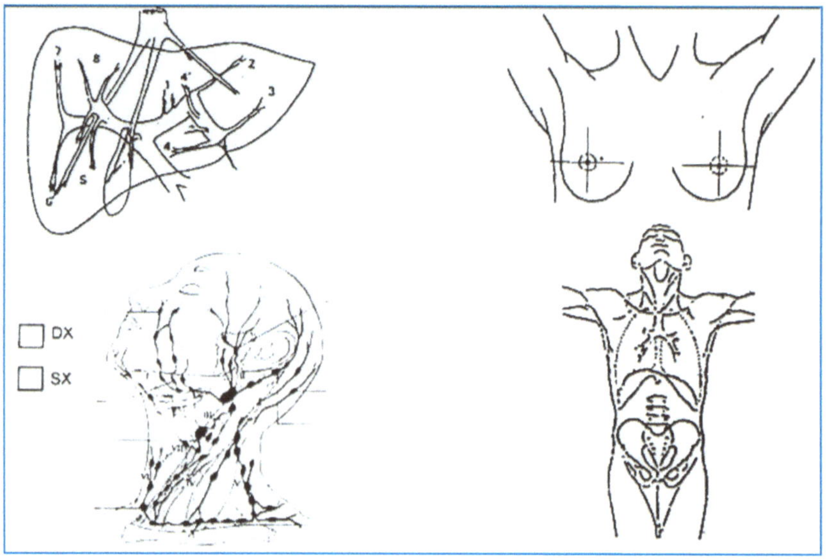

Fig. 1.1 Images printed on the request form help to better identify the site of the lesion

smears and a cell-block from needle rinse, and/or a core-needle tissue specimen) to fully satisfy the clinical need. Additional pre-FNB requirements are the results of coagulation tests and the acquisition of informed consent from the patient. Abnormal coagulation test results predict bleeding in the setting of FNB of deep-seated lesions and thus contraindicate the procedure.

Proper outline of the clinical problem can be obtained by using a detailed request form that includes basic information in terms of imaging or clinical data or regarding laboratory tests carried out prior to the procedure. A problem-oriented questionnaire can be set up locally and then systematically filled in for each case. Images printed on the request form help to better identify the site of the lesion(s) (Fig. 1.1). Accurate knowledge of the imaging features of the lesion is essential to anticipate whether the sample is expected to be semi-solid, liquid, hemorrhagic, or necrotic, in order to plan the site of needle sampling within the lesion and the best procedures for proper sample processing. It is also essential to plan the best and most appropriate procedure for additional sampling, if required. For example, in the investigation of a deep-seated mass, if a core-needle biopsy (CNB) is contraindicated due to anatomic reasons, one can decide to plan additional passes using fine needles to obtain a sample from the needle rinse that is sufficient for a cell-block preparation, which is a good alternative to a core-needle tissue specimen.

1.1.3 Needles

The caliber of needles used for collecting cellular samples to be processed for preparation of direct smears, smears from cytocentrifugation, or conventional centrifugation is between 23G and 27G (Figs. 1.2, 1.3) [15–18]. The external diameter of these needles varies, respectively, between 0.65 and 0.35 mm, and their internal lumina between 0.31 and 0.16 mm. The size of the needle is small enough to allow for its insertion without local anesthesia, which, however, is administered when needles of a larger caliber are used. The needle tract produced by a probe ≤23G is minute, inflicts minimal trauma, and avoids the induction of bleeding. The diameter of the internal

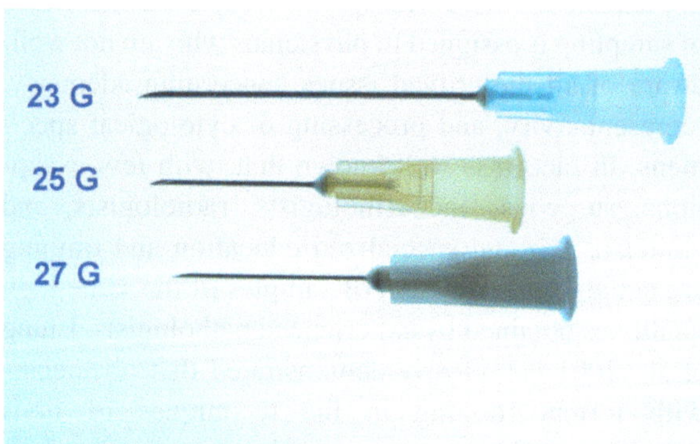

Fig. 1.2 Most commonly employed fine needles for sampling superficial masses

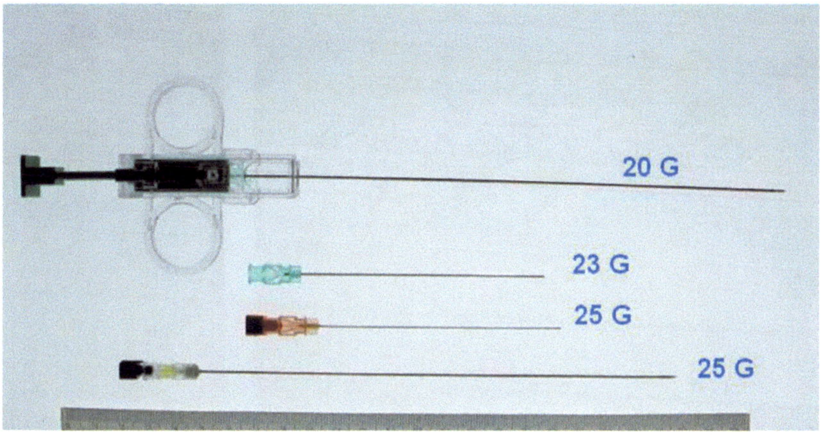

Fig. 1.3 Long fine needles employed for sampling deep-seated masses. A core-needle biopsy device is seen at the top

lumen of the needle is large enough to accommodate complex tissue structures without compromising their integrity (for example, a thyroid follicle whose diameter is, on average, not more than 200 µm) [18]. The needle used for biopsy sampling should be long and beveled, with a narrow angle. The narrower the angle (9° is an average value), the more effective the guillotine-like effect of the trailing edge with respect to tissue cells during harvesting while the needle is advanced forwards (Fig. 1.2). The cellular yield is maintained within the needle lumen by a combination of forward movement of the needle and the suction-like tension induced by capillary action. The smaller the diameter of the needle, the greater its suction effect. Moreover, the small angle of the bevel prevents the needle from becoming occluded during sampling. The smaller the caliber of the needle, the lower the risk of intralesional hemorrhage and blood contamination of the sample. Finally, the maneuver should be performed fast enough to allow expulsion of the cellular harvest before blood within the needle core starts to coagulate.

Proper needle choice is crucial to the success of the procedure. In general, for *superficial masses* small-caliber needles (27G) are used for the first pass, while larger-caliber needles (25G and 23G) are used for additional passes. *Deep-seated lesions* are best sampled using needles ranging between 25G and 22G. *Cystic lesions* are sampled and evacuated with a single pass using a 22G needle. The length of the needle is an additional crucial parameter, and it can vary between 1.5 and 20–25 cm (Fig. 1.3). Longer needles contain a removable mandrel that prevents penetration of tissue fragments or blood into the needle lumen before the target is reached. The mandrel is subsequently removed and the syringe inserted at the base of the needle.

1.1.4 Aspiration vs. Non-Aspiration Technique

Tissue sampling of a solid mass can be performed either with or without aspiration. Aspiration is carried out by connecting the needle to a syringe and by imparting a vacuum within it (Fig. 1.4). On average, a vacuum of no more than 2–5 mL is required for successful sampling. The amount of negative pressure should reach a maximum and remain unmodified during the procedure, then reduced to zero before needle removal. Various aspiration devices are commercially available. They allow the operator to direct the needle into the target and to supply negative pressure with one hand and, with the other hand, to immobilize the target, assess the depth of needle penetration, and feel the needle as it moves within the lesion [15–18]. Sampling of superficial masses, however, is better performed without aspiration using the so-called Zajdola technique [19]. In practice, the needle is directly inserted percutaneously by the operator into the target. A bare needle is used without a syringe or suction devices (Fig. 1.5). It is moved backward and forward and partly rotated like a screwdriver until the collected specimen appears in the hub of the needle (Fig. 1.5). This procedure provides a surprisingly abundant cellular harvest when employed to sample palpable nodular lesions of the breast, salivary glands, and enlarged lymph nodes [20–23].

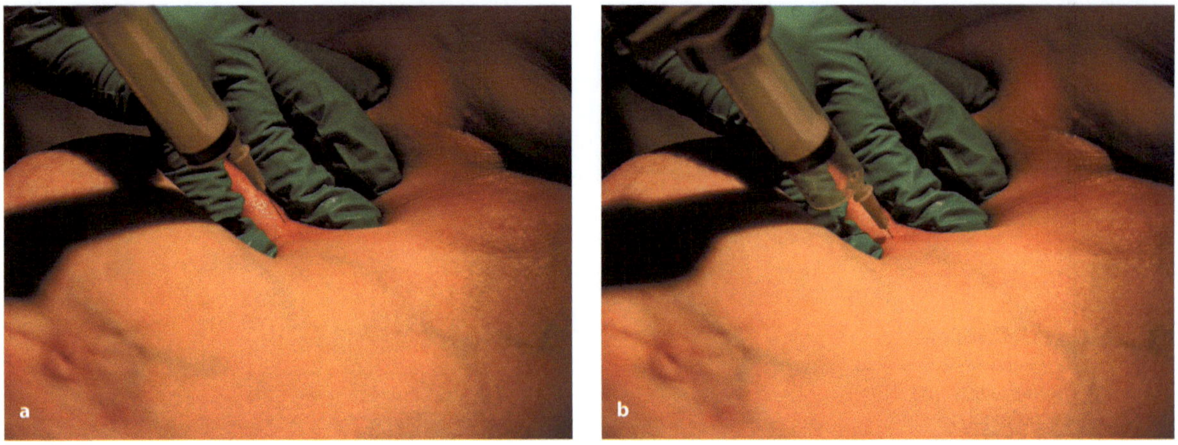

Fig. 1.4 **a** Sampling maneuver using the aspiration technique. The palpable nodule is immobilized between the operator's two fingers. **b** Once the needle has reached the target, vacuum is induced by retracting the plunger

In addition, blood contamination of the sample is minimal. At the end of the procedure, the needle is immediately removed from the target and quickly inserted into a syringe, which serves as an expulsion device for depositing the harvest onto the surface of a glass slide. The non-aspiration technique is slightly disappointing in terms of the amount of specimen recruited from thyroid lesions and, in general, from nodular lesions that contain a desmoplastic stroma (for example, lobular carcinoma of the breast, sclerotic lymph nodes due to lymphoma sclerosis, etc.). In sampling nodular masses of the breast or salivary glands or enlarged and palpable lymph nodes, the operator should start with the non-aspiration technique and, if required, change to the aspiration procedure. Generally, however, a thorough sampling of these lesions is accomplished by the non-aspiration technique and, in most cases, with two to three passes.

1.1.5 Core-Needle Biopsy Devices

A needle biopsy device comprises a suction source, an inner cannula having a biopsy reservoir, and an outer cannula (outer blade) that can be slid along the inner cannula (Fig. 1.3). The latter has a cutter at its distal end. The caliber of the needle is between 19G and 21G. An actuating mechanism is available for moving the outer cannula from the distal position to the proximal position and vice versa. Moving the outer cannula from the distal position to the proximal position causes the tissue sample to be pulled into the biopsy reservoir included in the inner cannula. Moving the outer cannula from the proximal position to the distal position causes the cutter to cut the tissue sample from the surrounding tissue and also captures the tissue sample within the biopsy reservoir. There are several types of spring-loaded, core biopsy, single-action or double action devices. Single-action spring-activated needle devices are believed to result in less trauma. It is also important that the stylet tip does not advance further into the specimen during the cutting action. The core-needle biopsy is obtained only for lesions 1–3 mm deeper than the pre-triggering cutting notch, which represents a limitation because the sampling of small and/or superficial lesions is precluded.

1.1.6 Sampling Procedures

The modalities for sample collection differ depending on whether the lesion is palpable or not. A palpable nodule can be readily immobilized between the forefinger and the middle finger of the operator by applying light pressure on the skin [15]. For thyroid lesions, the patient is asked to swallow several times before the procedure begins, thereby preventing involuntary movement of the lesion. Muscular relaxation is required for sampling superficial lymph nodes in the neck or axilla. It is best to talk to the patient and keep him/her informed of the progress of the biopsy. If the

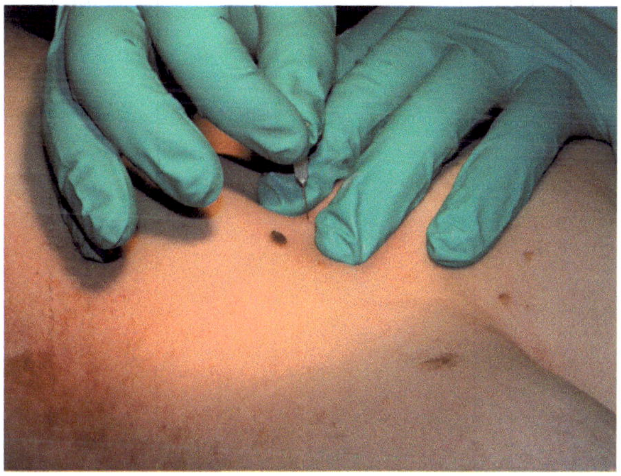

Fig. 1.5 Sampling maneuver using the non-aspiration technique

non-aspiration technique is employed, the needle should penetrate the lesion in a vertical position and moved within the lesion under the visual guidance of the operator (Fig. 1.5). The maneuver is immediately interrupted just about at the time when the sample appears at the hub of the needle. Generally, the best sample in terms of representativity and minimal fluid or blood contamination is obtained when this happens several seconds after needle insertion. The immediate appearance of blood is, instead, a sign of inadequate sampling due to blood contamination. If the aspiration technique is adopted (Fig. 1.4), and the lesion does not contain fluid, a vacuum of no more than 2–5 mL should be induced in the syringe by retracting the plunger. The maneuver is immediately interrupted as soon as the sample spills out into the hub of the needle. The plunger is rapidly released and the vacuum removed before the needle is withdrawn from the target. The immediate appearance of fluid at the needle hub suggests that the nodule is at least partially cystic in nature; in this case, suction is maintained and all the fluid is aspirated, possibly changing the syringe without removing the needle.

Sampling of non-palpable lesions in superficial or deep locations requires assistance by imaging techniques, namely, ultrasound or CT scan. The former is used to guide sampling of non-palpable lesions in superficial sites and for deep-seated lesions within the abdomen. The latter is best indicated for sampling intrathoracic lesions. In some cases, ultrasound can be used also for these lesions, provided that the tumor mass is adherent to the thoracic wall and can be visualized through the intercostal musculature. Ultrasound allows for real-time monitoring of the position of the needle shaft and for adjustment of the needle path to the target. It is used to assist FNB via percutaneous and endoscopic approaches. Collaboration between the radiologist and the pathologist is pivotal to the success of the procedure. In general, the cell yield is within the jurisdiction of the radiologist to provide and the pathologist to evaluate.

Several types of devices are available to assist percutaneous needle placement. These consist of special transducers with needle guide attachments. As an alternative, the "free hand method" [24,25] can be used as it allows the operator to work alone, using one hand to hold the ultrasound probe and the other to guide the needle. In general, however, the procedure is best performed by two operators, namely, the radiologist and the interventional pathologist. If the probe is maintained far from the sterile area of the puncture site, the needle may be introduced on a plane more perpendicular to the ultrasound beam (Fig. 1.6a). It is therefore possible to better visualize the progression of the needle to the target, thus avoiding cumbersome precautions for covering and sterilizing the probe. When the needle tip has reached the target, the mandrel is removed by the second operator and the syringe—which is inserted into the holder—is connected to the needle (Fig. 1.6b). The role of the second operator is to start suction and to impart a backward and forward movement to the syringe holder and the needle within the target under ultrasound guidance (Fig. 1.6c). This has to be done perfectly in tune with the first operator, who introduced the needle into the target and is still holding it. Once the sample spills out into the hub of the needle (Fig. 1.6d), the maneuver is immediately stopped and the needle gently removed. Undoubtedly, the "free hand technique" requires greater operator experience and perfect timing, but it is also time- and cost-effective. The echoendoscopic technique involves the use of an echoendoscope, which is placed into the stomach, duodenum, or trachea. Under the guidance of the high-frequency ultrasound transducer located on the tip of the echoendoscope, a small-gauge needle is passed through the wall of the above-mentioned viscera and into all possible surrounding solid masses. A number of different sized needles are used, ranging in caliber from 25G to 19G.

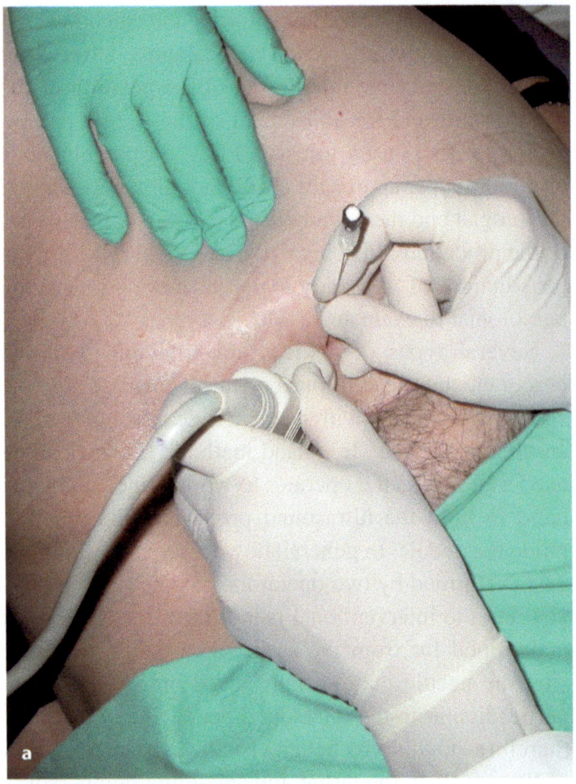

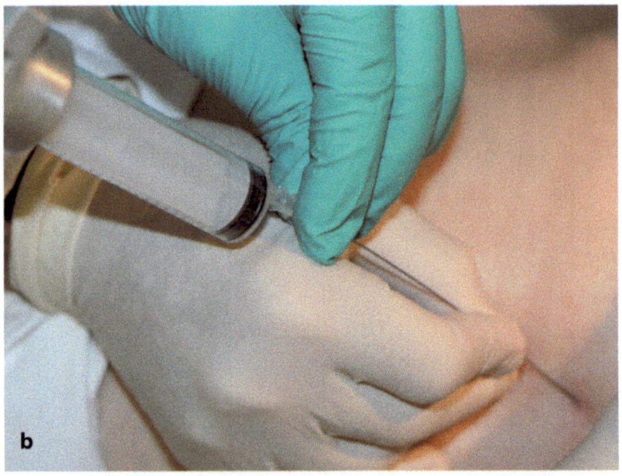

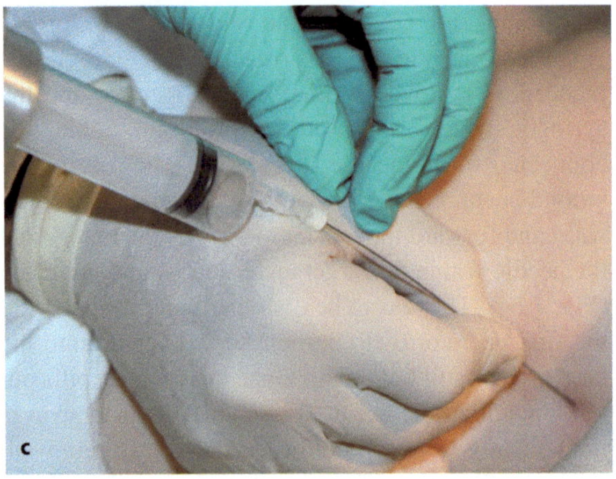

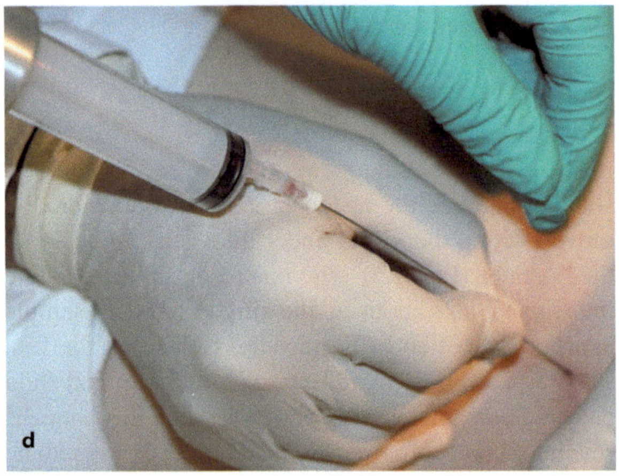

Fig. 1.6 **a** "Free hand" insertion of the needle into a deep mass (a right ovarian tumor in this case) under ultrasound guidance. **b** Once the needle tip has reached the target, the operator (his hand is shown wearing a green glove) connects the syringe to the needle. **c** Vacuum is induced by retracting the plunger and the needle is moved back and forth under ultrasound guidance. **d** Aspiration is interrupted and the plunger released as soon as a semi-solid drop appears in the needle hub

1.2 Specimen Triage

1.2.1 Direct Smears and Smearing Techniques

Optimal smearing is essential for subsequent cytomorphological evaluation. The goal of smear preparation is to spread a semi-solid cellular harvest over a slide, thus achieving a monolayer of isolated or aggregated cells. The smearing procedure should be delicate enough to maintain the semi-cohesive nature of the tissue fragments in order to preserve tissue-specific aggregation patterns; at the same time, it should produce the thinnest cellular monolayer possible.

Several different techniques are used to make smears from aspirates and they vary according to the dilution of the cellular material with fluid. The two-step, one-step, absorption, and watch-glass techniques have been comprehensively described by Abele et al.,

1985 [26]. An excellent explanation of these techniques is available on the internet at the Papanicolaou Society website, under the section "FNA video techniques", http://www.papsociety.org/fna.html. Some of these different procedures for smear preparation deserve a brief comment. With the conventional glass slides used for cytology, the *one-step* method allows a semi-solid drop to be smeared for a length of 20–40 mm and the shape of the smear is approximately oval. The semi-solid sample drop is deposited close to the frosted edge of the stationary slide (Fig. 1.7a), which is held in one hand and angled slightly downward, as seen in Figure 1.7b. The second slide (the smearing slide) is held in the other hand and is slowly moved from above towards the stationary slide and perpendicular to it. The former should touch the latter with its longer edge opposite the sample drop, with an angle of about 45° (Fig. 1.7b). This step of the procedure ends when the longer edge of the smearing slide leans completely against the surface of the stationary slide. At this point, the angle between the two slides is rapidly reduced and the drop begins to spread between the two slides (Fig. 1.7c). The contact between the two slides displaces the semi-solid droplet in a circular monolayer due to surface tension. When the slides are on parallel planes and the sample is spread almost completely, the smearing slide is moved opposite the frosted edge of the stationary slide (Fig. 1.7d) and finally removed. This technique allows for the examination of nearly all the harvest on one slide. The cells in the smears are concentrated within the half proximal to the frosted end of the stationary slide (Fig. 1.7e). A minor part of the harvest remains on the smearing slide and contains cells that are poorly preserved due to excessive smearing artifacts. The main drawbacks of this smearing procedure are the non-homogeneous distribution of the cells within the smear and the partial loss of the cellular harvest. The *pull-apart method* results in two mirror image preparations, one on the stationary slide and the other on the spreader slide, with no cellular loss. Droplets are released at about the center of the stationary slide. The smearing slide is placed in contact with the droplet until the surface tension displaces the liquid as a circular monolayer, thus concentrating the screening area to one side. The smears are separated in a perpendicular direction to avoid smearing the cells and then immediately immersed in 95% ethanol for fixation. The obtained smear appears as a round spot characterized by a higher concentration of cellular fragments at the center (Fig. 1.7f). The main drawback is that the smear may be too thick in some areas, thus precluding proper interpretation. This technique is therefore best applicable to compact semi-solid drops of small volume, such as those obtained by lymph node sampling.

1.2.2 Fixation

Fixation is one of the most crucial aspects of processing the specimen for proper cytomorphological evaluation. Ideal fixation requires that the tissue specimen is fixed immediately after removal and that the interaction of all its components with the fixative is simultaneous and instantaneous. Fixation procedures of smears may consist of immediate immersion in 95% ethanol (Fig. 1.8) or rapid air-drying. Ethanol fixation is followed by staining of the smear using a modified Papanicolaou method, while the air-dried smear is stained with a Romanowsky stain. Ethanol fixation can be accomplished by spray fixation, which is dependent on the alcohol content in the spray, but in no way does it provide the same results as obtained with immersion in liquid ethanol solution for 5–10 min. Air-drying of smears does not require expertise but it must be instantaneous and its effectiveness is inversely proportional to the thickness of the smear.

1.2.3 Cytospin Preparation

Cytocentrifugation of the residual needle rinse is a convenient procedure to be performed when possible after the preparation of direct smears. It provides additional slides that can be used immediately or frozen banked [27]. We do not cytocentrifuge the harvest as a primary procedure because the preparation of direct smears bears the advantage of speed and convenience. The procedure of cytocentrifugation is responsible for a delay in fixation and a partial modification of cellular aggregation patterns. While the former disadvantage is minimized by rinsing the harvest in appropriate tissue culture medium, any modification of the image quality of the cells in their arrangement and in their spatial relationship to each other can preclude correct cytomorphological interpretation of the harvest.

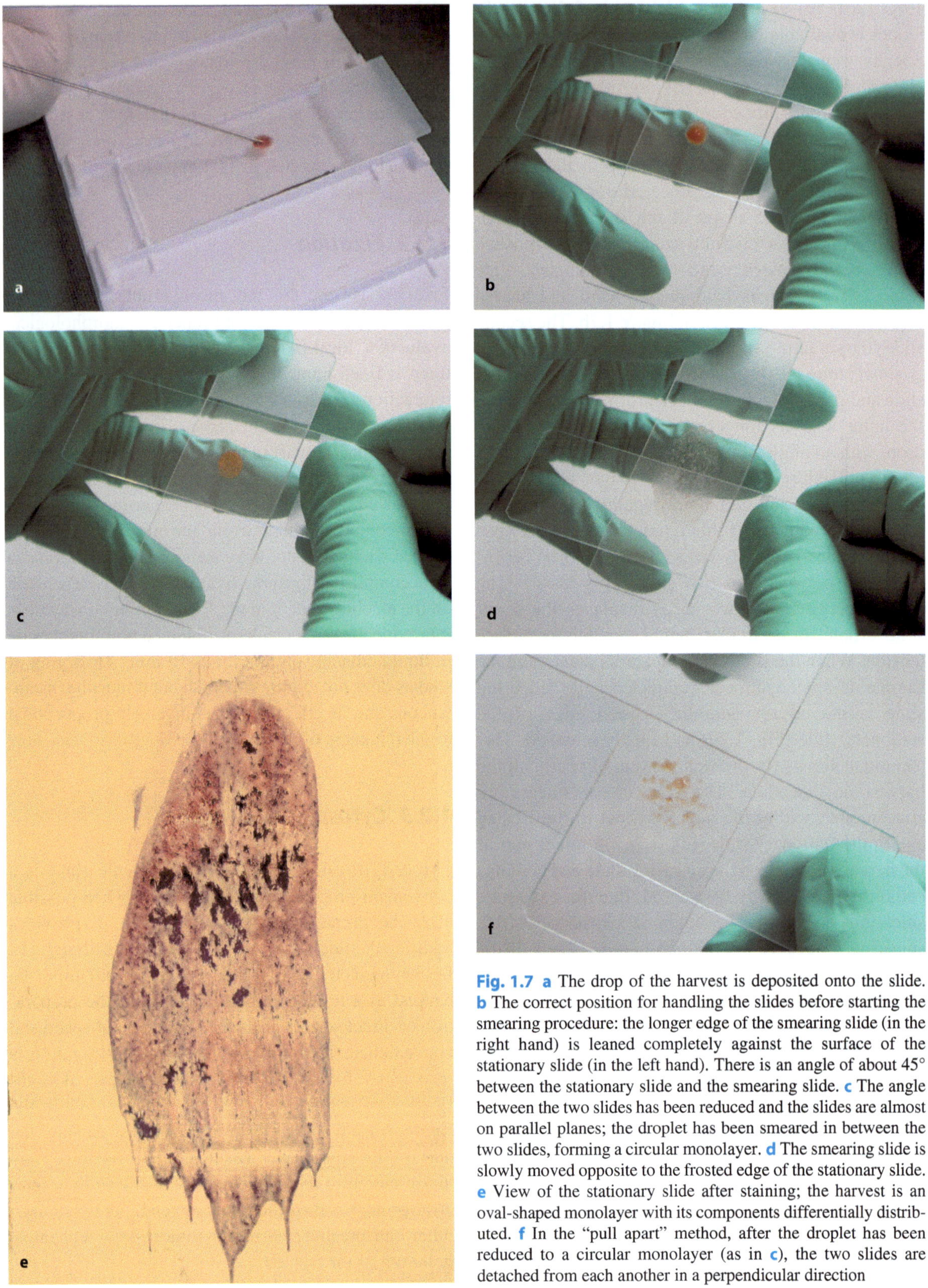

Fig. 1.7 **a** The drop of the harvest is deposited onto the slide. **b** The correct position for handling the slides before starting the smearing procedure: the longer edge of the smearing slide (in the right hand) is leaned completely against the surface of the stationary slide (in the left hand). There is an angle of about 45° between the stationary slide and the smearing slide. **c** The angle between the two slides has been reduced and the slides are almost on parallel planes; the droplet has been smeared in between the two slides, forming a circular monolayer. **d** The smearing slide is slowly moved opposite to the frosted edge of the stationary slide. **e** View of the stationary slide after staining; the harvest is an oval-shaped monolayer with its components differentially distributed. **f** In the "pull apart" method, after the droplet has been reduced to a circular monolayer (as in **c**), the two slides are detached from each another in a perpendicular direction

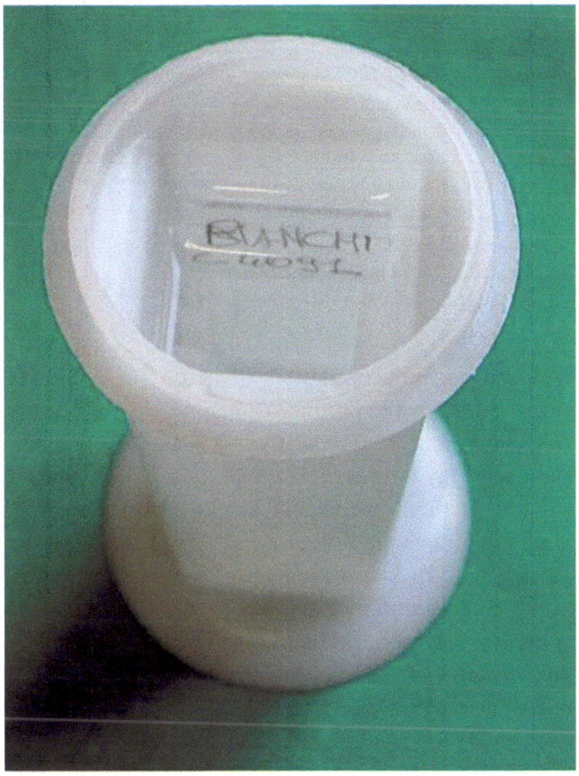

Fig. 1.8 The slide should be immediately immersed in ethanol

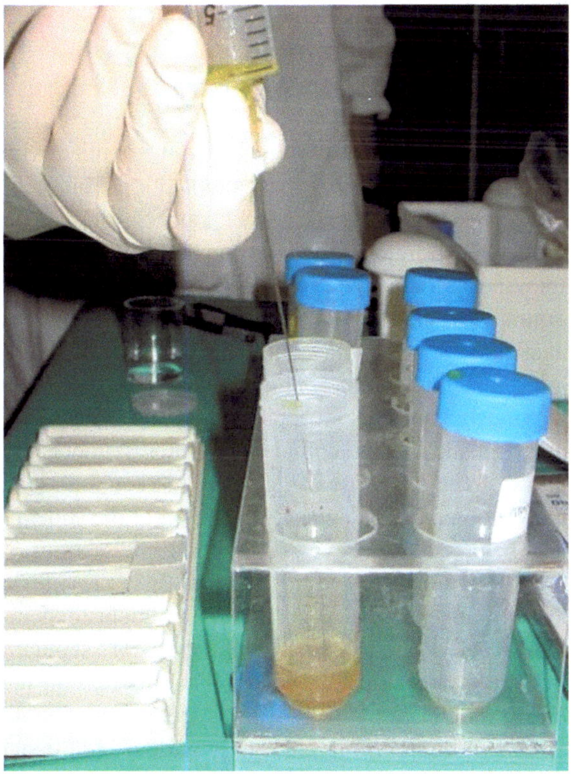

Fig. 1.9 The residual material within the needle is rinsed using saline or diluted Bouin's fixative

1.2.4 Cell-Block Preparation

Preparation of a cell block from a needle rinse is highly advisable and absolutely indicated when sampling deep-seated masses. This type of sample provides an invaluable substrate for multiple immunostains, and in some cases it is a source of additional data for morphological evaluation [27]. After the sample has been deposited on the slide for smearing, the residual material within the needle is rinsed using saline or diluted Bouin's fixative (Fig. 1.9). The cell block is prepared after the cells have been concentrated in a small volume sample by centrifugation and by the additional coagulative and precipitating effect of methanol-acetic acid or Bouin's fixative. Fixation in 10% buffered formalin provides optimal results as well. Evaluation of the gross features of the harvest after the first pass should govern the most proper triage for further specimen processing. In fact, if the harvest looks frankly contaminated by blood, the needle content of the second pass should be entirely rinsed in saline solution and treated for a cell-block preparation. In sampling deep-seated lesions, the operator should plan at least one pass for smear preparation and one for needle rinse, in addition to performing a CNB (Fig. 1.10).

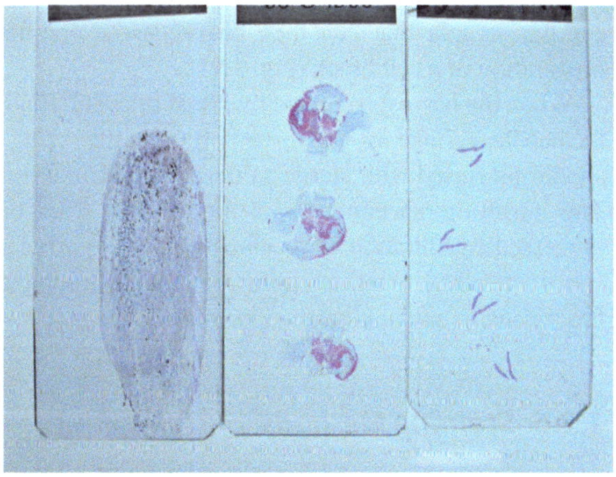

Fig. 1.10 In sampling deep-seated masses, the goal is to obtain smeared material for cytological evaluation (*left*), paraffin sections from the cell block of the needle rinse (*middle*), and paraffin sections from a core biopsy (*right*)

1.2.5 Direct Smear vs. Cell-Block Preparation for Immunohistochemistry

Immunocytochemical techniques can be applied with optimal results to both smear preparations and cell-block paraffin sections. Direct smears provide an excellent substrate, qualitatively and quantitatively, for immunostaining. The preservation of antigenicity is optimal and the complete content of cellular antigen is available for immunodetection, because the entire cell is present for immunostaining. Immunostaining of a previously Papanicolaou-stained direct smear is easily accomplished using automatic immunostainers and allows for the detection of a given marker following conventional morphological evaluation of the slide. In routine practice, however, cutting multiple sections of a cell block prepared from a needle rinse provides a larger number of slides for testing immunohistochemical reactivities and the application of standard immunohistochemical protocols. For this reason, the preparation of a cell block from a needle rinse should always be attempted in order to provide an additional cellular substrate for immunohistochemistry studies. This protocol promotes simplicity, reproducibility of the test, and maximization of the diagnostic yield. Preliminary and immediate examination of direct smears stained with the preferred rapid stain allows for judicious selection of those cases that require clarification by immunological testing. If the need for immunoprocessing is anticipated, additional passes may also be performed to obtain a more abundant cellular sample that can then be processed for the preparation of a cell block (Fig. 1.9).

When the harvest is diluted by blood or cystic fluid, the needle, syringe tip, and distal portion of the syringe should be rinsed with sterile saline or liquid fixative. The resulting specimen is a liquid that can be processed by filtration, cytocentrifugation, or whole-specimen centrifugation followed by histological processing to obtain paraffin mini-blocks.

1.2.6 Staining Methods

The best staining methods for routine conventional cytomorphological evaluation of smears are the Romanowsky and the Papanicolaou methods. *Romanowsky stains* are a mixture of methylene blue with varying concentrations of azure A, B, and C. Eosin Y is added to produce a "neutral" dye. The most frequently used Romanowsky type stains are Wright's stain and May Grünwald Giemsa stain. The respective staining methods are widely employed in hematological preparations and require fixation of the smear by air-drying [27]. The reagents used provide differential staining of acidophilic and basophilic substances. In addition, polymeric macromolecules such as proteoglycans induce a purple tone to basophilic substances due to metachromasia. The classical May Grünwald Giemsa stain is included in Table 1.1 [27].

Table 1.1 Modified May-Grünwald Giemsa stain for air-dried smears[a]

Step	Reagent/procedure	Time (min)
1	May-Grünwald solution	5
2	Running water	1
3	Giemsa solution	15
4	Running water	1–2
5	Air dry and mount	

[a]The staining procedure may vary somewhat and testing is recommended for optimal results.

The *Papanicolaou stain* has been adopted from exfoliative cytology and requires ethanol fixation of the sample. The substrate is stained pink or blue, respectively, according to acidophilia and basophilia. The reagents are similar to those employed in the hematoxylin and eosin (H&E) protocol for paraffin sections of tissue histological samples–except for the addition of EA50, which stains some protein substances orange, such as keratin. The classical Papanicolaou staining procedure and its modified rapid version are included in Table 1.2 [28].

Selection of one of the above staining procedures is based on the observer's own preferences, depending on his or her scientific or professional education. In general, the May Grünwald Giemsa stain is preferred by cytopathologists with hematological training while the Papanicolaou stain is preferred by surgical pathologists. Nonetheless, there are significant differences between the two methods (Table 1.3). Specifically, in air-dried smears there is a relative expansion of the nuclear and cytoplasmic compartments and perfect preservation of the intracellular and extracellular chemical components. Cells thus appear larger than in Papanicolaou-stained smears, and both the cytoplasmic details and the morphological features of the extracellular substances are well seen. Nuclear

Table 1.2 Papanicolaou stains for ethanol-fixed smears

Step	Reagent	Time/procedure
Papanicolaou stain		
1	95% ethanol	Minimum 15 min
2	80% ethanol	10 dips
3	70% ethanol	10 dips
4	50% ethanol	10 dips
5	Tap water	1 min
6	Gill's hematoxylin	2 min
7	Tap water	Rinse until clear
8	0.05% HCl	Rinse until yellow
9	Tap water	Rinse
10	Scott's tap water	Rinse until blueing
11	Tap water	Rinse
12	50% ethanol	10 dips
13	70% ethanol	10 dips
14	80% ethanol	10 dips
15	95% ethanol	1 min
16	Orange G stain	90 s
17	Ethanol 95% (3 dishes)	10 dips each
18	EA stain	2 min
19	95% ethanol (3 dishes)	10 dips each
20	100% absolute isopropyl alcohol (2 dishes)	1 min each
21	Xylene	Minimum 10 min
Rapid Papanicolaou stain		
1	95% ethanol	Minimum 3 min
2	70% ethanol	10 dips
3	Running tap water	5 dips
4	Gill II hematoxylin	30 s
5	Running tap water	5 dips
6	70% ethanol	10 dips
7	95% ethanol	10 dips
8	Orange G stain	15 s
9	95% ethanol	10 dips
10	95% ethanol	10 dips
11	EA 50 stain	15 s
12	95% ethanol	10 dips
13	95% ethanol	10 dips
14	100% ethanol	10 dips
15	100% ethanol	10 dips
16	Xylene	Minimum 30 s

modifications induced by air-drying, however, result in different morphological details in smears stained according to the May Grünwald Giemsa method vs. Papanicolaou-stained preparations. In the latter, moreover, the nuclear morphology is more akin to that seen in tissue sections from formalin-fixed and paraffin-embedded samples. Thus, May Grünwald Giemsa preparations provide nuclear morphological details that are less suitable for proper cytohistological correlation with respect to samples prepared with Papanicolaou stain. In addition, cellular details in three-dimensional aggregates are better evaluated in Papanicolaou-stained smears; this represents a major drawback to the May Grünwald Giemsa method. However, ethanol fixation, which is required for Papanicolaou staining, is responsible for the removal of most of the lipid and lipoprotein substances in the smear. The morphological details of the cytoplasm and extracellular compartment are therefore less discernible in Papanicolaou-stained smears than in smears stained with the May Grünwald Giemsa method. Table 1.4 describes the different appearances of several cytological components in smears stained with Papanicolaou vs. May Grünwald Giemsa stain.

The above considerations explain why two sets of smears, one stained with May Grünwald Giemsa and

Table 1.3 Difference in overall smear examination

Air-drying fixation and Romanowsky stain	Ethanol fixation and Papanicolaou stain
Usually larger number of cells	Cell loss, especially in bloody aspirates
Cells more isolated	Cell cohesion greater
Original architecture less well-preserved	Original architecture better preserved
Cells larger due to air drying and spreading on slide	Cells slightly smaller due to shrinkage artifact
Tendency of the cells to round up	Original cell shape better preserved
Cytoplasmic outline less well-defined	Cytoplasmic delineation superior
Poor cell preservation in inflammatory and necrotic material	Overall cell preservation superior in inflammatory or necrotic material
Cytoplasmic and extracellular products easier to identify	Less differential staining of cytoplasmic products and extracellular material with background
Thick specimens difficult to examine due to heavy staining of nucleus and cytoplasm	Thick specimens easier to examine due to transparent cytoplasm
Bloody smears easier to scan for small tumor cell groups or isolated cells	Bloody smears more difficult to scan for small tumor cell groups or isolated cells
Naked nuclei frequent due to rupture of cytoplasm (e.g., lymphoma, small cell carcinoma, endocrine tumors, etc.,	Better preservation and delineation of cytoplasm, and fewer naked nuclei
Nuclear characteristics inferior	Nuclear characteristics (chromatin distribution, parachromatin visualization, nuclear membrane thickness, nuclear irregularities) superior
Cytoplasmic granules or secretory products and extracellular material well-visualized	Cytoplasmic granules or secretory products and extracellular material less well-visualized
Keratin not well-stained (poor differential staining)	Differential staining of keratin (in Papanicolaou stain) excellent
Keratin and thick cytoplasm in necrotic cells may be difficult to differentiate	Keratin and thick cytoplasm in necrotic cells easier to differentiate in Papanicolaou stain

Table 1.4 Different microscopic appearances in May Grünwald Giemsa vs. Papanicolaou stains

Cellular component	May Grünwald Giemsa	Papanicolaou
Thin colloid	Pink-blue-purple	Shades of green
Thick colloid	Dark blue-purple	Shades of green
Neuroendocrine granules	Bright red-magenta	Faint granularity
Amyloid	Glassy, pink-blue-purple	Glassy-green, green-brown
Mucin	Pink-bluish-purple	Shades of green
Collagenous ground substance	Bright purple-magenta	Green
Adenoid cystic carcinoma matrix	Bright purple-magenta	Clear
Lymphoglandular bodies	Bluish globules	Greenish globules (difficult to appreciate)

the other with Papanicolaou stain, should be made available for a detailed cytomorphological evaluation of direct smears, as together they provide the best visualization of all the different cellular and extracellular compartments, albeit on different slides. For several reasons, however, this is not always possible in daily practice. Accordingly, fixing all or almost all the slides in ethanol with subsequent Papanicolaou staining seems a reasonable option to warrant the most complete cytomorphological evaluation of the sample. This strategy is best applicable for samples collected from the breast and the lymph node, and from deep-seated lesions. Nevertheless, the concomitant availability of smears stained with Papanicolaou stain and with May Grünwald Giemsa is an important requisite for evaluating FNB samples of thyroid and pulmonary lesions.

1.3 Microscopic Evaluation

1.3.1 Pattern Recognition Approach

This book classifies tumors based on their distinctive cytological patterns. By definition, a pattern, from the French *patron*, is "a type of theme of recurring events or objects, sometimes referred to as elements of a set. These elements repeat in a predictable manner. It can be a template or model which can be used to generate things or parts of a thing, especially if the things that are created have enough in common for the underlying pattern to be inferred, in which case the things are said to exhibit the unique pattern" [29]. Pattern recognition in FNB cytopathology is no different than in other scientific fields.

The approach to diagnosis by pattern analysis is, likewise, not new in Pathology, as it has been used with optimal results, for example, in the histopathological classification of inflammatory skin disease. To quote from Bernard Ackerman's "Histologic diagnosis of inflammatory skin diseases" [30], the identification of cytological patterns "is firmly rooted in morphology" and "the morphologic method requires accurate observation and orderly classification." In addition, "once the major pattern has been identified, the diagnostic possibilities are dramatically reduced. The next step is to home in on the exact diagnosis."

In cytopathology, as in dermatopathology, while an "exact diagnosis" cannot always be reached, pattern analysis enables the observer to place the set of morphological changes, i.e., the pattern, found in the sample within a well-circumscribed category of reasonable diagnostic hypotheses. Starting from this point, it should be possible to build up a diagnostic algorithm based on clinical correlation and on further data obtained by ancillary techniques, according to a rigorous methodology of deductive reasoning. The end result is not always a conclusive diagnosis but can provide a restricted list of possible diagnoses sharing the same cytomorphological pattern. In this latter case, further clinical work-up or a surgical pathology approach is required to reach a conclusive diagnosis.

The approach to the morphological evaluation of FNB smears is quite similar to that employed in classical histopathology. It starts from a survey of the sample at low magnification using the scanning objective of the microscope. This evaluation must cover the entire smear, starting from the portion closest to the frosted end and containing most of the cellular aggregates, if present. Moving away from the frosted end, the smear should be evaluated in its entirety in order to define the extent of *cellularity* of the sample and the type of *prevailing aggregation*. These are two major features of the sample and they are pivotal to subsequent pattern recognition. The observer should be trained to estimate the approximate number of cells in the smear at low-power magnification. Cellularity is measured semi-quantitatively as poor, moderate, or abundant. It is difficult to provide any reproducible criteria to define the limits for this assessment. In general, cellularity is inadequate if in several adjacent fields it is possible to observe, overall, no more than 200 cells. The range for poor cellularity is approximately 200–500 cells, while the upper limit for moderate cellularity is typically 1000 cells. Using the scanning objective of the microscope, one should then examine the tendency of cells to aggregate, thus recognizing the relative proportion of non-cohesive and cohesive elements. Some smears may contain only aggregates of cohesive cells, and others only non-cohesive cells, and still others significant amounts of both components.

Before the smear is examined at high magnification, the aggregation patterns should be defined. A first distinction is made between two-dimensional and three-dimensional aggregates. Two-dimensional aggregates are flat and laminar; they vary in width and length in addition to shape. Three-dimensional aggregates are characterized by overlapping cellular layers, with thickness thus representing their third dimension. Aggregates may vary in size and shape; obviously, two- and three-dimensionality can coexist in the same aggregate. Additional characterization of the aggregates is based on the evaluation of their external outlines (cords, trabeculae, acini) and internal architecture (papillae, tubules, sieve-like, "solid" appearance).

Further cytomorphological evaluation is performed at higher magnification. The aim is to determine the cell types and fine cellular features, including cytoplasmic and nuclear morphology, cellular interaction with stromal components, and extracellular ground substance. Measurement of the size of the entire cells, or the nucleus, or other cellular structures, is an essential requirement in this phase, and it is expressed in terms of fold difference with a diameter of a red blood cell (RBC), for example 1.5xRBC, or 3xRBC, etc.

1.3.2 Diagnostic Accuracy

By no means is a FNB cytological diagnosis equivalent to a conventional histopathological diagnosis, even if both are "tissue" diagnoses. The features distinguishing the two are the different extent of cellular sampling and the different approach to microscopic evaluation of the cellular morphology. As a matter of fact, the validity of a cytological diagnosis is measured by means of its potential to predict a histological diagnosis, obtained following excisional biopsy of the lesion and conventional histopathological processing and preparation. Histological diagnosis of the lesion is thus considered the "gold standard" of the diagnostic process. Due to several factors intrinsic to the structure of the lesion and the sampling procedure, the potential of a FNB cytological diagnosis to predict a histological diagnosis of the same lesion can be very high, thus indicating with absolute certainty the nature of the lesion; however, it may be less than optimal and in these cases the final report is to be expressed in terms of the "probability" that the given cytological picture corresponds to one or more disease entities.

One should become familiar with the parameters that measure the accuracy of FNB as a medical test. Sensitivity and specificity indicate the *effectiveness* of a medical test and are used for tests that have only two outcomes, i.e. "positive" and "negative." The significance of sensitivity and specificity is easily understood if the reader examines the "2×2" table illustrated in Fig. 1.11. Given a population of samples with and without the disease, the test result may fall into one of four categories: true positive, false positive, true negative, and false negative. A perfect test gives only true positive and true negative results, and the worst possible test would be the same as guessing. Sensitivity describes the proportion of samples showing signs of the disease that have a positive test, while specificity refers to the proportion of samples without the disease that have a negative result. Sensitivity and specificity are calculated by viewing the "2×2" table vertically (Fig. 1.11) and are meaningful only when the studied population has undergone an acceptable "gold standard" investigation used to "rule in" or "rule out" the disease of interest. In the field of FNB, the gold standard is represented by the histological examination of a surgically excised sample of the lesion. Two additional parameters of the test are the positive and negative predictive values, which are calculated by viewing the "2×2" table horizontally. The positive predictive value of a test expresses the proportion of samples with a positive test that are found to show signs of the disease. The negative predictive value expresses the proportion of samples with a negative test that are disease-free.

From a practical point of view, the closer the sensitivity is to 100%, the more likely a positive result actually means that the sample is diseased. The closer the specificity is to 100%, the more likely a negative result means that the sample is truly disease-free. Similarly, the closer the positive predictive value is to 100%, the more likely the test can serve to make a "positive" diagnosis. The closer the negative predictive value is to 100%, the more likely the test can serve to exclude

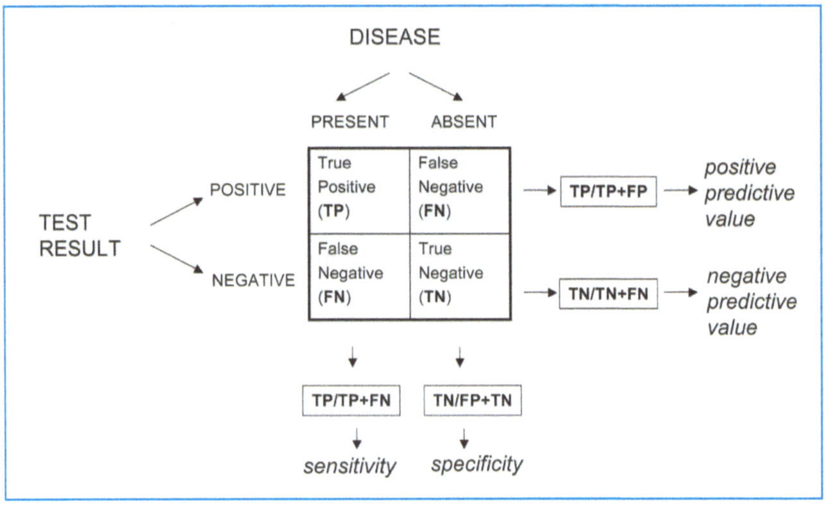

Fig. 1.11 The "2×2" table

the disease, i.e., to make a "negative" diagnosis. While many medical tests are highly accurate, none are 100% sensitive and 100% specific. In general, FNB is expected to bear a significant risk of false negative results but by definition should not lead to false positive results. In other words, the positive predictive value of FNB is very high but its negative predictive value is less than optimal. Thus, when confronted with a positive result, for example, the diagnosis of malignancy, one can rely on the test and proceed to the following steps of patient management; conversely, when confronted with a negative result, for example, a diagnosis that is negative for malignancy, one cannot rely on the test and, instead, alternative tests with a higher negative predictive value must be used. The measure of to what extent a negative FNB result should not be relied on is given by the results of preanalytical tests. For example, in the case of a breast nodule with a high risk of suspicion of malignancy by imaging techniques, a negative FNB result should not be used to rule out malignancy; instead, further investigation is needed using diagnostic procedures with a higher negative predictive value. These procedures essentially consist of an incisional or excisional biopsy leading to histological examination of the sample. Thus, only on the basis of histological examination of a representative sample can a lesion that appears suspicious on imaging be diagnosed as benign. Conversely, in the case of a breast nodule that looks benign on imaging but is malignant on FNB examination, histological confirmation would not be required due to the very high positive predictive value of cytology in this particular context. In conclusion, the FNB procedure, which is less harmful and less expensive than incisional or excisional biopsy, can be conveniently placed first in the diagnostic evaluation of a breast nodule, provided that the imaging features of the lesion are concomitantly evaluated. The same reasoning applies to several other FNB applications, including the lymph nodes, thyroid, and lung.

References

1. Ljung BM, Drejet A, Chiampi N et al (2001) Diagnostic accuracy of fine-needle aspiration biopsy is determined by physician training in sampling technique. Cancer 93: 263–268.
2. Dray M, Mayall F, Darlington A (2000) Improved fine needle aspiration (FNA) cytology results with a near patient diagnosis service for breast lesions. Cytopathology 11:32–37.
3. Mayall F, Denford A, Chang B, Darlington A (1998) Improved FNA cytology results with a near patient diagnosis service for non-breast lesions. J Clin Pathol 51:541–544.
4. Florentine BD, Staymates B, Rabadi M et al (2006) Cancer Committee of the Henry Mayo Newhall Memorial Hospital. The reliability of fine-needle aspiration biopsy as the initial diagnostic procedure for palpable masses: a 4-year experience of 730 patients from a community hospital-based outpatient aspiration biopsy clinic. Cancer 107:406–416.
5. Florentine BD, Staymates B, Rabadi M et al (2006) Cancer Committee of the Henry Mayo Newhall Memorial Hospital. Cost savings associated with the use of fine-needle aspiration biopsy (FNAB) for the diagnosis of palpable masses in a community hospital-based FNAB clinic. Cancer 107: 2270–2281.
6. Anne S, Teot LA, Mandell DL (2008) Fine needle aspiration biopsy: role in diagnosis of pediatric head and neck masses. Int J Pediatr Otorhinolaryngol 72:1547–1553.
7. Abele JS (2008) The case for pathologist ultrasound-guided fine-needle aspiration biopsy. Cancer 114:463–468.
8. Brown LA, Coghill SB (1991) Fine needle aspiration cytology of the breast: factors affecting sensitivity. Cytopathology 2:67–74.
9. Brown LA, Coghill SB, Powis SA (1991) Audit of diagnostic accuracy of FNA cytology specimens taken by the histopathologist in a symptomatic breast clinic. Cytopathology 2:1–6.
10. Bandyopadhyay S, Pansare V, Feng J et al (2007) Frequency and rationale of fine needle aspiration biopsy conversion to core biopsy as a result of onsite evaluation. Acta Cytol 51:161–167.
11. Suen KC (2002). Fine-needle aspiration biopsy of the thyroid. Can Med Ass J 167:491–495.
12. Brown LA, Coghill SB (1992) Cost effectiveness of a fine needle aspiration clinic. Cytopathology 3:275–280.
13. Kim A, Lee J, Choi JS et al (2000) Fine needle aspiration cytology of the breast. Experience at an outpatient breast clinic. Acta Cytol 44:361–367.
14. Padel AF, Coghill SB, Powis SJ (1993) Evidence that the sensitivity is increased and the inadequacy rate decreased when pathologists take aspirates for cytodiagnosis. Cytopathology 4:161–165.
15. Stanley MW, Lowhagen T (1993) Fine needle aspiration of palpable masses. Butterworth-Heinemann, Boston.
16. Jeffrey PB, Miller TR (1996) Fine-needle aspiration cytology of the thyroid. In: Ljung BM (ed) Pathology: State of the art reviews. Hanley and Belfus, Philadelphia, p 320
17. Koss LG, Woyke S, Olszewski W (1996) Aspiration biopsy. Cytologic interpretation and histologic bases. 2nd Ed. Igaku-Shoin, New York.
18. Bishop Pitman M, Abele J, Ali SZ et al (2008) Techniques for Thyroid FNA: A Synopsis of the National Cancer Institute Thyroid Fine-Needle Aspiration State of the Science Conference. Diagn Cytopathol 36:407–424.
19. Zajdela A, de Maublanc MA, Schlienger P, Haye C (1986) Cytologic diagnosis of orbital and periorbital palpable tumors using fine-needle sampling without aspiration. Diagn Cytopathol 2:17–20.

20. Cajulis RS, Sneige N (1993) Objective comparison of cellular yield in fine-needle biopsy of lymph nodes with and without aspiration. Diagn Cytopathol 9:43–45.
21. Haddadi-Nezhad S, Larijani B, Tavangar SM, Nouraei SM (2003) Comparison of fine-needle-nonaspiration with fine-needle-aspiration technique in the cytologic studies of thyroid nodules. Endocr Pathol 14:369–373.
22. Rizvi SA, Husain M, Khan S, Mohsin M (2005) A comparative study of fine needle aspiration cytology versus non-aspiration technique in thyroid lesions. Surgeon 3:273–276.
23. Pothier DD, Narula AA (2006) Should we apply suction during fine needle cytology of thyroid lesions? A systematic review and metaanalysis. Ann R Coll Surg Engl 88:643–645.
24. Matalon TAS, Silver B (1999) US guidance of interventional procedures. Radiology 174:43–47.
25. Caturelli E, Giacobbe A, Facciorusso D et al (1996) Free-hand technique with ordinary antisepsis in abdominal US-guided fine-needle punctures: three-year experience. Radiology 199:721–723.
26. Abele JS, Miller TR, King EB, Lowhagen T (1985) Smearing techniques for the concentration of particles from fine needle aspiration biopsy. Diagn Cytopathol 1:59–65.
27. Koss LG (1992) Diagnostic Cytology and its histopathologic bases. Cytologic Techniques. Lippincott, Philadelphia, pp 1503–1504.
28. Kaminsky DB (1981) Aspiration Biopsy for the Community Hospital. In: Johnston WW (ed) Masson Monographs in Diagnostic Cytopathology, Masson Publishing USA, New York, pp 12–13.
29. Wikipedia contributors (2009) Pattern. In: Wikipedia, The Free Encyclopedia. Permanent link: http://en.wikipedia.org/w/index.php?title=Pattern&oldid=295609960
30. Ackerman AB (1978) Histologic Diagnosis of Inflammatory Skin Diseases. A Method by Pattern Analysis. Lea & Febiger, Philadelphia, pp 157–168.

2 Breast

2.1 Introduction

Despite the alarming worldwide increase in the incidence of breast cancer in the last 30 years, especially in highly developed countries, we have witnessed a parallel decrease in mortality and a longer disease-free survival of breast-cancer patients, both of which can be ascribed to increasingly early diagnosis and the use of drugs that are highly effective in large subgroups of patients.

The earlier breast cancer is detected, the more likely it can be successfully treated. In fact, the overall 15-year survival of women treated for breast cancer is inversely proportional to the size of the tumor at the time of diagnosis, varying between 86 and 46% for tumors, 10–14 and 30–39 mm, respectively, in their largest diameter [1,2].

Since women with breast cancers of small size can benefit from greater treatment choices and have a more favorable prognosis, diagnosing the tumor as early as possible has become a primary goal in breast-cancer care [3]. Early breast cancers generally consist of in situ carcinomas of any size, or of unifocal, small tumors of low-grade invasiveness (classified as ductal or lobular type), or of invasive tumors with histologies associated with a more favorable prognosis.

Early invasive tumors do not show significant peritumoral angioinvasiveness and are either not associated with metastatic deposits in regional nodes or there may be only micrometastatic involvement of the sentinel node. Moreover, the biological markers detected in these tumors are predictive of a good response to conventional treatment.

2.2 Non-Operative Diagnosis of Breast Cancer

Non-operative procedures for the diagnosis of breast cancer are far less expensive than traditional surgery and more applicable to screening campaigns. In addition, they promote anatomic conservation and integrity of the breast and warrant the patient's right to participate in the process of treatment decision. These procedures consist of *fine-needle biopsy* (FNB), *core-needle biopsy* (CNB), and mammotome type *vacuum-assisted core-needle biopsy* (VACNB). They differ from one another with respect to the caliber of the needle employed, the sampling modalities, and the type of post-sampling processing for microscopic evaluation.

FNB is carried out with 27-gauge (0.4 mm) to 23-gauge (0.6 mm) needles, while CNB is performed with 19-gauge (1.27 mm) and 14-gauge (2.10 mm) needles, and VACNB with needles no larger than 11-gauge (3.1 mm). FNB sampling is done with or without aspiration, and the harvested material consists of a cellular sample that is generally smeared on a glass slide and then examined cytologically. By contrast, the diagnostic yield of CNB is a core of tissue that is removed through the cutting edge at the tip of the needle and then examined after conventional histological processing. The VACNB device allows for the removal of multiple tissue samples with a single insertion of the needle; the samples are then similarly processed for histological examination.

FNB offers several advantages [4–8]. The procedure is simple, easy to perform, quick, very well-tolerated by the patient, immediately repeatable, and practically never followed by complications. Moreover, it is a highly cost-effective diagnostic procedure. The only contraindication is a hemorrhagic diathesis. The biopsy sample can be ready for definitive diagnostic evaluation after a very short time (20–30 min). In experienced hands, the diagnosis of malignancy is reliable and the procedure has a very high positive predictive value. There are limitations, however. FNB is an operator-dependent technique and its accuracy is strongly related to the experience, training, and approach of both the physician performing the biopsy and the pathologist interpreting the cellular sample. A high degree of accuracy is obtained only when the same pathologist performs the puncture and assesses the adequacy of the specimen. FNB is characterized by a suboptimal negative predictive value and is not the method of choice in the investigation of lesions detected solely by X-ray mammography, such as microcalcifications. Finally, even in the most experienced hands, not less than 5–10% of FNB samples are inadequate.

CNB has the advantage of minimal sample inadequacy. The sampling procedure is easier and the diagnostic approach more reproducible than is the case for FNB, due to the greater inclination of pathologists to interpret histological sections rather than cytological smears. CNB is indicated in the investigation of non-nodular and non-palpable lesions detected as mammographic microcalcifications and is more accurate in the differential diagnosis of borderline breast lesions. However, since a representative sample consists of at least 4–5 tissue cores, the procedure is much more expensive and invasive than FNB. In addition, the need for histological processing of tissue cores renders the procedure more time-consuming. It is also generally less well-tolerated by the patient and can induce minor complications, such as bleeding or infections. Furthermore, post-sampling tissue changes are potential pitfalls in subsequent histological interpretation of the surgically removed lesion [9–13]. CNB shares the same risk of sampling errors as FNB and there is emerging evidence that it bears a significant risk of a false-negative or false-positive diagnosis as well as underestimation of invasive carcinoma [13].

Due to the high cost of the material and instrumentation, VACNB is indicated as the first-choice modality only in the investigation of mammographic microcalcifications [14,15]. It allows the sampling of multiple specimens and provides a larger volume of breast tissue for histological examination. VACNB requires local anesthesia and a cutaneous incision. It is used under stereotaxis but can also be guided by ultrasound. Overall, it is significantly more invasive than FNB or CNB and is not used in large-scale screening programs.

2.3 Fine-Needle vs. Core-Needle Sampling

The above considerations explain why FNB and CNB compete for primacy as the first-choice procedure in the primary diagnosis of breast cancer. The former gained great popularity worldwide in the 1980s and 1990s in recognition of its practical advantages and low cost but in recent years there has been a reversal in this trend, especially in the USA [16]. This change was triggered by the declining willingness of pathologists to carry out image-guided fine-needle aspiration (FNA) biopsy for the continuously increasing number of patients with non-palpable breast lesions, due to the meager reimbursement for assistance in on-site specimen adequacy assessment and interpretation. The consequence was the introduction of the more expensive, risky, and time-consuming procedure of CNB, which is performed by a radiologist without the need for the assistance of a pathologist. The result has been a progressive and rapid decrease in the number of pathologists who are expert on the cytopathology of breast lesions and, in particular, of early carcinomas, the evaluation of which is considered difficult due to paucicellular samples and highly subtle cellular diagnostic alterations [16]. In the meantime, private surgeons and primary-care clinicians began performing breast FNAs and this has resulted in a dramatic increase in the number of non-diagnostic specimens, with accompanying delays in diagnosis and treatment. CNB became the easiest alternative–encouraged by a significant increase in the income of radiologists performing the procedure. Not unexpectedly, the same decline in the popularity of FNB has occurred in European countries, even if cost-efficient health care is a priority in most of them. The involvement of the pathologist in sampling palpable and non-palpable breast lesions is no longer encouraged in academic training programs, despite the general recognition that pathologist-performed breast sampling provides a cellular harvest that correlates better with histopathology, minimizes the number of inconclusive and unsatisfactory specimens, and allows for the procurement and proper work-up of additional material for ancillary techniques, if required.

In conclusion, neither FNB nor CNB alone seems optimal, entirely faultless, or a convincingly superior procedure for the primary diagnosis of early breast carcinoma [10–13,17]. An evidence-based approach should include the use of both techniques. In fact, lesions that are palpable at clinical examination or easily detected upon ultrasound as a nodular target should be distinguished from lesions that are detected solely at mammography as microcalcifications or that appear as an indefinite density upon ultrasound. FNB represents the best procedure for investigating lesions of the first category (Fig. 2.1). In experienced hands, multiple passes are obtained literally within a few seconds and the sample is ready for microscopic interpretation in 10–20 min. Immediate staining and evaluation of the specimen allows for a definite diagnosis in at least 60–80% of cases involving these palpable or easily detectable lesions. CNB is best indicated for evaluation of those cases in which FNB did not provide a conclusive diagnosis and for lesions belonging to the second category, i.e., mammographic microcalcifications or indefinite ultrasound densities lacking nodular features. CNB sampling is similarly performed within minutes under stereotactic or ultrasound guidance; microscopic diagnostic evaluation includes the time required for histological processing, sectioning, and routine staining or immunostaining. Considering that in daily practice the lesions of the first category represent about 90% of cases, the initial use of FNB provides a conclusive diagnosis in about two-thirds of the total number of cases while CNB is used for the remaining ones. This promotes cost containment, reduced time for diagnosis, and significant improvement in terms of general organization. A highly accurate diagnosis can thus be made in the majority of cases within one hour of sampling and, for the remaining cases, the day after. Cases requiring additional investigation by VACNB are selected on the basis of radiological appearance of the lesion and the FNB or CNB results.

Strong involvement of the pathologist in the preanalytical discussion of the case, in the puncture of the lesion, and in the rapid evaluation of the specimen is pivotal to the success of this multidisciplinary diagnostic approach. A breast clinic [18,19] is the best environment for this model of organization as it promotes close cooperation between the radiologist, the pathologist, and, in selected cases, the breast surgeon. The end result is the expeditious and reliable selection among patients requiring clinical follow-up only, additional sampling by VACNB, immediate surgical intervention, or systemic neoadjuvant chemotherapy.

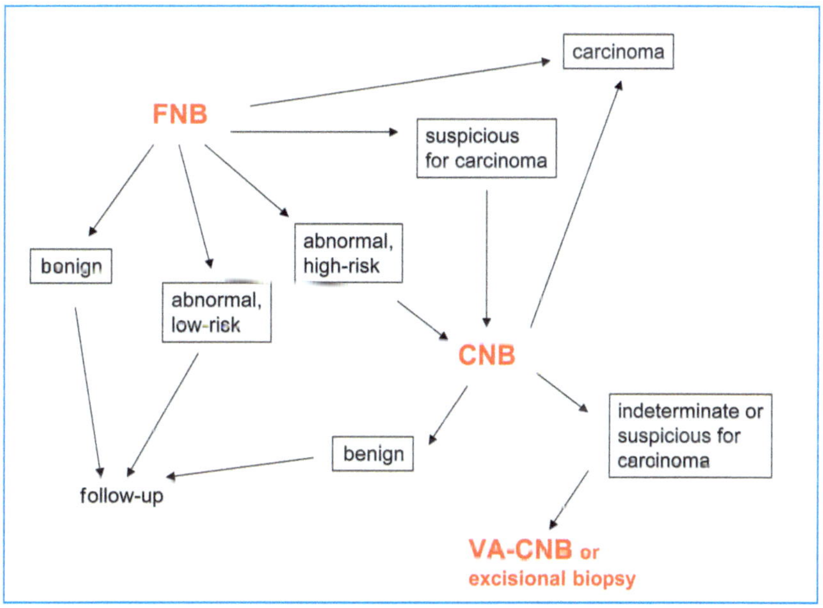

Fig. 2.1 Diagnostic algorithm for breast nodular lesions that are palpable or easily detected upon ultrasound

2.4 Diagnostic Terminology

The purpose of diagnostic terminology in non-operative cytological and microhistological procedures is to allow classification of the lesion within a clear-cut diagnostic category in order to facilitate further care of the patient and therapeutic decision-making. In general, cytological diagnostic categories for adequate samples can be divided into benign, malignant, and "abnormal" categories. By definition, samples judged "abnormal" are characterized by morphological features that are not atypical enough to be considered diagnostic or "suspicious" of carcinoma but also cannot be considered as benign. In breast cytopathology, the limits of this diagnostic category are rather blurred and its use traditionally has been governed by great subjectivity. The relative incidence of cases falling into the "abnormal" category has increased over the years, paralleling the increased detection of premalignant lesions and early breast cancer. Since there may be a qualitative overlap in the cytological morphology of premalignant and malignant samples, in this category a distinction between low-risk and high-risk cases is pivotal in order to further assist clinical decision-making, which ranges, respectively, from a conservative "watch and wait" approach to an immediate further investigation by CNB or even surgical excision.

In the 1990ies, several articles focusing on the issue of the best terminology for breast cytological samples were published in the medical literature. Masood et al., 1991 [20], and Sneige et al., 1994 [21], introduced similar reporting formats, which consisted of the following five categories: inadequate, benign lesion, proliferative lesion, suspicious for carcinoma, and malignant (Table 2.1). A second reporting format, shown in Table 2.2, was introduced by the European Community (EC) Working Group on Breast Screening [22–24], which also consisted of five categories but only somewhat analogous to the above scheme. The two classification systems coincide as far as the categories of inadequate (C1), benign (C2), suspicious for carcinoma (C4), and malignant (C5) are concerned but differ for samples falling in the "abnormal". In fact, for lesions classified as "proliferative" in the scheme of Masood et al., 1991 [20] and Sneige et al., 1994 [21], there is a further grading into two groups according to the presence and extent of atypia. In the scheme proposed by the EC Working Group on Breast Screening [22–24], all abnormal lesions fall in the all-embracing concept of C3 or "atypical, probably benign." In summary, the aim of further subdivision in the first system is to provide a clear indication of the risk of the lesion being malignant, to facilitate subsequent decision-making. In the second model, any further indication regarding the actual extent of atypia is lacking; this adversely affects both the accuracy and the clinical impact of the procedure. It is no surprise that even in the most experienced hands the incidence of carcinoma (in situ and invasive) in samples diagnosed cytologically as "C3 atypical, probably benign" can reach 55.7% [25], implicitly contradicting the formulation itself. The question remains, how can we define as "probably benign" a lesion that is expected to be malignant in more than half the cases? For such lesions, there is absolutely no room for a conservative "watch and wait" approach, which would be justified only if the risk of malignancy was no higher than 20–30%.

In summary, a grading category of abnormal or atypical findings, defined according to reproducible criteria that allow low-risk lesions to be differentiated from high-risk ones, is pivotal to maintaining a role for FNB in the diagnosis and management of breast nodular lesions in daily clinical practice [26]. Consistent with this point of view, the approach offered by Masood et al., 1991 [20], in which, within the category of borderline breast lesions, low-risk lesions are differentiated by means of a score system from those that are high-risk (respectively, "proliferative lesions without atypia" and "proliferative lesions with atypia"), introduced several highly standardized and reproducible criteria, thus representing a milestone in the history of FNB of the breast. According to this author's experience, strict adherence to these criteria results in a significantly higher positive predictive value of cytological interpretation of breast FNB samples falling within the "abnormal" category. A scheme for reporting FNB breast aspirates is provided in Table 2.3 and represents both a revision and a simplification of the M.D. Anderson Cancer Center proposal [21], with integration of the cytological score to grade proliferative breast lesions. The use of this simple reporting format is strongly suggested and has been adopted in this chapter as an alternative to the scheme proposed by the EC Working Group on Breast Screening [22–24].

Table 2.1 Reporting terminology. The M.D. Anderson Cancer Center proposal [21]

Adequacy/diagnostic category

Specimen adequacy
- Satisfactory for evaluation (see diagnostic categories 1–4)
- Insufficient for evaluation due to scant cellularity (<4–6 cell groups)
- Unsatisfactory for evaluation due to distortion artifact/obscuring blood

(1) Benign

Specify as to lesion type (e.g., fibroadenoma, fibrocystic change, adenosis, papilloma)

(2) Proliferative

A. Identified by cytological atypia (e.g., crowded, enlarged, pleomorphic, overlapping nuclei, three-dimensional groups or sheets, loss of cohesion, few single cells, homogeneous cell population, hyperchromasia)
B. Identified by cytological features combined with the architectural pattern. Proliferative lesions may be further classified as:
  a. Ductal hyperplasia
  b. Atypical or lobular hyperplasia/low-grade carcinoma in situ

(3) Suspicious for carcinoma

Includes cases with:
- Insufficient cellularity for diagnosis of carcinoma
- Low-grade carcinomas that are admixed with benign ductal elements or detected on one slide only

(4) Malignant

- Breast carcinoma; specify as to the type (e.g., ductal, lobular, mucinous) and nuclear grade (1–3); in situ carcinoma cannot be distinguished from invasive carcinoma on fine-needle aspiration
- Others (sarcoma, lymphoma, metastasis, etc.)

Table 2.2 E.C. Working Group on Breast Screening: diagnostic terminology [22-24]

C1. Unsatisfactory	Inadequate sample due to one or more of the following: - Hypocellularity - Error in aspiration, spreading, and/or staining - Excessive blood
C2. Benign	Adequate sample showing no evidence of malignancy; if representative, a positive diagnosis of a specific condition (e.g., fibroadenoma, fat necrosis) can be rendered
C3. Atypia probably benign	Adequate sample with all the characteristics of a benign aspirate, showing, in addition, one or more of the following: - Nuclear pleomorphism - Some loss of cellular cohesiveness - Nuclear and cytoplasmic changes resulting from proliferative changes, involutionary changes, pregnancy, or treatment influences - High cellularity
C4. Suspicious of malignancy	Adequate sample with highly atypical features but a confident diagnosis of malignancy cannot be rendered due to one or more of the following: - Scant, poorly preserved, or poorly prepared smear - Detection of some malignant features without the presence of overtly malignant cells - Occasional cells showing distinctly malignant features within an otherwise benign-looking sample
C5. Malignant	Adequate sample containing cells characteristics of carcinoma or other malignancy

Table 2.3 Proposed reporting terminology

Adequacy/diagnostic category	Recommendation
Specimen adequacy - Satisfactory for evaluation (see diagnostic categories 1–4) - Insufficient for evaluation due to scant cellularity - Unsatisfactory for evaluation due to distortion artifact/obscuring blood	 CNB or surgical excisional biopsy, if clinically indicated Repeat FNB
(1) Benign Specify as to lesion type (e.g. fibroadenoma, fibrocystic change, adenosis, papilloma)	Correlation with clinical/mammographic findings is needed
(2) Proliferative A. Proliferative without atypia (low-risk lesion) B. Proliferative with atypia (high-risk lesion): a distinction based on the cytological score according to Masood et al., 1991 [20], is advisable	Correlation with clinical/mammographic findings is needed - Follow-up is indicated for low-risk lesions - CNB or surgical excisional biopsy is indicated for high-risk lesions
(3) Suspicious for carcinoma Includes cases with: - Insufficient cellularity for diagnosis of carcinoma - Low-grade carcinomas that are admixed with benign ductal elements or present on one slide only	Excisional biopsy or CNB to confirm carcinoma
(4) Malignant - Breast carcinoma; specify as to the type (e.g. ductal, lobular, mucinous) if possible - Others (sarcoma, lymphoma, metastasis, etc.)	Surgery or preoperative chemotherapy according to clinical indication

CNB Core-needle biopsy, *FNB* fine-needle biopsy

2.5 Diagnostic Approach

In daily practice, the most common indications demanding FNB sampling and evaluation are, for a solid nodular lesion, verification of a clinical and/or radiological suspicion of malignancy and confirmation of a clinical and/or radiological supposition of benignancy. Palpable nodular solid lesions are sampled by FNB using the aspiration (Fig. 2.2a) and non-aspiration technique (Fig. 2.2b). Non-palpable lesions are best sampled under ultrasound guidance using the "free hand" procedure and without aspiration (Fig. 2.2c). For cystic or partly cystic (mixed) lesions, FNA is required to characterize the parietal cellular component exfoliated within the cystic fluid or an intracystic vegetating cellular component detected at ultrasound examination. Mammographic microcalcification aggregates with suspicious features and lacking any corresponding clinical and/or ultrasound findings should be investigated by CNB or by VACNB under stereotactic guidance.

All patients should undergo a thorough preliminary work-up, including clinical examination and imaging, to assess the pre-analytical probability of malignancy. The latter should be expressed according to a score system in which 0 is used if the lesion is considered benign, 1 if it has suspicious features, and 2 if it appears to be malignant. Thus, the clinical score and the imaging score should be expressed clearly before FNB or CNB sampling as they will be included together with the microscopic assessment in the triple-test final score [27,28]. This is a time-honored and accurate approach in which all three score components are considered, and it represents a reliable basis to support subsequent clinical decision-making (Table 2.4). In fact, if all three components point to the lesion being benign (0-0-0), or malignant (2-2-2), the negative and positive predictive value, respectively, of the triple-test approach is very high. If, however, the components are not in agreement, then different actions must be taken. For example, the positive predictive value of imaging techniques and cytological findings is very high; thus, if at least one of them has a score of 1, the lesion is to be considered at risk and further investigation is immediately advisable. Conversely, if only clinical findings are considered

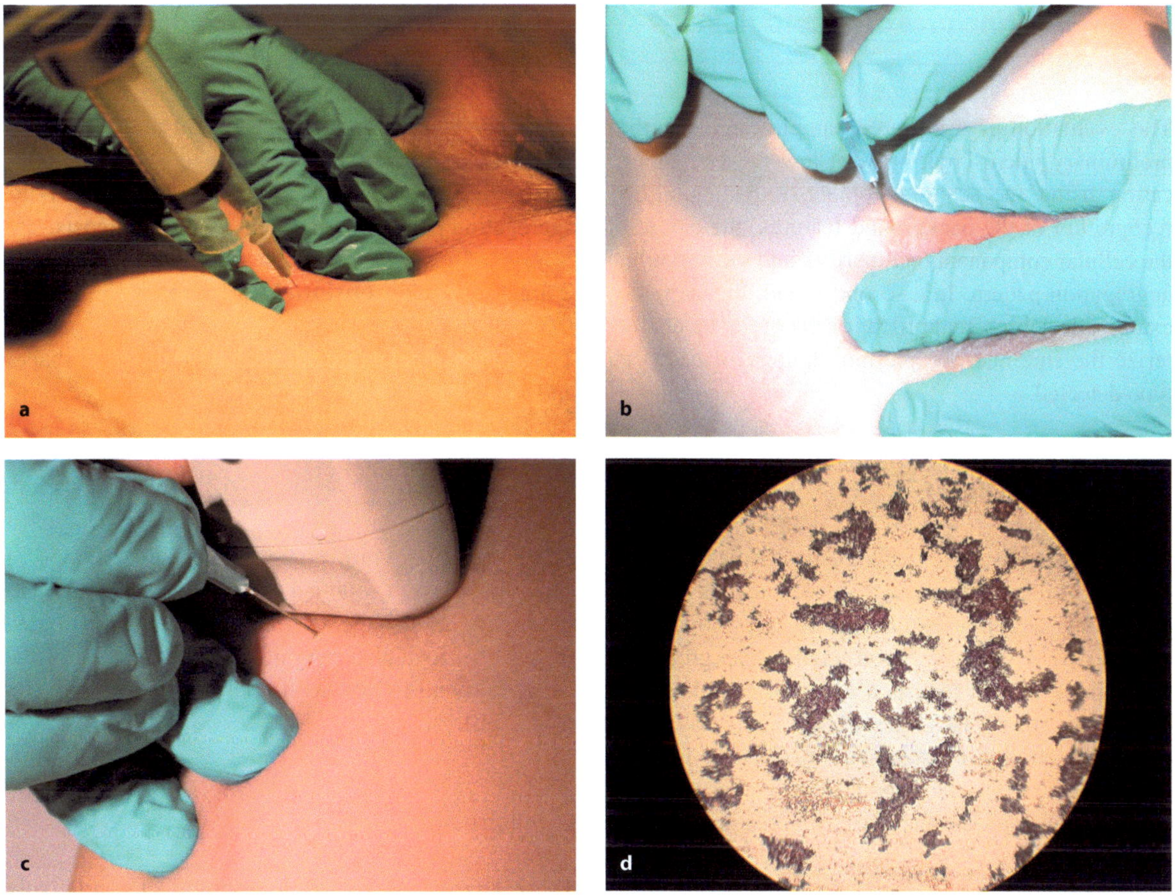

Fig. 2.2 **a** Sampling procedure of a palpable breast lump using the **a** aspiration technique and **b** non-aspiration technique. **c** Sampling procedure of a non-palpable breast lump using the non-aspiration technique under free-hand ultrasound guidance. **d** Low-power "panoramic" view of a FNB harvest with a high cellularity; the background is clear and proteinaceous with occasional red blood cells; epithelial parenchymal cells appear in two- or three-dimensional clusters of variable size and shape. Papanicolaou (P) stain, ×40

Table 2.4 Triple-test approach

Clinical	Imaging	FNB	Conclusion or further decision
0	0	0	Definitely benign
1 or 2	0	0	Most probably benign, follow-up indicated
0	1 or 2	0	Indefinite, CNB required
0	0	1	Indefinite, CNB required
0	0	2	Definitely malignant

CNB Core-needle biopsy

suspicious, then follow-up of the patient is justified. Finally, if both clinical findings and imaging techniques indicate that the lesion is benign but the cytology results are clearly in favor of malignancy, the lesion is considered to be malignant due to the very high positive predictive value of cytology in this context. A relevant example of the latter situation is represented by malignant tumors that simulate clinically and radiologically benign breast lesions and are unexpectedly discovered only by means of cytology.

2.6 Basic Principles of Cytological Evaluation

The evaluation of a smeared sample begins with a preliminary microscopic view at low-power magnification using the scanning objective, which allows recognition of the background features, the extent of the cellular component (cellularity), and the prevailing aggregation pattern. In a second round, the sample is examined at high magnification in order to characterize the fine microscopic morphology of each cell type detected.

2.6.1 Background

The background of a cytological sample generally consists of a transparent proteinaceous matrix containing a variable number of red blood cells (Fig. 2.2d). Excessive blood in the background is undesirable and, in fact, is a cause of sample inadequacy. In other cases, the background may show a variable amount of mucinous material or necrotic debris. Thus, the background is described as proteinaceous, blood-stained, mucinous, or necrotic.

2.6.2 Cellularity

Quantifying the amount of cells in the harvest is an essential prerequisite for diagnostic evaluation. Cellularity is evaluated semi-quantitatively as low, moderate, and high based on the examination of several areas of the smear. It is calculated by quantifying the concentration of cells per low-power microscopic field and in several fields. The number of fields to be evaluated is not fixed and depends on the type of sample. A smear with high cellularity is shown in Fig. 2.2d. The evaluation should start in those areas with the highest cellular concentration. Cellularity is considered adequate when more than 6–8 aggregates each containing at least 20 epithelial glandular cells are detected in several different fields [22–24]. However, this number of cells is too small for any diagnostic formulation; thus, the importance of examining smears containing a much larger number of cells cannot be overemphasized.

2.6.3 Aggregation Patterns of Epithelial Glandular Cells

Epithelial glandular cells may be clustered in aggregates or dissociated and non-cohesive. When aggregates are seen, the evaluation and definition of the aggregation pattern is important for the diagnosis.

2.6.3.1 Two-Dimensional Aggregates

Two-dimensional aggregates can have different shapes and structures.

Laminar Sheets

These aggregates are composed of several tens of cells; they have a rounded or polygonal (rectangular, rhomboid, etc.) shape and often appear partly folded (Fig. 2.3a). At higher magnification, the nuclei of the cells are round to oval with finely granular chromatin (Fig. 2.3b).

Digitiform Aggregates

These aggregates are also composed of a relatively large numbers of cells that have an elongated and finger-like shape and a rectilinear or curvilinear profile (Fig. 2.3c). Frequently, several aggregates appear to radiate from a common origin.

Elongated Aggregates

These aggregates are composed of no more than 20–30 cells and are characterized by the prevalence of length over width. They sometimes consist of two parallel lines of cells and may show minor overlapping of the cell nuclei (Fig. 2.4).

Indian Files

These are aggregates composed of generally less than 10 cells, which are linked one behind another to form a chain, or an "Indian file" pattern (Fig. 2.5).

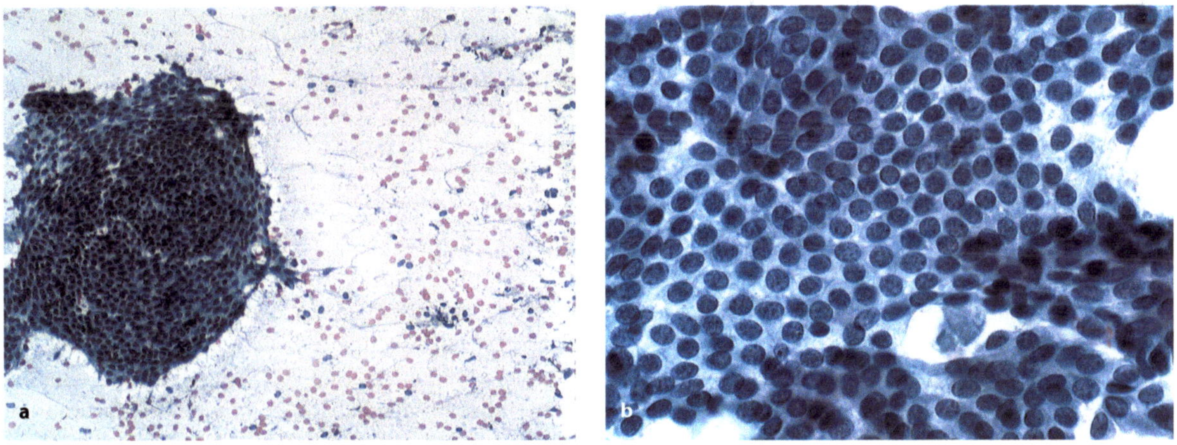

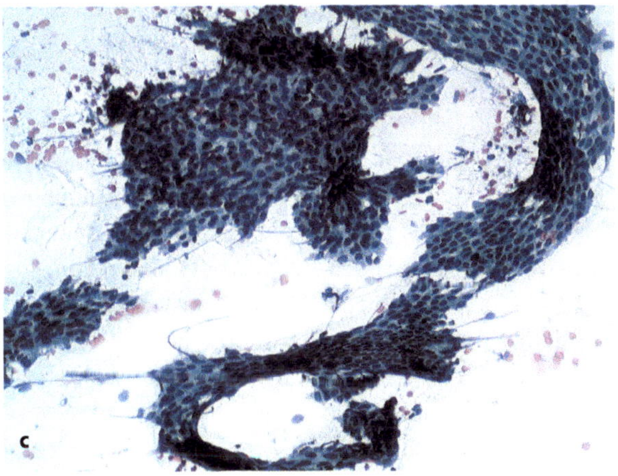

Fig. 2.3 **a** Round laminar aggregate is seen on the *left* side of the image; the background is proteinaceous and contains bipolar bare nuclei and red blood cells. P stain, ×400. **b** High-power view of a two-dimensional aggregate; nuclei appear monotonous and round in shape; the chromatin is finely granular and shows occasional chromocenters. P stain, ×1000. **c** Two-dimensional clusters of variable shape, some of which are partially twisted. P stain, ×400

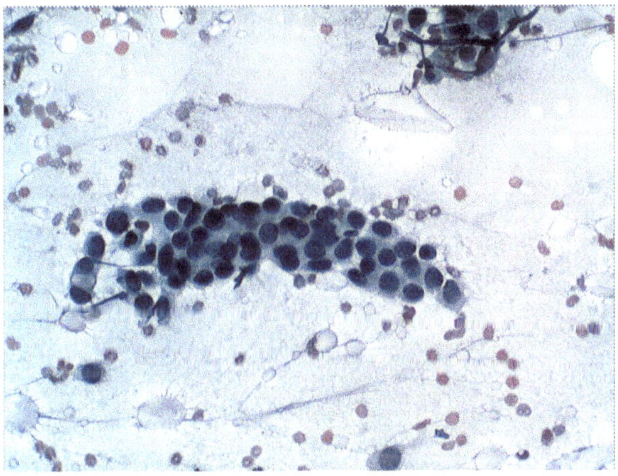

Fig. 2.4 Two-dimensional cluster of elongated shape shows focally overlapping nuclei; the chromatin texture is coarsely granular. P stain, ×800

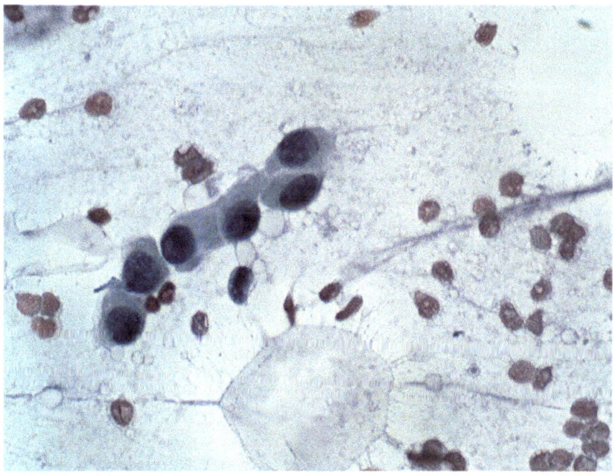

Fig. 2.5 Cells form an "Indian file" and are characterized by hyperchromatic nuclei. P stain, ×1000

2.6.3.2 Three-Dimensional Aggregates

The great structural variability of three-dimensional aggregates makes their classification difficult. Other than large aggregates, consisting of multiple layers of cells that appear patternless, it may be important to identify the following.

Trabecular Aggregates

They have a somewhat rectangular or oval shape and are characterized by marked cellular overlap (Fig. 2.6).

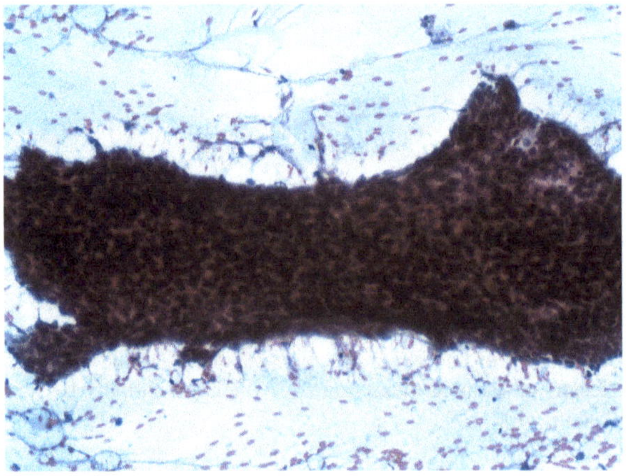

Fig. 2.6 Trabecular aggregates are three-dimensional clusters containing multiple nuclear layers and are rectangular or oval in shape. P stain, ×400

Tubular Aggregates

These have an elongated shape with only minor nuclear overlap and a central, seemingly empty core that suggests the presence of a lumen (Fig. 2.7).

Papillary Aggregates

Papillae are peculiar three-dimensional aggregates characterized by cuboid or cylindrical cells radiating from a connective-tissue stalk (Fig. 2.8). The latter is sometimes absent but the cells maintain an unusual pattern (pseudopapillae).

2.6.4 Cellular Dissociation

Dissociated and non-cohesive epithelial cells are, by definition, round or oval-shaped elements that contain a variable amount of cytoplasm and appear singly in the smear. Truly dissociated cells should not retain any spatial relationship to each other, instead appearing absolutely non-cohesive. Thus, loose cellular aggregation cannot be classified as true dissociation. Loosely cohesive cells (Fig. 2.9) are frequently observed in association with true dissociation–a finding that should prompt a more extensive search for truly non-cohesive cells. Cellular dissociation may be minimal, partial, or total. The latter is depicted in Figure 2.10. It is important to measure the percentage of epithelial glandular

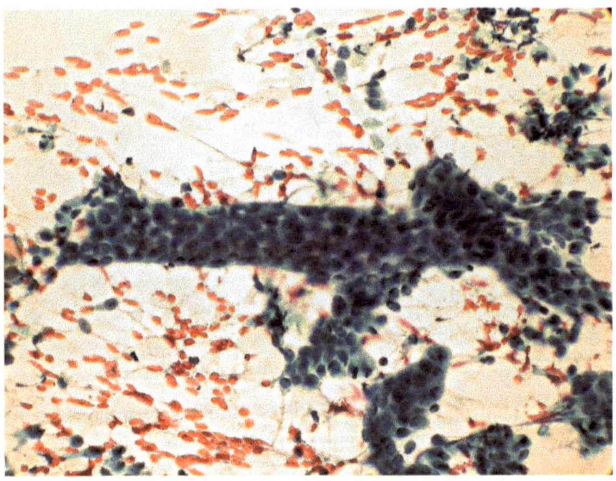

Fig. 2.7 Tubular aggregates are elongated and rectilinear and may be ramified, as in this image; they are sharply outlined and may appear to contain a central lumen. P stain, ×400

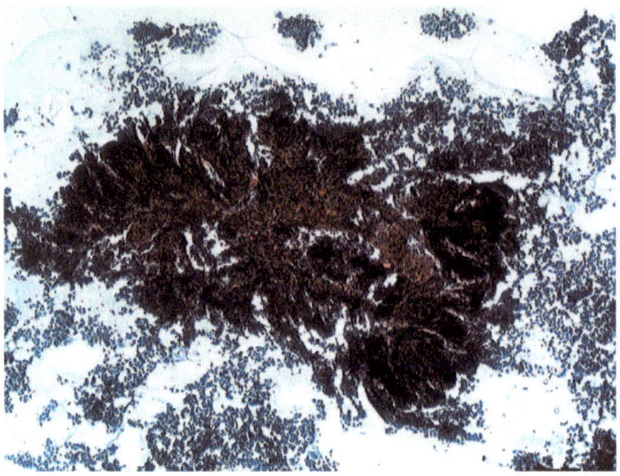

Fig. 2.8 A complex papillary aggregate is shown; papillae appear to radiate from a central core and consist of a connective-tissue stalk. P stain, ×250

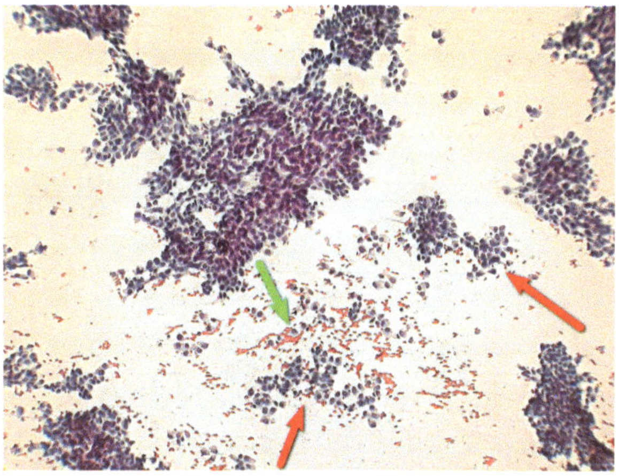

Fig. 2.9 Epithelial cells are seen in large three-dimensional clusters or appear loosely cohesive (*red arrows*), or occasionally totally non-cohesive (*green arrow*). P stain, ×400

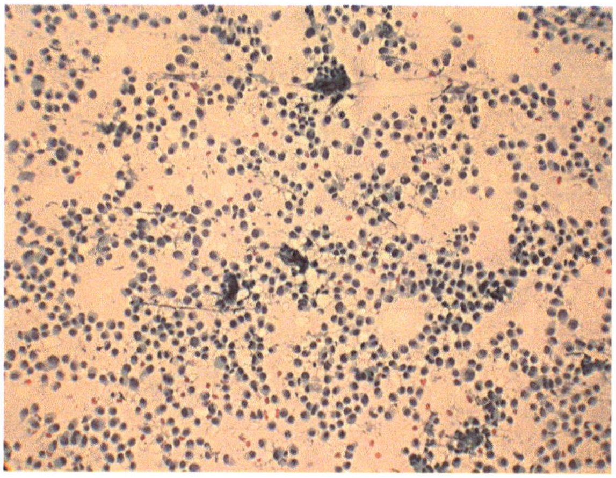

Fig. 2.10 Highly cellular smears with totally non-cohesive cells. P stain, ×400

cells dissociated within the harvest. Dissociation is classified as minimal if involving <10% of the glandular cells, moderate if involving up to 30% of these cells, and elevated if involving >30%.

2.6.5 Ancillary Elements

2.6.5.1 Bipolar Bare Nuclei

Bipolar bare nuclei are single nuclei devoid of their cytoplasmic envelope and dispersed in the background. They show a distinct and characteristic oval shape, a dense and patternless or finely granular chromatin, and terminate with two sharp extremities (Fig. 2.11). They are small (<1.5 RBC) and concentrate in areas that are sparse in erythrocytes.

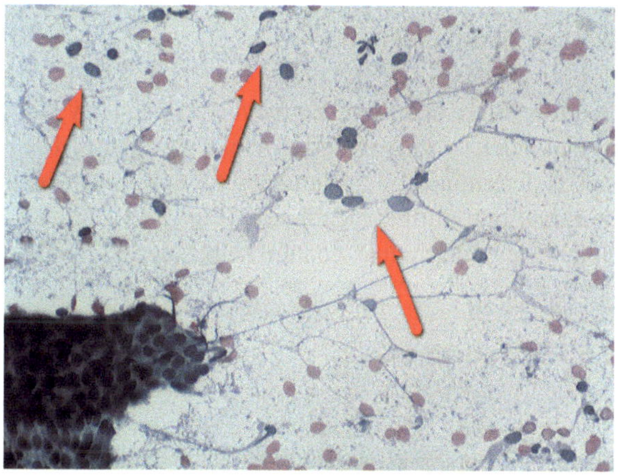

Fig. 2.11 Bipolar bare nuclei (*arrows*) have an elongated shape and their largest diameter is equal the size of a red blood cell or slightly larger; the chromatin is homogeneous and patternless. P stain, ×1000

2.6.5.2 Fibrous Stromal Fragments

These aggregates of variable size and shape are made up of elongated fibrocytes displaying a thin and elongated nucleus and admixed with a pale-staining collagenous matrix (Fig. 2.12). Fibrous stromal fragments may also contain endothelial cells and/or capillary vessels. Fibrocytes may appear to have detached from the fragments or occur as isolated elements in the background and can coexist with bipolar bare nuclei (Fig.2.12).

2.6.5.3 Adipocytic Stromal Fragments

These aggregates of adipocytes, i.e., round cells with abundant optically clear cytoplasm and a peripherally displaced elongated nucleus, are admixed with both a variable amount of fibrocytes within a pale-staining connective-tissue matrix and endothelial cells. Adipocytes may appear to have detached from such fragments and are seen scattered in the background.

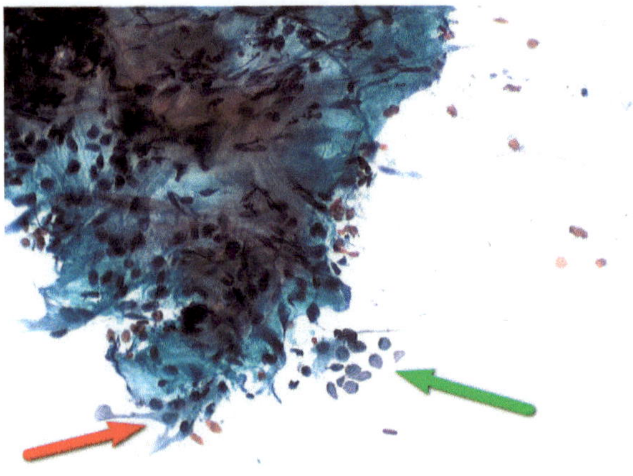

Fig. 2.12 Fibrous stromal aggregate containing fibrocytes and dense collagen matrix; at the periphery, spindled fibrocytes appear to detach from the aggregate (*red arrow*); a few bare bipolar nuclei are seen in the background (*green arrow*). P stain ×800

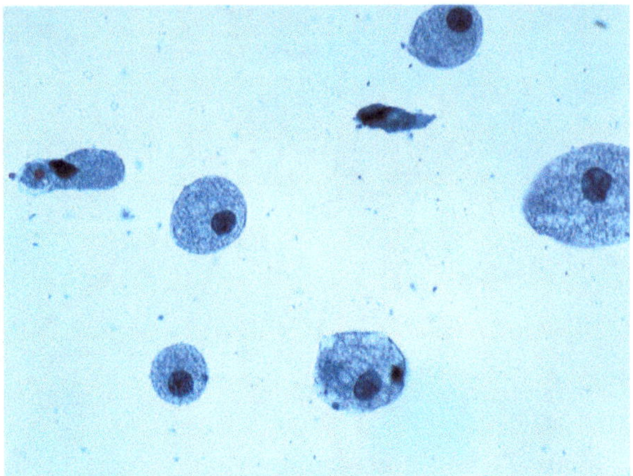

Fig. 2.13 Foam cells are round and have a microvacuolated cytoplasm. P stain, ×800

2.6.5.4 Foam Cells

Foam cells are mainly of histiocytic origin. They have a small nucleus with a finely granular chromatin. Their size is determined by the amount of cytoplasm, which is foamy due to fine vacuolation (Fig. 2.13). In addition, the cytoplasm may contain hemosiderin granules.

2.6.5.5 Apocrine Cells

Apocrine cells are metaplastic glandular cells that occur in sheets or as isolated elements. Their shape is oval to polygonal, and their size medium to large. The cytoplasm is granular, acidophilic, and generally abundant (Fig. 2.14). The nuclei are of variable size and occasionally contain prominent nucleoli.

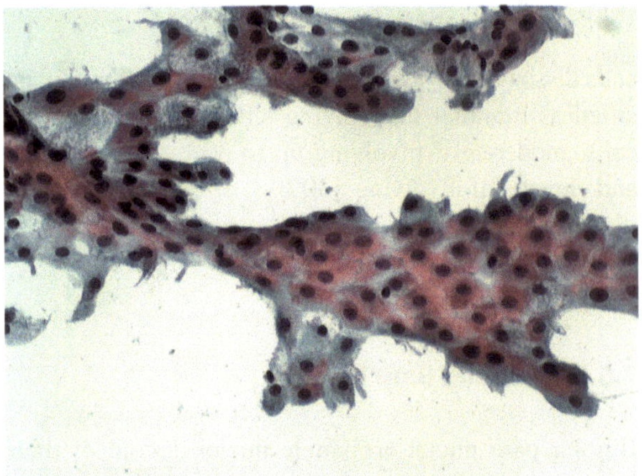

Fig. 2.14 Sheet of epithelial cells with apocrine features; the cells are medium-sized and oval to polygonal in shape; the cytoplasm is granular and eosinophilic. P stain, ×800

2.6.6 Fine Cytomorphological Features of Epithelial Glandular Cells

2.6.6.1 Nuclear Size and Shape

Epithelial cells can show nuclear enlargement as well as a variable nuclear shape. The largest diameter of nuclei in resting and normal epithelial cells does not exceed 1.5–2.0× RBC; nuclear enlargement above that limit is thus considered abnormal (Fig. 2.15). Nuclear pleomorphism (Fig. 2.16), i.e., significant variability in nuclear shape, is an additional abnormal finding to be recorded and possibly quantified.

2.6.6.2 Chromatin Texture

There are at least three patterns of chromatin texture: (a) dense and homogeneous (hyperchromasia), (b) finely granular, and (c) coarsely granular. Hyperchromasia is normal in resting cells, which by definition have a small nucleus, while it is definitely abnormal if seen in larger nuclei (Figs. 2.15, 2.16). Finely granular chromatin is present in proliferative and hyperplastic

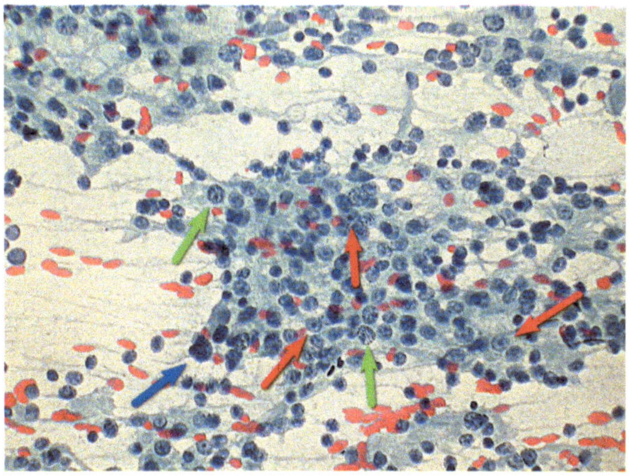

Fig. 2.15 Large three-dimensional cluster showing significant nuclear pleomorphism. Some nuclei are >2×RBC in diameter (*blue arrow*), others contain prominent nucleoli (*red arrows*), and still others show premitotic changes (*green arrows*). P stain, ×400

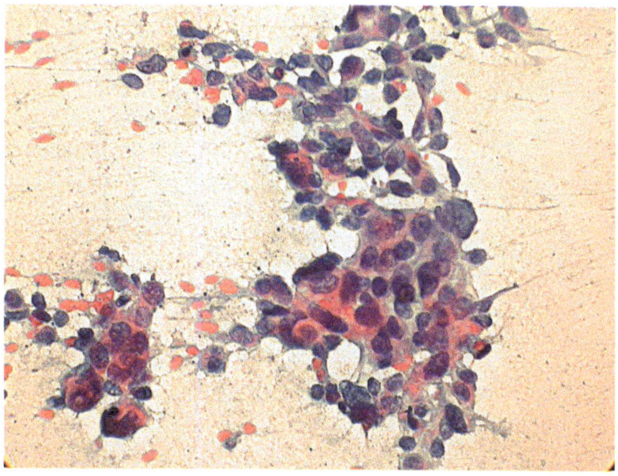

Fig. 2.16 Nuclei in this cluster vary significantly in shape and their size is significantly >2×RBC; the chromatin texture is coarsely granular. P stain, ×400

conditions (Fig. 2.3b), while a coarsely granular texture (Fig. 2.15) should be considered abnormal.

2.6.6.3 Nucleolus

A single and small nucleolus is generally seen only in a minor proportion of cells in the resting state and the nuclear texture is finely granular. Prominent nucleoli represent an abnormal finding in epithelial cells, especially if they are large (Figs. 2.15, 2.17). They generally coexist with a coarsely granular chromatin texture.

2.6.6.4 Mitotic Figures

Mitoses are very rarely seen in smears of benign lesions and their presence is to be considered highly suggestive of malignancy (Fig. 2.17).

2.6.6.5 Non-Bipolar Bare Nuclei

These are essentially the pre-apoptotic or apoptotic nuclei of epithelial cells, which are usually dispersed in the background. They are round and hyperchromatic or have stippled chromatin (Fig. 2.18). Non-bipolar bare nuclei are an abnormal finding, especially when their presence is more than occasional and their size

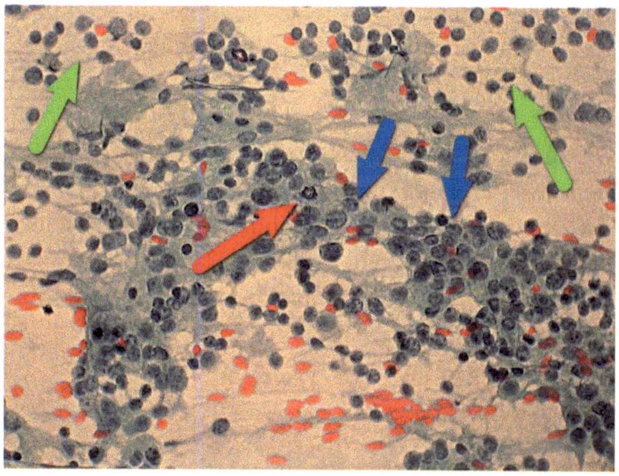

Fig. 2.17 A mitotic figure is indicated by the *red arrow* and non-bipolar bare nuclei by *green arrows*; these nuclei show significant pleomorphism and their size is often >2×RBC; the other nuclei in the smear contain prominent nucleoli and have a coarsely granular chromatin (*blue arrows*). P stain, ×400

>2×RBC. They should not be confused with bipolar bare nuclei, which have a different shape and size.

2.6.6.6 Cytoplasmic Changes

The cytoplasm of epithelial cells can be variable in appearance and in its staining features. Sometimes a large vacuole in the cytoplasm displaces the nucleus eccentrically in a signet-ring fashion. The vacuolar

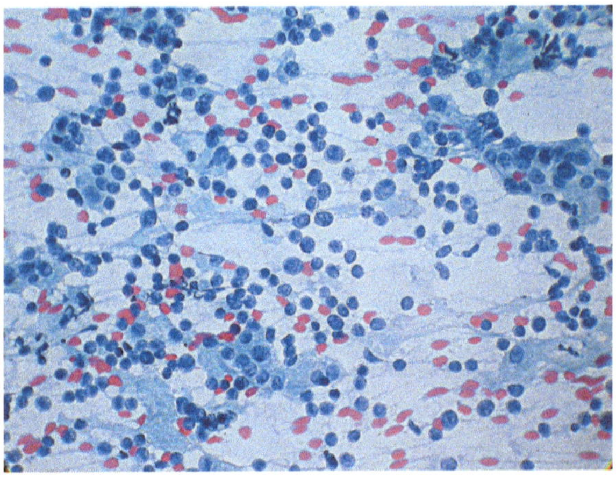

Fig. 2.18 The image is dominated by abundant non-bipolar bare nuclei that are mostly round in shape and have a coarsely granular chromatin. P stain, ×400

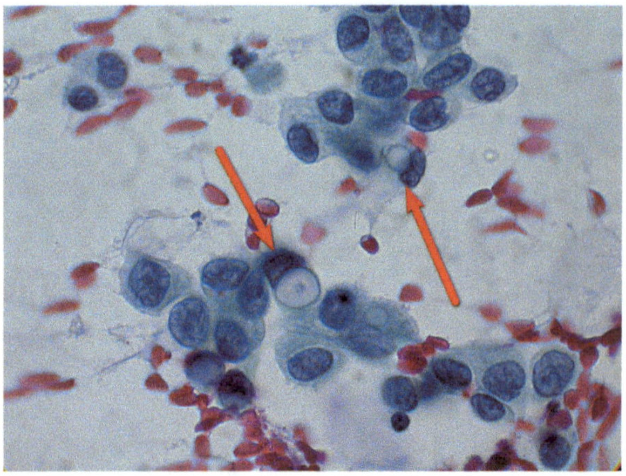

Fig. 2.19 Prominent cytoplasmic vacuoles with an optically clear content; the larger ones contain an inclusion-like structure ("targetoid" appearance) indicated by the *arrows*. P stain, ×1000

content can be optically clear due to mucin accumulation. Alternatively, the vacuole may contain a centrally located structure and have a targetoid appearance (Fig. 2.19). This is due to the presence of intracytoplasmic lumina and is an unequivocal sign of malignancy. Finally, the detection of cellular cannibalism, i.e., the phagocytosis of an entire cell by a glandular cell (the "cell-in-cell" phenomenon), is practically never a feature of benign conditions and is thus highly suspicious for malignancy (Fig. 2.20).

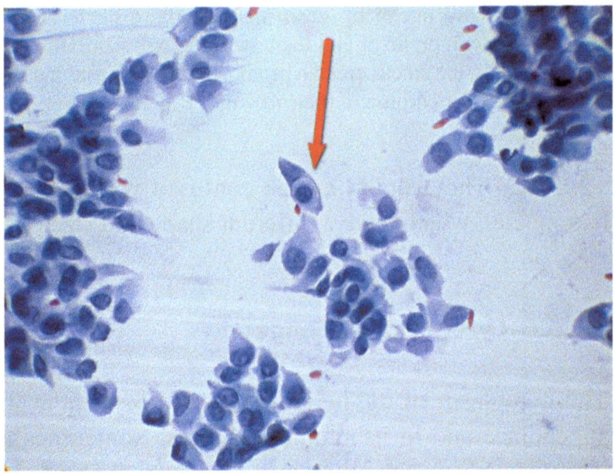

Fig. 2.20 The "cell-in-cell" phenomenon. P stain, ×1000

2.7 Primary Diagnosis of Common Benign or Premalignant Breast Lesions

2.7.1 Benign Fibroepithelial Lesions

The concomitant proliferation of both an epithelial and myoepithelial cell components and a fibroblastic connective-tissue component give rise to nodular fibroepithelial breast lesions. These constitute a spectrum of lesions ranging from the usual fibroadenoma with all its variants at one end to phyllodes tumor, with benign, borderline, and malignant variants, at the opposite end.

2.7.1.1 Fibroadenoma and its Variants

Fibroadenoma mostly occurs in women between the ages of 25 and 35, usually as a nodular lesion that is frequently palpable and often detected by the patient herself [29]. A history of rapid growth is typically reported. The size of the lesion rarely exceeds 3 cm in its largest diameter. The nodule is easily palpable, easily moved, and has a smooth surface. Fibroadenoma rarely develops in women 40 years and older. Since the ultrasound appearance of fibroadenoma can closely simulate that of mucinous carcinoma, tubular carcinoma, or low-grade invasive ductal carcinoma, the detection in this latter age group of a lesion with imaging features suggesting fibroadenoma should always be considered with great caution. Fibroadenomas typically undergo regressive changes, such as massive sclerosis and possible dystrophic calcification, which are easily detected at mammography or ultrasound especially in patients age 50 and older.

The cytological appearance of the usual variant of fibroadenoma is typically characterized by:

- A clear proteinaceous, sometimes myxoid background with abundant bipolar bare nuclei (Fig. 2.3a,b, Fig. 2.11).
- Two-dimensional, elongated, and finger-like or "stag-horn" epithelial cell aggregates, with possible ramifications and/or folding (Fig. 2.3a). At higher magnification, these cells tend to have regular nuclei with a finely granular texture chromatin and nuclei that rarely overlap (Fig. 2.3b).
- Stromal fragments of fibrous tissue (Fig. 2.12).

At variance with this picture are lesions in which the background is massively myxoid or the epithelial aggregates are also three-dimensional, but the presence of abundant bare bipolar nuclei represents an unequivocal finding allowing the reliable diagnosis of fibroadenoma. Other variants enter the differential diagnosis of carcinoma and are discussed later in this chapter.

2.7.1.2 Benign and Borderline Phyllodes Tumor

Phyllodes tumor is generally observed in women age 40 and older and appears as a nodule >3 cm in its broadest diameter. The clinical appearance is that of usual fibroadenoma [29]. The diagnostic cytological pattern of this lesion is characterized by:

- Bipolar or spindly bare nuclei abundant in the background, with possible necrotic debris and isolated fibrocyte-like or histiocyte-like cells (Fig. 2.21a).
- A variable component of two- and three-dimensional epithelial cell aggregates (Fig. 2.21b), comprising cells characterized by slight anisonucleosis and occasional nucleoli.
- Thick stromal fragments with a vague leaf-like morphology and containing multiple layers of spindle cells (Fig. 2.21a).

The clue to the diagnosis is the presence of bare nuclei with a bipolar and spindly morphology coexisting with leaf-like stromal fragments [30]. Additional findings that favor the diagnosis of phyllodes tumor are aggregates of epithelial cells with squamous metaplasia and the presence of adipocytes in the stromal component. The fibroadenoma variant in which there is stromal hypercellularity can present on FNB with overlapping cytological features, but only phyllodes tumor is characterized by squamous

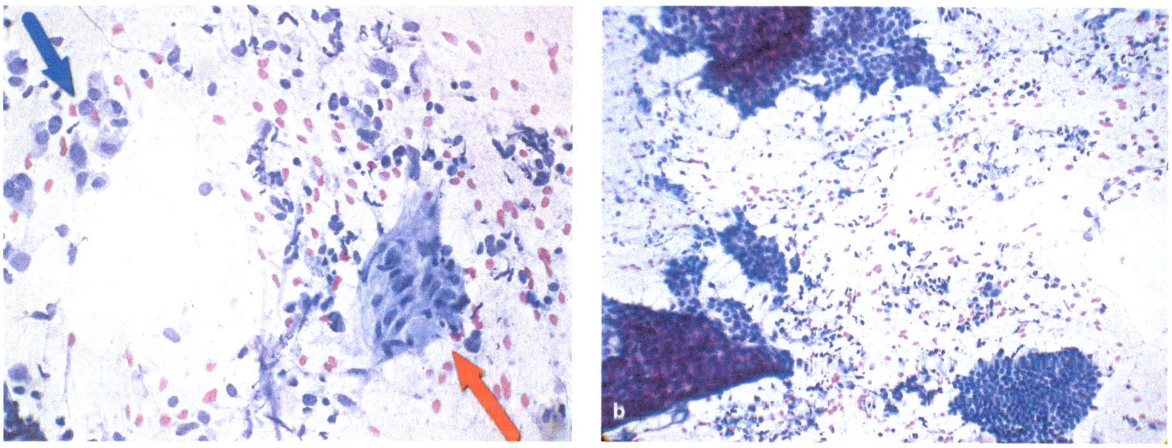

Fig. 2.21 **a** In FNB samples from phyllodes tumor, the background is characteristically dominated by bipolar and spindly bare nuclei, histiocyte-like cells (*blue arrow*), and stromal fragments containing somewhat pleomorphic fibrocytes (*red arrow*). P stain, ×400. **b** Low-power view of the same case as in **a**, showing epithelial clusters of variable size and shape as well as bipolar and non-bipolar bare nuclei with histiocyte-like cells in the background. P stain, ×250

metaplasia of epithelial cells and adipocytic metaplasia in the stromal component. Cellular pleomorphism with enlarged and hyperchromatic nuclei and the detection of mitoses in the stromal fragments is a clear indication of a malignant phyllodes tumor.

2.7.1.3 Intraductal/Intracystic Papilloma

Papillomas can occur in women between the fourth and sixth decades of life and arise at any level in the mammary ductal tree, from the ductular-lobular terminal unit (peripheral papillomas) to the large ducts of the nipple (central papillomas) [29]. They can be single or multiple. In addition, they can arise within a cystic cavity, filling it partially or completely. Segmental dilation of the ductal system due to an expanding papilloma or intracystic papilloma can produce a palpable or non-palpable breast lump that is otherwise readily visible at US examination. Bloody discharge from the nipple is, however, the main clinical manifestation of a papilloma.

The cytological picture is dominated by the presence of papillary fronds of epithelial ductal cells with a well-defined connective-tissue stalk (Fig. 2.8). These fronds are variably arranged and variably ramified. The epithelial cells are columnar in shape. The outline of the papillary vegetation is marked by the external membrane of epithelial cells, which occasionally shows examples of decapitation secretion (Fig. 2.22). Nuclei form palisades and are regular in shape and size (Fig. 2.22). The background is rich in red blood cells, foamy histiocytes, or histiocytes containing hemosiderin pigment granules, and sometimes small lymphocytes or bare bipolar nuclei. Isolated cylindrical duct cells are also easily detected in the background due to their exfoliation and detachment. Apocrine metaplasia is commonly seen. The unexpected detection of papillary fronds in a FNB sample from a breast lump should always prompt a careful re-consideration of the ultrasound and mammographic images as well as the patient's clinical history. Provided that: (a) the lesion has been adequately sampled, (b) cytology provides unequivocal evidence establishing the benign nature of the lesion, and (c) imaging data support this contention, then surgical excision can be avoided but the patient should enter careful clinical surveillance. However, if there is any element of doubt with respect to the cytology or imaging findings, the lesion should be excised for a definitive and more reliable histological evaluation [31,32]. CNB, especially VACNB, represents a valid option for further diagnostic evaluation and even the complete excision of small lesions. In general, the ambiguous diagnosis of "proliferative and papillary breast lesion with atypia: malignancy cannot be excluded" is preferred for lesions showing atypical changes.

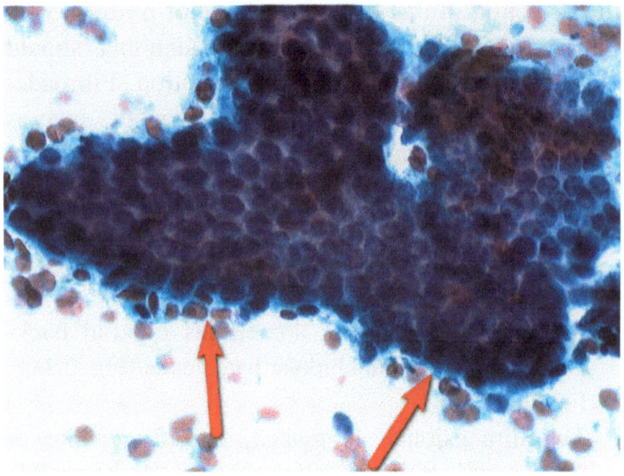

Fig. 2.22 A papillary cluster showing peripheral palisading of nuclei (*arrows*). P stain, ×1000

2.7.2 *Sclerosing Lesions Following Fat Necrosis*

Fat necrosis of breast parenchyma is rather common in elderly patients or at least in women with large breasts, due to adipose involution. Predisposing conditions are contusive traumas and recent surgical manipulation of the breast. Radiologically, the lesion can closely simulate a carcinoma, especially in the phase of early florid development in that it assumes a characteristic stellate or spiculated configuration. FNB discloses a characteristic picture and quickly resolves any questions as to the diagnosis. On FNB, the background contains cellular detritus as well as lipoid droplets, adipocytes with vacuolated cytoplasm, foamy histiocytes sometimes in the form of multinucleated giant cells, and stromal fragments. Epithelial cells are not seen.

2.7.3 Intramammary Lymph Nodes

Lymph nodes can occur in the breast parenchyma, mostly in the upper external quadrants. They simulate a fibroadenoma at mammography and at ultrasound examination. FNB shows a lymphoid harvest consisting of small to medium-sized lymphocytes, a variable number of the characteristic tingible bodies, macrophages, and stromal fragments containing endothelial cells. There are no epithelial cells.

2.7.4 Proliferative Breast Lesions

There is a wide group of benign breast lesions that on FNB present a non-characteristic or non-specific picture that does not correspond to any of the above-described benign lesions. This group comprises proliferative lesions affecting the lobular units or, conversely, the ductal cavities and they are defined under the headings of adenosis, various types of adenoma, lobular neoplasia, and intraductal proliferative lesions. Their main feature is the concomitant proliferation of epithelial and myoepithelial cellular components and the possibility that the epithelial compartment assumes a florid or atypical morphology. In daily practice, these represent the large majority of benign lesions included in the differential diagnosis of carcinoma.

Lesions of the adenosis group are classified histologically as sclerosing adenosis, apocrine adenosis, blunt duct adenosis, and microglandular adenosis [29]. They most frequently occur in women between the ages of 30 and 50. The proliferative process mainly affects the lobular component of the breast parenchyma. Epithelial proliferation leads to the formation of a complex aggregation of acinar and tubular structures, always with a fairly distinct myoepithelial cellular component. The extent of concomitant myoepithelial cellular proliferation is variable and strongly influences the overall morphology and architecture of the lesion. Different types of epithelial proliferations belonging to the adenosis group can coexist with a complex sclerosing process in the so-called radial scar/complex sclerosing lesion. This is a benign lesion that resembles invasive carcinoma both mammographically and on gross examination. Histologically, it consists of a mixture of adenosis, mainly of the sclerosing type, ductal epithelial hyperplasia of solid or cribriform type, apocrine metaplasia, and papillomas.

The proliferative conditions of the ductal epithelium also called borderline ductal proliferations are mainly located in the ductulo-lobular unit and show a variable degree of cellular atypia but no stromal invasion [33]. They are divided into three categories: typical (usual) duct hyperplasia, atypical duct hyperplasia, and low-grade ductal carcinoma in situ (DCIS) [29,34]. These lesions share several morphological features that are variably expressed but differ with respect to their potential transformation into invasive carcinoma. Histologically, usual and atypical duct hyperplasia are characterized by an intraductal proliferation of cells with variable morphological features filling, partially or completely, the lumen of the ductulo-lobular units. Atypical duct hyperplasia is an obligate precursor to DCIS which in turn is a precursor to invasive carcinoma. The reproducibility of histopathological criteria in the distinction and grading of these lesions is poor.

Basically, the cytological sample of a proliferative breast lesion is moderately to highly cellular and consists of aggregated epithelial glandular cells in a clear to proteinaceous background containing bare bipolar naked nuclei (Fig. 2.24). Despite the heterogeneity in the histological picture, the cytopathology of proliferative breast lesions on FNB can be reduced to the evaluation of a few parameters that refer to the aggregation pattern of epithelial cells, their morphology in terms of cellular pleomorphism and nuclear features, and, most importantly, the concomitant proliferation

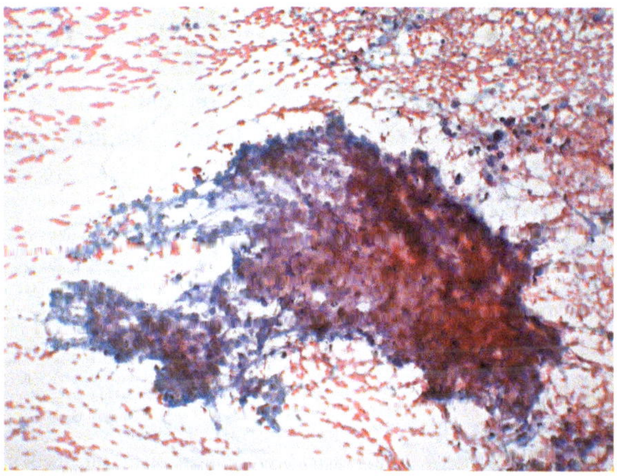

Fig. 2.23 A coagulative necrotic cluster wherein nuclear "shadows" are seen. P stain, ×400

Table 2.5 Cytological score for classification of proliferative breast lesions adapted by Masood et al., 1991 [20]

Score	Bipolar naked nuclei (myoepithelial cells)	Cellular arrangement	Cellular pleomorphism	Anisonucleosis	Nucleoli	Chromatin clumping
1	Abundant	2-dimensional	Absent	Absent	Absent	Absent
2	Moderate	2- and 3-dimensional	Slight	Slight	Sparse	Slight
3	Sparse	3-dimensional	Moderate	Moderate	Micronucleoli	Moderate
4	Absent	Minor non-cohesiveness	Conspicuous	Conspicuous	Micro- and macronucleoli	Conspicuous

Total score: 6–10 = non-proliferative, 11–14 = proliferative without atypia, 15–18 = proliferative with atypia, 19–24 = carcinoma

of myoepithelial cells. The cytological picture of florid hyperplastic lesions and premalignant or low-grade malignant conditions can overlap on FNB samples, at least qualitatively; however, significant quantitative differences in the above parameters can be observed. In this regard, the score system developed by Masood et al., 1991 [20], distinguishes among these alterations according to a semi-quantitative approach and allows for the distinction between low-risk and high-risk cases. The system is based on the evaluation of six cytological parameters (Table 2.5), each of which is scored separately along a scale of 1 to 4, with the total yielding the cytological score. Samples from borderline breast lesions generally have a score of 12–18. In this author's experience, scores <15 and >16 are indicative of, respectively, low-risk and high-risk lesions. In fact, the cytohistological correlation discloses cases of usual florid hyperplasia in the former group, and atypical ductal hyperplasia, low-grade in situ ductal carcinoma, and invasive ductal carcinoma in the latter. A score of 15 and 16 represents the gray zone of the system, where usual florid and atypical ductal hyperplasia and in situ carcinoma all can occur. The combined DNA and image analysis of the cytological sample from this group of patients shows that a hypoproliferative diploid pattern is more often associated with low-risk lesions while hyperproliferative diploid or aneuploid lesions are at increased risk of being malignant [35].

2.8 Diagnosis of Carcinoma

The diagnosis of breast carcinoma is primarily based on a pattern-analysis approach. Examination of the cytological specimen requires the systematic evaluation of several criteria in order to construct a diagnostic algorithm according to a rigorous methodology of deductive reasoning. The specimen should be firstly evaluated for its cellularity and secondly according to several major and minor diagnostic criteria that concur to yield a final diagnostic formulation, which may be totally conclusive for carcinoma or express the diagnosis of malignancy or premalignancy in probabilistic terms. In other words, since a diagnosis of carcinoma is not always possible, lesions with suspicious features or with cytological alterations suggesting a high-risk proliferative lesion should be properly identified based on reproducible criteria that convey the most appropriate clinical information.

In the diagnosis of a lesion as malignant, the cellularity of the specimen should be at least moderate to high (Fig. 2.2). Conversely, a low or sparse cellularity is an indication for a more cautious approach.

2.8.1 Specimens with Adequate Cellularity

The analytical approach should take into account the evaluation and classification of several major and minor criteria whose presence contributes to the development of a diagnostic algorithm (Table 2.6). The

Table 2.6 Major and minor cytological criteria of malignancy

Major criteria
- Extent of cellular dissociation
- Prevailing aggregation pattern
- Presence of bipolar bare nuclei

Minor criteria
- Anisonucleosis
- Non-bipolar bare nuclei
- Mitoses
- Cytoplasmic targetoid vacuoles
- Necrotic background
- High cellularity

distinction between major and minor criteria is based on the different "weights" of the former with respect to the latter in the context of the decision-making process. Major criteria are detected and evaluated by microscopy, by observing the smear at low-power magnification, while minor criteria are mostly assessed at high-power magnification.

2.8.1.1 Major Criteria

Dissociation of Epithelial Cells

This parameter should be quantified as absent (score 0), present but ≤10% (score 1), or present and >10% (score 2). It is important not to mistake non-cohesive epithelial cells for fibroblasts or histiocytes, as the appearances of the latter cell type may resemble that of dissociated elements. The extent of cellular non-cohesion is a powerful and robust predictive criterion for malignancy.

Prevailing Aggregation Pattern

Scrutiny of the cellular smear at low or medium magnification should allow the pathologist to determine whether there is a prevalence of two- or three-dimensional aggregates. In addition, it is useful to identify a possible prevailing tendency for the formation of distinct types of aggregates fulfilling the morphological features previously described (cords, tubules, papillae, two-dimensional sheets, etc.). The aggregation pattern has no predictive value in terms of a diagnosis of malignancy but is essential to the construction of the diagnostic algorithm.

Presence of Bipolar Bare Nuclei

Evaluation of the smear at low- and medium-power magnification should be completed by a careful search for bipolar bare nuclei with their characteristic morphology. This parameter should be quantified as absent (score 0), or present (score 1). A score of 1 is used if bipolar bare nuclei are seen not only occasionally but with an abundance of 4–5 per high power field and in different fields throughout the smear. Their shape and size should be rigorously congruent with the above-described criteria. The presence of this feature is a powerful and robust criterion in favor of the benignancy of the specimen.

2.8.1.2 Minor Criteria

Anisonucleosis

Atypical nuclear features should be carefully searched mostly within aggregates of epithelial cells and consist of the following: (a) increased nuclear size and pleomorphism, (b) changes in chromatin texture, and (c) the presence of prominent nucleoli (Figs. 2.4, 2.5, 2.15, 2.16, 2.17). Nuclear size is assessed by comparison to the RBC diameter; if the limit of 1.5–2.0×RBC diameters is exceeded in most cells, this is a significantly atypical finding. Atypical chromatin patterns consist of hyperchromasia in enlarged nuclei and a coarsely granular chromatin texture. Well evident nucleoli are an atypical feature in epithelial glandular cells of the breast and the nucleolus may sometimes become very prominent. Each of the above changes should be confirmed in a significant proportion of cells. Generally, increased nuclear size, abnormal chromatin texture, and the presence of prominent nucleoli occur together but a wide repertoire of combinations is observed. In particular, in carcinoma of low-grade malignancy, nucleoli may be completely lacking or inconspicuous whereas a significant increase in nuclear size and the presence of coarsely granular chromatin are generally easily recognized.

Non-bipolar Bare Nuclei

Non-bipolar, roundish nuclei devoid of a cytoplasmic envelope and present in the background of the smear represent a definitely atypical finding, especially if the size of these nuclei exceeds the limit of 1.5–2.0×RBC (Fig. 2.18). The hyperchromatic and/or coarsely granular pattern contrasts with the finely granular pattern of bipolar bare nuclei, seen in benign conditions.

Mitoses

Mitotic figures should be searched for within the cellular aggregates. While their detection is rare, their presence strongly favors a diagnosis of malignancy even if their morphology is typical (Fig. 2.17).

Targetoid Cytoplasmic Vacuoles

These are single large vacuoles that displace and sometimes compress the nucleus. They are empty-looking and characterized by a prominent external membrane. The targetoid appearance is due to the presence of a centrally placed eosinophilic globule (Fig. 2.19). Targetoid vacuoles have a distinct morphology and are not to be confused with other types of cellular vacuoles. The detection of these cellular modifications, even if only occasional, is highly suggestive of malignancy, especially of lobular carcinoma.

Hypercellular Smear

The detection of high cellularity in a FNB sample from a breast nodule in an elderly woman who is not receiving hormone therapy, and the detection in the sample of two- or three-dimensional aggregates of epithelial cells lacking any significant nuclear atypical features strongly support a diagnosis of low-grade invasive or in situ ductal carcinoma. In other words, high cellularity in a specimen from a nodular lesion in an elderly patient is definitely to be considered as abnormal despite the otherwise benign appearance of the cells.

Necrosis

Necrotic detritus in the background of a cellular smear is unusual in benign conditions and should be considered a hint for possible malignancy (Fig. 2.23). In general, careful inspection of the smear discloses more significant and confirmatory features.

2.8.1.3 Construction of the Diagnostic Algorithm

Major and minor criteria should to be evaluated and scored separately in the first step, while in the second step they are assimilated to construct the diagnostic algorithm. The extent of dissociation is scored as 0 (absent), 1 (≤10%), or 2 (>10%). The prevailing pattern of aggregation is identified and defined as "two-dimensional" or "three-dimensional." The presence of bare bipolar nuclei is scored as 1 according to the above-described criteria, and their absence as 0. The detection of at least one of the minor criteria is scored as 1, otherwise as 0.

Evaluation of the extent of cellular dissociation is the first requirement and it allows for the preliminary delineation of three categories. Within each one, the additional consideration of other major and minor criteria points to different algorithms and the role of individual criteria can vary in the different categories. Implementation of the algorithms leads to the most probable diagnosis and the best diagnostic formulation of the case.

Pattern with Cellular Dissociation Score = 0

Cellular dissociation is a robust predictive factor in terms of malignancy but it can be completely lacking in a significant proportion of carcinomas. In the latter situation, other major and minor criteria should be considered in the process of problem solving; the diagnostic conclusions are listed in Table 2.7. It is important to underscore that in this group of cases a prevailing three-dimensional aggregation pattern is more predictive for malignancy than a prevailing two-dimensional pattern. Thus, in practice, in the presence of the same scores for bare bipolar nuclei and minor criteria, a three-dimensional aggregation pattern indicates a higher risk of malignancy. This category typically includes proliferative breast lesions with or without atypia (Fig. 2.24), as well as "in situ" ductal carcinoma and low-grade invasive ductal carcinoma. The detection of nuclear alterations with a prevailing three-dimensional aggregation pattern in the absence of bipolar bare nuclei delineates the highest risk of the lesion being malignant. At the opposite end of the spectrum, the detection of a prevailing two-dimensional aggregation pattern, with the presence of bare bipolar nuclei and the absence of minor criteria, is an indication that the lesion is most probably benign. Rarely, aggregates of highly atypical large and bizarre epithelial cells are seen but with no sign of dissociation. The cellularity of the sample is high and characterized by necrotic debris. Cells in aggregates appear

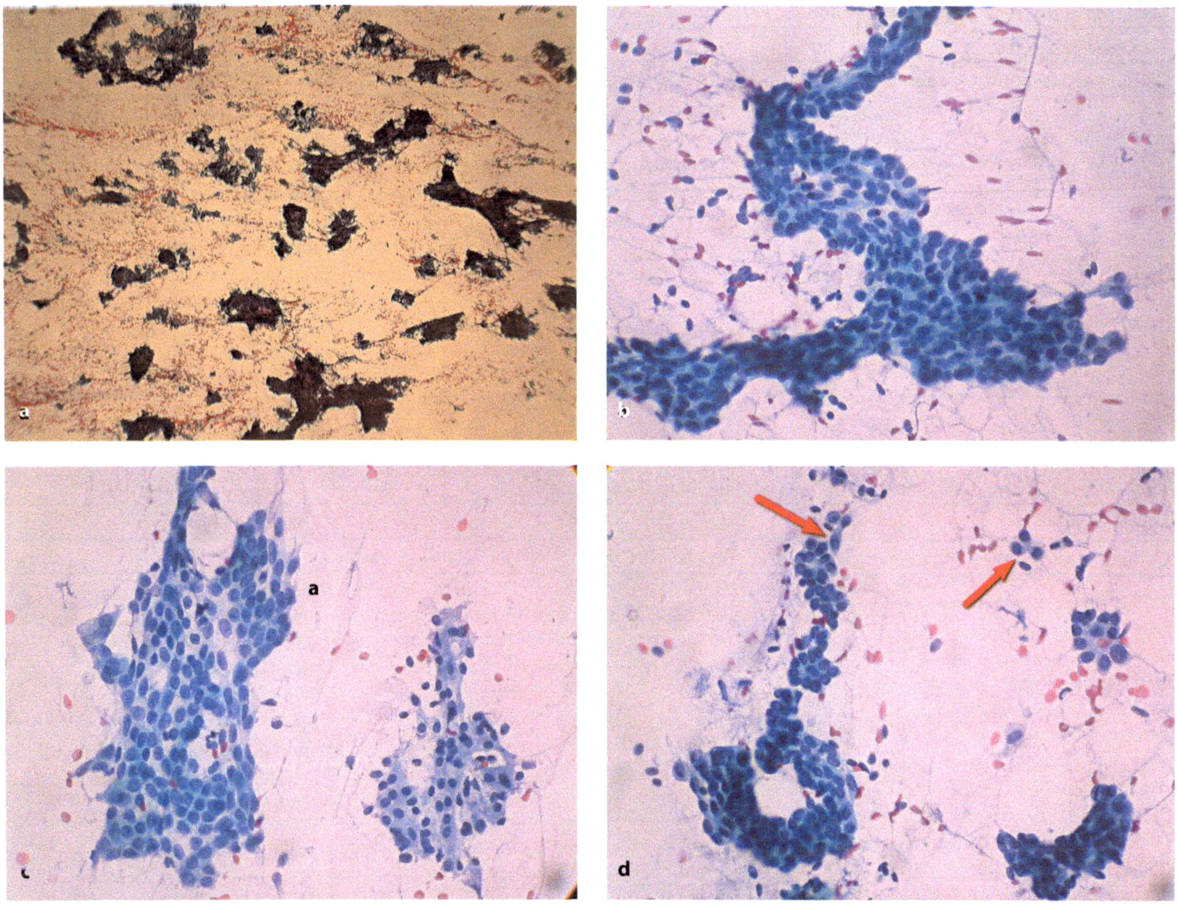

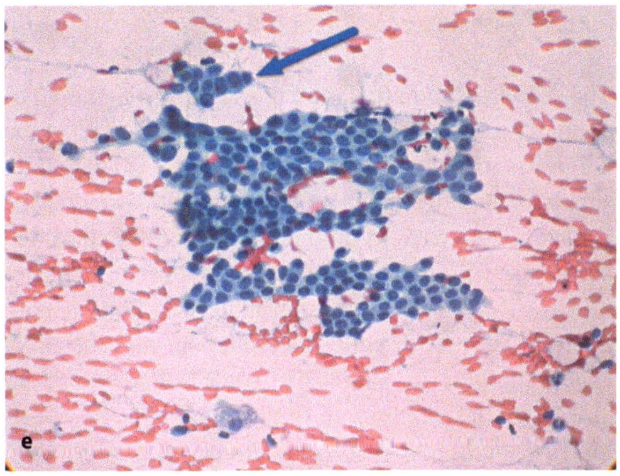

Fig. 2.24 **a** Characteristic low-power view of a FNB sample obtained from a patient with a proliferative breast lesion consisting of clusters of variable size and shape in a background rich in red blood cells. P stain, ×100. **b** Two-dimensional and elongated cluster of epithelial cells shows significant nuclear pleomorphism while bare bipolar nuclei are abundant in the background. P stain, ×400. **c** Significant anisonucleosis is evident in the cluster on the *left* as compared to that on the *right* side of the image. P stain, ×400. **d** Tubular and acinar aggregates with initial non-cohesiveness (*arrows*); bipolar bare nuclei are seen in the background. P stain, ×400. **e** Two-dimensional aggregate of epithelial cells showing empty spaces (cribriform appearance); the *arrow* indicates a small cluster with a definite “Indian file” configuration and chromatin clumping. P stain, ×400

very large, with pleomorphic nuclei and prominent nucleoli, and mitotic activity is easily detected. This cytological picture is typically seen in medullary carcinoma or in highly aggressive tumors in young women.

Pattern with Minimal Cellular Dissociation Score = 1

The presence of cellular dissociation, even of minimal extent (Fig. 2.9), is a marker of the increased risk that the lesion is malignant rather than benign. The diag-

Table 2.7 Different diagnostic possibilities with cellular dissociation = 0

Major criteria			Minor criteria	Diagnosis
Cellular dissociation	Aggregation pattern	Bipolar bare nuclei		
0	2-dimensional	1	0	Proliferative without atypia
0	2-dimensional	1	1	Proliferative with atypia
0	2-dimensional	0	0	Proliferative without atypia
0	2-dimensional	0	1	Proliferative with atypia/suspicious for carcinoma
0	3-dimensional	1	0	Proliferative without atypia
0	3-dimensional	1	1	Proliferative with atypia/suspicious for carcinoma
0	3-dimensional	0	0	Proliferative with atypia
0	3-dimensional	0	1	Suspicious for carcinoma/carcinoma

Table 2.8 Different diagnostic possibilities with cellular dissociation = 1

Major criteria			Minor criteria	Diagnosis
Cellular dissociation	Aggregation pattern	Bipolar bare nuclei		
1	2-dimensional	1	0	Proliferative with atypia
1	2-dimensional	1	1	Suspicious for carcinoma
1	2-dimensional	0	0	Proliferative with atypia
1	2-dimensional	0	1	Suspicious for carcinoma
1	3-dimensional	1	0	Proliferative with atypia
1	3-dimensional	1	1	Proliferative with atypia/suspicious for carcinoma
1	3-dimensional	0	0	Proliferative with atypia
1	3-dimensional	0	1	Carcinoma

nostic algorithm is strongly influenced by this finding, as shown in Table 2.8, and the diagnostic suggestions are very different from those in the absence of dissociation (score = 0, Table 2.7), other parameters being equal. However, as in lesions not showing cellular dissociation, the tendency of the cells to form a two-dimensional aggregation pattern favors a benign proliferative lesion while the prevalence of a three-dimensional aggregation suggests a malignant lesion. Similarly, the presence of bipolar bare nuclei and the absence of any minor criteria favors a benign proliferative lesion while in the opposite case a malignant lesion should be suspected. The main difference is that a documented tendency to cellular dissociation enhances the weight of the above negative criteria, thus calling for a stronger suspicion of malignancy. In summary, the finding of minimal cellular dissociation together with a prevailing three-dimensional aggregation pattern, the absence of bare bipolar nuclei, and the presence of any minor nuclear changes leads to a definite diagnosis of carcinoma (Fig. 2.25).

Pattern with Dissociation Score = 2

The detection of dissociation in a significant amount of epithelial cells (Fig. 2.10) is an important clue to the diagnosis of carcinoma. This finding is generally supplemented by other observations, such as increased nuclear size, coarsely granular chromatin texture, the presence of prominent nucleoli, and–possibly but not necessarily–a necrotic background, non bipolar bare nuclei, the "cell in cell" phenomenon, and the presence of targetoid vacuoles in some cells (Figs. 2.15 to 2.20). These additional findings are a useful corollary for the diagnosis of carcinoma, especially when moderate cellular dissociation is seen as well (10–30% of the cell population). The presence of cellular dissociation >30% is a definite indication that the lesion is malignant. The pattern of cellular aggregation has no influence on the diagnosis of carcinoma but a prevailing two-dimensional pattern correlates well with low-grade "in situ" or invasive ductal carcinoma and, conversely, a prevailing three-dimensional pattern

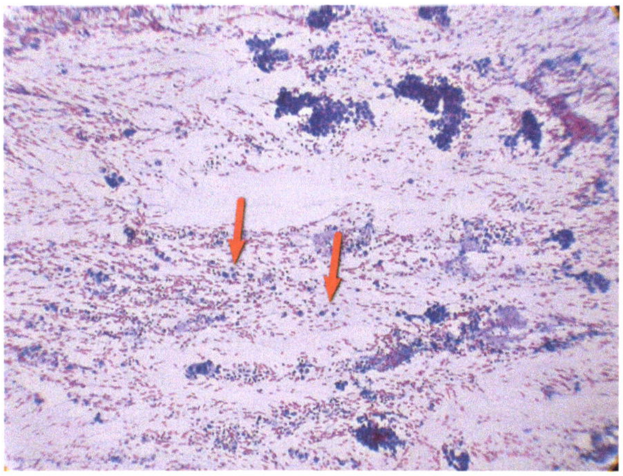

Fig. 2.25 The finding of minimal cellular dissociation (*arrows*), the absence of bare bipolar nuclei in the background, and the presence of anisonucleosis lead to a definite diagnosis of carcinoma. P stain, ×250

correlates with high-grade DCIS and moderate- to high-grade invasive ductal carcinoma. When dissociation is observed in >50% of the cell population, the tumor is most probably a high-grade DCIS or an invasive ductal carcinoma grade 2 or 3. The detection of numerous cytoplasmic vacuoles with a characteristic targetoid appearance strongly correlates with a diagnosis of invasive lobular carcinoma, pleomorphic or alveolar variants.

2.8.2 Samples with Minimal to Low Cellularity

If the diagnostic yield is adequate but sparse, the diagnosis of carcinoma should be considered with great caution. It is for this reason that additional biopsy passes should be performed, to ensure that a representative sample is obtained, especially from lesions characterized by a high index of suspicion at the pre-analytical evaluation. In a significant proportion of patients, however, the harvest remains sparse despite additional sampling due to features intrinsic to the tumor. This is particularly the case for invasive lobular carcinoma, classical variant, and is probably due to a marked desmoplastic reaction that surrounds the neoplastic cells infiltrating the stroma as single elements, thus hindering their mobilization through the biopsy needle. Moreover, some tumors are characterized by massive sclerosis, especially in central areas; this is especially true for scirrhous carcinoma or tumors of very large size detected in elderly patients. In these latter cases, sampling should be repeated and concentrated on the peripheral portion of the tumor nodule.

Low cellularity in the harvest modifies the diagnostic algorithm in the sense that the level of cellular dissociation required for a definite diagnosis of carcinoma should not be <30% (Table 2.9). Below this level, the preferred diagnosis should be "suspicious for carcinoma" unless other criteria of malignancy are present, especially cytoplasmic targetoid vacuoles and/or major nuclear atypia. The detection of targetoid vacuoles in this context is of great help in the diagnosis of lobular carcinoma. The pattern of cellular aggregation plays no decisive role in samples with low cellularity. When confronted with samples that are adequate albeit hypocellular and show only minor cellular dissociation as well as bare bipolar nuclei and no minor criteria, the pathologist is better off reporting the lesion as inconclusive, thus advising a repeat FNB or CNB. Nonetheless, on subsequent evaluation, many of these lesions turn to be malignant.

2.8.3 Limitations and Pitfalls

The above-described approach allows for the identification of most but not all malignant epithelial tumors of the breast. Indeed, a significant proportion of

Table 2.9 Diagnostic possibilities in hypocellular samples

Dissociation (%)	Bare bipolar nuclei	Minor criteria	Diagnosis
0	0–1	0	Benign/inadequate
0	0	1	Inconclusive/suspicious for carcinoma
0	1	1	Inconclusive, probably proliferative
1–30	0–1	0	Suspicious for carcinoma
1–30	0 1	1	Carcinoma
31–100	0–1	0–1	Carcinoma

0 = absent, 1 = present

tumors cannot be diagnosed by FNB cytology alone because of several heterogeneous factors concerning both the architecture of tumor growth and the degree of cellular differentiation. The former greatly influences the adequacy and representativity of the sample, and the latter the extent of cellular modification and atypia. Some limitations may be encountered when FNB is used in the diagnosis of the following variants of invasive carcinoma.

Invasive Ductal Carcinoma (NOS), Well-Differentiated (G1)

In many cases, the pattern of cellular aggregation and cellular modifications in samples from these tumors does not allow for a clear-cut distinction from a borderline breast proliferation; consequently, the diagnosis falls into the category of "atypical" but there is no definite diagnosis of malignancy.

Invasive Lobular Carcinoma, Classical Variant

A characteristic feature of this tumor variant is an extensive stromal desmoplasia that surrounds and envelops tumor cells that mostly infiltrate as single elements. These factors prevent needle aspiration of the cells in significant amounts and the sample is frequently diagnosed as inadequate. An immediate repeat pass is often followed by intralesional hemorrhage and blood contamination of the sample.

Invasive Ductal Carcinoma, Desmoplastic Variant (Scirrhous) of Large Size

Tumor nodules of large size (>3 cm in diameter) or those characterized by marked intralesional desmoplasia contain vast areas devoid of epithelial cells. This is particularly true in the central portion of the tumor nodule and is a cause of poor cellularity in the sample. Thus, paradoxically, the larger the tumor, the higher the chance of a poorly cellular or even inadequate sample. For this reason, needle sampling should be concentrated on peripheral areas, at the interface with normal tissue, where cellularity is expected to be more abundant.

Inflammatory Carcinoma ("Carcinomatous Mastitis")

This is an especially aggressive variant of carcinoma that occurs in women at any age, including the elderly. It is characterized by diffuse edematous swelling of the breast, which is painful and warm to the touch. There is no tumor lump and swelling is reported as having appeared suddenly, possibly with a nipple discharge. The nipple may be flattened or inverted. Persistent itching can occur and the overall picture is first interpreted as mastitis and treated as such. Although no tumor lump is palpated in the breast, palpable lymph nodes can be readily detected in the axilla or supraclavicular area. This clinical appearance is explained by an early, diffuse, and marked tendency of the tumor cells to invade lymphatic vessels, eventually impairing lymphatic drainage. Since there is no nodular target within the breast parenchyma, needle biopsy fails to collect a sample of sufficient cellularity and frequently the harvest is contaminated by blood. In these cases, lymph node sampling in axillary areas provides a better chance of collecting a representative amount of tumor cells.

2.9 Variants of Carcinoma

2.9.1 Mucinous Carcinoma

Mucinous carcinoma is a rather frequent variant of invasive carcinoma, especially in elderly patients, but it is often encountered in young and middle-aged women [29]. Clinically and radiologically, mucinous carcinoma can simulate a fibroadenoma or a benign cyst. The cytological sample is generally hypocellular, with a variable amount of mucoid ground substance in the background (Fig. 2.25). There are no bare bipolar nuclei. Epithelial cells are found in small two- or three-dimensional aggregates that have a round contour and are sharply outlined. Nuclear atypia is mild with small, prominent nucleoli [36]. The cytoplasm is homogeneous and glassy in appearance and sometimes shows vacuolar changes. Cytoplasmic borders are sharp. Non-cohesive cells are sparse and may be completely absent (Fig. 2.26). The diagnosis of mucinous carcinoma is based on detection of the characteristic cellular aggregates within a diffusely mucinous background while the presence of cellular dissociation is not required. The differential diagnosis includes fibroadenoma with a

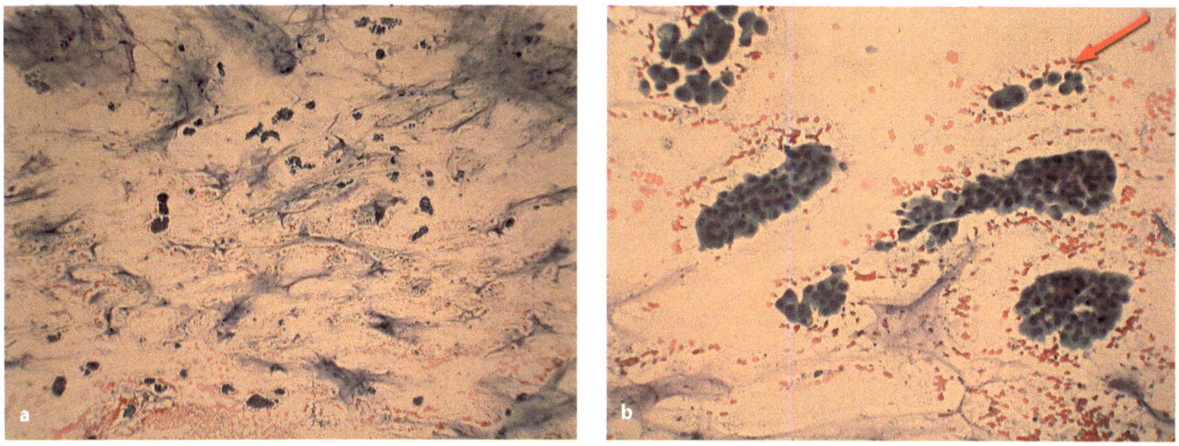

Fig. 2.26 a Low-power view of a typical FNB sample from mucinous (colloid) carcinoma showing sparse cellularity within a mucoid background. P stain, ×250. b High-power view of the same case as in a; small laminar or acinar clusters are seen and are characterized by moderate anisonucleosis; non-cohesion is minimal (*arrow*) or may be absent. P stain, ×400

mucinous background, mucocele-like lesions, and the mucinous variant of DCIS. The possibility of fibroadenoma should always be taken into consideration in patients between the ages of 25 and 40 years but not in those in older age groups. Aspirates from fibroadenoma with a mucinous stroma contain the characteristic two-dimensional aggregates of cells lacking any relevant nuclear atypia and, most importantly, a significant component of bare bipolar nuclei. These features help to rule out mucinous carcinoma but sometimes the differential diagnosis is not so obvious. In fact, bipolar bare nuclei can be obscured by massive mucinous change; epithelial cells within aggregates may show mild nuclear atypia due to hyperplasia; and a focal nuclear stratification can occur, all of which can make the distinction from carcinoma difficult or impossible. A CNB is the procedure of choice to solve this problem. Mucocele-like lesions develop as a consequence of extravasated mucin from dilated ductal structures [29]. In FNB samples, the background contains fibrocytes and histiocytes, in addition to mucin, and the cellularity is generally poor [37]. Epithelial cells are seen in aggregates and appear normal or atrophic, thus distinguishing these lesions from mucinous carcinoma [38]. It is important, however, to remember that mucocele-like lesions may develop in the proximity of mucinous carcinoma. For this reason, a careful scrutiny of possible epithelial atypia within aggregates is warranted. The mucinous variant of in situ carcinoma is a rare tumor entity characterized by a significant component of signet-ring cells [29]. Samples from this lesion are easily diagnosed as malignant and the distinction from conventional mucinous carcinoma at the time of needle-biopsy evaluation is of little or no practical impact.

2.9.2 Tubular Carcinoma

Classical, pure tubular carcinoma generally refers to a small tumor (<1 cm) that mammographically appears as a spiculate opacity with a characteristic stromal reaction [29]. Sometimes, however, tubular carcinoma is characterized by a regular and sharp outline and can be confused with a fibroadenoma. It is seen in elderly patients but is not rare in younger age groups. Moreover, it can be associated with a low-grade DCIS or develop within a radial scar. The FNB sample of a pure tubular carcinoma may show a significant component of bare bipolar nuclei in the background together with fibrocytes and a granular or fibrillary substance. The cellularity is frequently abundant and consists of a mixture of two- and three-dimensional aggregates in variable proportions (Fig. 2.27). Nuclear atypia is not a feature of this tumor. Three-dimensional aggregates with a tubular morphology and an angulated profile are considered a diagnostic feature of tubular carcinoma [39,40] but in this author's experience they are rarely detected even in otherwise typical cases. In fact, three-dimensional aggregates mostly display a rectilinear or curvilinear profile (Fig. 2.28) and their morphology is no different from that of similar

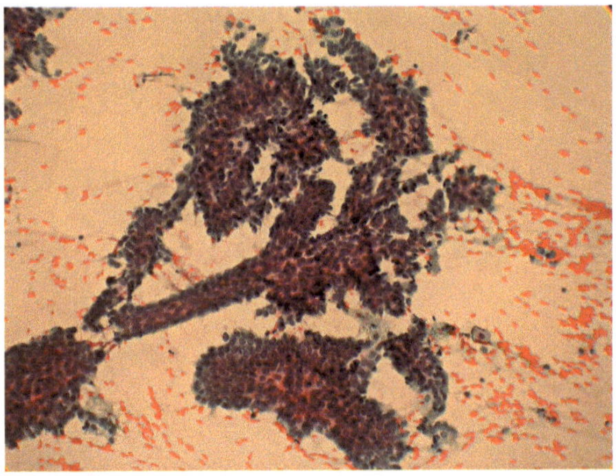

Fig. 2.27 The FNB sample from tubular carcinoma may consist of rectilinear and branching tubular clusters containing epithelial cells characterized only by minimal atypia. P stain, ×250

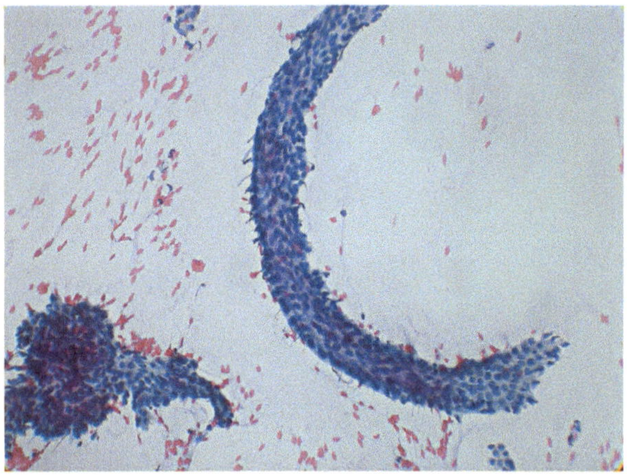

Fig. 2.28 In FNB samples of tubular carcinoma, clusters sometimes assume a peculiar curvilinear profile. P stain, ×400

aggregates in borderline proliferative lesions. In summary, the overall picture is that of a proliferative borderline lesion, and FNB does not allow diagnosis of the tumor as such unless a significant component of non-cohesive cells is detected.

2.9.3 Medullary Carcinoma

On mammography, medullary carcinoma characteristically appears as a well-delineated nodule with a distinct round profile. It can sometimes undergo central cavitation. Due to these features it can be confused clinically with fibroadenoma or a benign cystic lesion. The tumor is characteristically detected in women in the fifth and sixth decades of life [29]. The FNB sample of solid tumors is generally quite cellular and shows a distinct necrotic background [36]. Large three-dimensional cellular aggregates prevail and contain large cells with large and irregular nuclei. Nucleoli are often prominent and mitoses are readily detected. The cellular contours are indistinct and the overall appearance is that of a syncytium. Cellular non-cohesion may not be a prominent feature (Fig. 2.29). A component of small lymphocytes is seen within the aggregates and in the background but the number of cells is quite variable (Fig. 2.30). In tumors showing central cavitation, the sample appears grossly fluid, turbid, and brown-stained. Cytologically, the background is diffusely necrotic with many histiocytes. Cellular aggregates containing the above described pleomorphic cells are less well-represented but easily detected.

2.9.4 Triple-Negative "Basal-Like" Carcinoma

There is a restricted number of tumors that have in common the fact that they are negative for the expression of ER, PgR, and HER2 (triple-negative tumors) as well as for the expression of a "basal-like" profile, i.e., positivity for CK5/6 and EGFR. Morphologically, these tumors represent a heterogeneous group as they may be diagnosed as high-grade ductal invasive carcinoma, medullary carcinoma, or pleomorphic lobular carcinoma [41]. Interestingly, the FNB sample in most of these tumors is characterized by large three-dimensional aggregates containing highly atypical and pleomorphic cells (giant nuclei, macronucleoli, atypical mitoses) in a necrotic background with little or no cellular dissociation. Thus, despite a rather heterogeneous morphology at histopathology, these tumors share an unusual cytological feature, i.e., a low tendency to cellular non-cohesion.

2.9.5 Micropapillary Carcinoma

Micropapillary carcinoma is a rare and peculiar variant of low-grade invasive ductal carcinoma [42]. Cytologically, the FNB sample is characterized by moderate to abundant cellularity with little cellular non-cohesion.

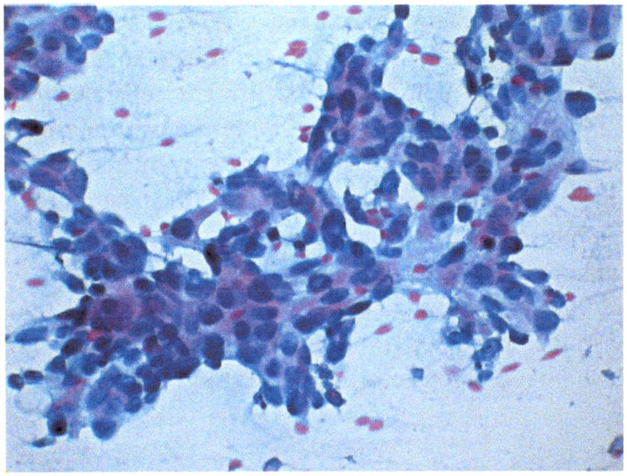

Fig. 2.29 In FNB samples of medullary carcinoma, tumor cells may appear only in clusters, with minimal or no non-cohesion; tumor cells are characteristically large in size and pleomorphic. P stain, ×450

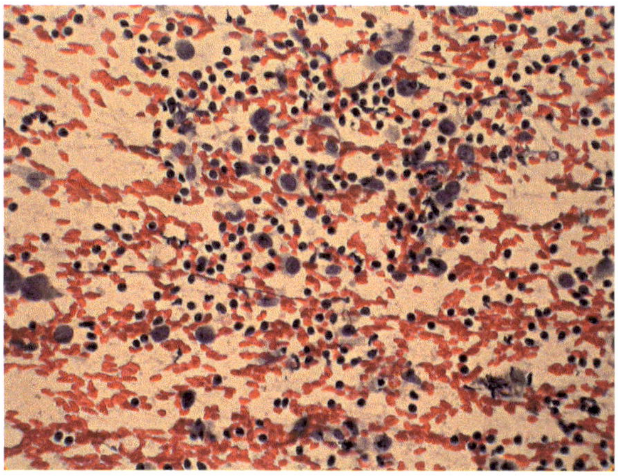

Fig. 2.30 In FNB samples of medullary carcinoma, small lymphocytes sometimes dominate the picture. P stain, ×400

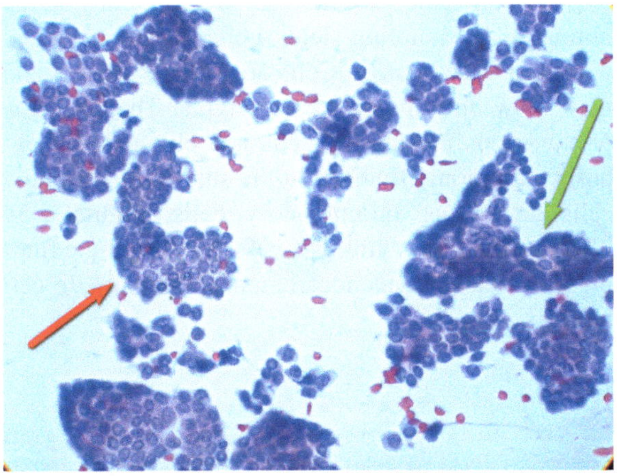

Fig. 2.31 FNB sample from a micropapillary invasive carcinoma showing two-dimensional cellular sheets (*red arrow*) and micropapillary aggregates lacking a connective-tissue stalk (*green arrow*), often with an angulated profile. Nuclei are round with minimal pleomorphism. P stain, ×400

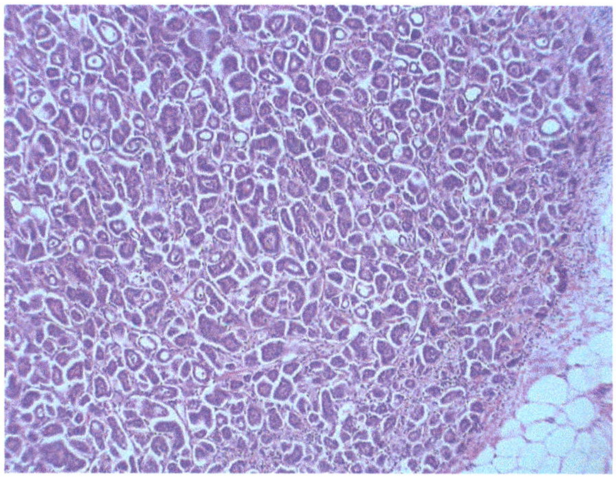

Fig. 2.32 Histopathology of invasive micropapillary carcinoma. Hematoxylin and eosin (H&E) stain, ×250

The picture is dominated by the presence of two-dimensional cellular sheets containing few cells, or micropapillary aggregates lacking a connective-tissue stalk, often with an angulated profile [43,44]. Nuclei are round with minimal pleomorphism, and the cells are small (<3×RBC). The chromatin texture is marked by a coarsely granular pattern and the nucleoli are small or absent (Fig. 2.31). Figure 2.32 illustrates the typical histopathological appearance of the tumor, which is dominated by micropapillary invasive growth.

2.9.6 Carcinoma with Apocrine-Type Differentiation

Apocrine carcinoma represents a rare variant of invasive ductal carcinoma [45]. Upon FNB sampling, the tumor yields a large number of medium-sized to large cells present in three-dimensional aggregates or as non-cohesive elements within a generally necrotic background (Fig. 2.33). These cells contain an abundant and homogeneous eosinophilic cytoplasm, large

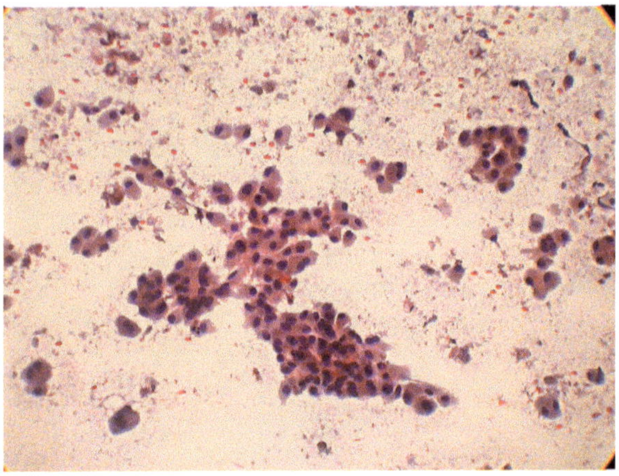

Fig. 2.33 Cytological appearance of an apocrine carcinoma of the breast displaying the typical oncocytic appearance of tumor cells. P stain, ×400

nuclei, and sometimes a prominent nucleolus. The overall appearance is that of an oncocytic malignancy.

2.9.7 Adenoid Cystic Carcinoma

Adenoid cystic carcinoma of the breast does not differ from its counterparts arising in the major or minor salivary glands or in other anatomic sites [46] (see Chapter 5). Cytologically, the FNB sample is characterized by three-dimensional aggregates with the morphology of cords and trabeculae and an abundant component of non-cohesive cells. The cells are typically basaloid in appearance, with scant cytoplasm, a round or elongated nucleus that is typically hyperchromatic, and the absence of nucleoli. The most unusual finding is globular accumulations of an amorphous and apparently mucinous substance within aggregates of proliferating basaloid cells. These accumulations may also be dispersed in the background, which may contain red blood cells but not necrotic debris.

2.9.8 Metaplastic Spindle Cell Carcinoma

Spindle cell lesions of the breast are rare but include metaplastic spindle cell carcinoma, nodular fasciitis, phyllodes tumor, and inflammatory pseudotumor [47]. Metaplastic carcinomas are generally large tumors. FNB sampling yields a highly necrotic smear with sparse cellularity. Cells are spindle shaped and may show only minor nuclear atypia. The detection of squamous metaplastic cells is a clue to the diagnosis. Additional findings in the smear are lymphoid cells and acute inflammatory cells. Figure 2.34 illustrate the FNB cytologic and CNB histologic findings in a case of adenocarcinoma with spindle cell metaplasia.

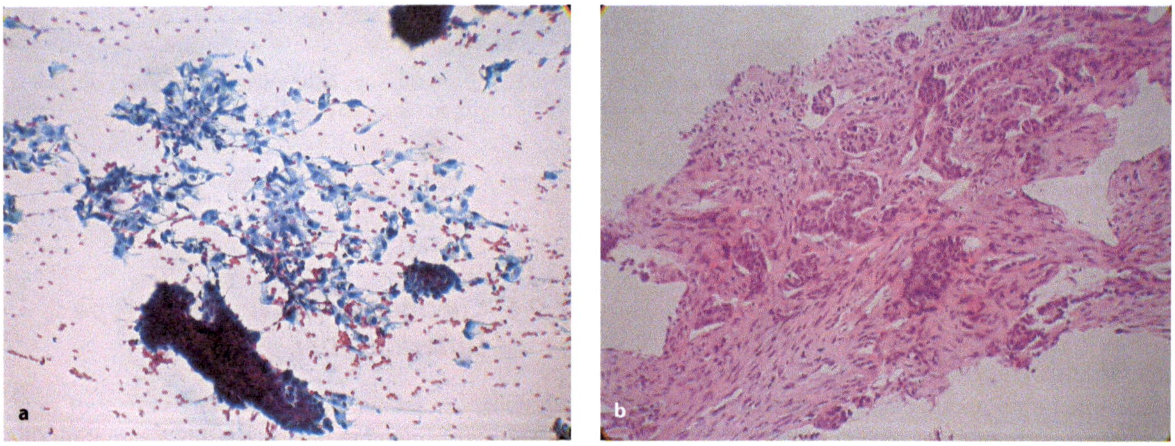

Fig. 2.34 a Cytological appearance of a FNB sample obtained from a patient with adenocarcinoma with spindle cell metaplasia; atypical medium-sized to large spindle cells are clustered in the background. P stain, ×400. b Core-needle biopsy of the same case as in a; histology reveals a biphasic proliferation of tubular structures admixed with spindle cells. H&E stain, ×400

2.10 Differential Diagnosis and Possible Misdiagnoses

2.10.1 *Fibroepithelial Lesions*

Fibroadenoma and its variants can enter the differential diagnosis of carcinoma in the following situations:

1. The epithelial cell component shows significant anisonucleosis or the presence of prominent nucleoli. This phenomenon occurs mainly in young patients and mostly during early development of the lesion. The concomitant finding of a huge component of bare bipolar nuclei is a clear indication that the lesion is a florid but benign fibroadenoma, despite cellular atypia. Surgical excision of the lesion for diagnostic purposes is not indicated in this age group. It is worth noting that a typical fibroadenoma may harbor foci of florid and/or atypical hyperplasia and even DCIS. This is a rare occurrence and is more often seen in patients older than 35–40 years of age. In these cases, the component of bare bipolar nuclei is sparse or even absent and the cytological picture falls in the category of breast borderline lesions.
2. The bare bipolar nuclear component is sparse and replaced by epithelioid fibroblasts. Fibroadenomas commonly undergo regressive changes consistent with fibrous tissue proliferation, with hyalinization of the stromal component. This is observed in patients older than 35–40 years of age. Moreover, fibroblasts with round to oval nuclei and scant cytoplasm can simulate dissociated and malignant epithelial cells. The picture may become even more complicated in the presence of ischemic changes, such that in FNB samples there is concomitant detection of necrotic debris in the background [48]. The presence of these changes often warrants surgical excision of the lesion but histopathology usually confirms a conventional fibroadenoma with regressive changes.
3. The stromal component undergoes diffuse myxoid change, which causes the bare bipolar nuclei to disappear in the smear while the epithelial component persists [49]. The cytological picture can thus simulate that of mucinous carcinoma [50]. Adequate sampling by multiple needle passes usually documents at least a small amount of bare bipolar nuclei; nonetheless, the presence of abundant mucin in the background is an indication for CNB sampling to rule out mucinous carcinoma, especially in patients over the age of 35–40 years.

Benign phyllodes tumors can enter the differential diagnosis of a borderline breast lesion if in the FNB sample the bare bipolar nuclei are sparse and the epithelial component is represented by large three-dimensional or papillary aggregates containing pleomorphic nuclei [51]. As an alternative, sampling of a malignant phyllodes tumor can yield a pleomorphic population of spindle and epithelioid cells that simulate metaplastic carcinoma or a spindle cell carcinoma. The distinction between malignant phyllodes tumor and carcinoma is of utmost importance due to a possibly different therapeutic approach.

2.10.2 *Intraductal/Intracystic Papilloma*

The detection of papillary fronds with nuclear atypia (anisonucleosis and presence of nucleoli) associated with necrotic debris, blood, and isolated cylindrical ductal cells in the background is worrisome as it increases the likelihood of papillary carcinoma [52]. Histological examination can, however, provide evidence of a completely benign intraductal or intracystic papilloma; thus, the presence of the above-described findings should be considered as "indefinite" rather than "suspicious" for carcinoma and a definitive diagnosis should be deferred to VACNB sampling. Papilloma can also undergo subtotal or total coagulative necrosis, and the FNB cellular sample of these lesions is an important cause of a misdiagnosis of carcinoma [53,54]. In fact, following necrosis, the cytological sample may document the presence of atypical cells that are seen in papillary fronds but also as isolated elements featuring a high nuclear cytoplasmic ratio, with coarsely granular chromatin and prominent nucleoli. The background contains a variable amount of necrotic debris and inflammatory cells with admixed degenerative cells showing coagulated and smudged nuclei. The detection of sheets of bland squamous cells is a clue to the benign nature of the lesion [55], as squamous metaplasia occurs in the late stage of papilloma infarction [54]. In practice, however, this is an inconsistent finding and the definitive diagnosis of these lesions is often deferred to core biopsy or open biopsy.

2.10.3 Mucocele-Like Lesions

Mucocele-like pseudotumors, i.e., the accumulation of extravasated mucin within mammary stroma, may be induced by a relatively wide spectrum of pathological lesions. Based on the FNB findings, the lesion enters the differential diagnosis of mucinous carcinoma and fibroadenoma with massive mucinous transformation (see above) [37,56,57]. In general, FNB samples of mucocele-like lesions display a scant cellularity, no or rare intact single epithelial cells, few if any two-dimensional aggregates of epithelial cells showing no nuclear atypia, and sparse histiocytes. By contrast, fibroadenomas show a minor component of easily detected bare bipolar nuclei and a sparse component of two-dimensional aggregates with the characteristic finger-like configuration. Finally, mucinous carcinoma is of high cellularity, consisting of non-cohesive epithelial cells with intact cytoplasm and cellular aggregates with marked nuclear atypia. Significant exceptions to these rules do, however, occur, such as the detection of low cellularity with only mild nuclear atypia and the absence of non-cohesive cells in colloid carcinoma—which may be an important diagnostic pitfall. In general, when confronted with a picture suggestive of a mucocele-like lesion, one should rely upon the clinical history and the imaging characteristics of the lesion, and this diagnosis made only if all of the findings are consistent with a benign lesion.

2.10.4 Retroareolar Abscess

Retroareolar or subareolar abscess (or Zuska's disease) [58] is an uncommon inflammatory condition that can also present with a bilateral involvement; it also has been described in the male breast. The condition is induced by a squamous metaplasia of the terminal lactiferous ducts, which causes plugging and obstruction of the ducts. An inflammatory reaction is thus elicited and subsequent infection can cause local and general symptoms. Nipple retraction, recurrent episodes of erysipelas, and the presence of painful nodules under the areola are characteristic findings. Not infrequently, the clinical suspicion is that of breast cancer. The FNB sample is quite characteristic and consists of sheets of bland squamous cells admixed with inflammatory cells that include foreign-body-type histiocytes. The clinician should be familiar with this cytological picture in order to promptly diagnose the lesion, which is best treated by nipple excision.

2.10.5 Hypercellular Sample in the Elderly

Benign proliferative breast lesions generally do not occur in the elderly woman. Sometimes, FNB sampling of a nodule shows a moderately to abundant cellular yield characterized by two- and three-dimensional aggregates of small, rather monotonous cells with a round and small nucleus lacking any atypical feature. The background is clear and proteinaceous and lacks bipolar bare nuclei. Isolated epithelial cells are not seen. The overall picture suggests a benign condition and, in fact, the imaging features of the nodule upon ultrasound or X-ray mammography often confirm this contention. However, despite its bland appearance the above cytological picture is most likely to be ascribed to a low-grade in situ or invasive ductal carcinoma. The only hint to a possible malignancy is the lack of bipolar bare nuclei in the background and the abundant cellularity of the sample, while the intrinsic nuclear and cytoplasmic features are by no means suggestive of carcinoma. This is an important pitfall in breast cytology and stresses the importance of a prudent and detailed correlation with clinical findings when the smear is examined.

2.10.6 Complex Sclerosing Lesion/Radial Scar

The detection of complex sclerosing lesions has become increasingly frequent with the advent of mammographic population screening. On X-ray mammography and ultrasound, these benign lesions simulate the stellate or spiculated morphology of breast carcinoma. On histology, they consist of adenosis with a central hyalinized and markedly elastotic stroma. Distortion by the scleroelastotic process is responsible for the overall stellate outline. Various patterns of concomitant intraepithelial typical or atypical proliferation are frequently present in larger lesions. The FNB sample is no different from that of other adenosis lesions and, unless a concomitant atypical hyperplasia or DCIS is present, these lesions are best classified using the criteria of Masood et al. [20] (Table 2.5).

2.10.7 Angiosarcoma After Breast-Conserving Therapy

Patients who have been treated conservatively for limited-stage breast cancer are at increased risk for the development of angiosarcoma of the breast skin and/or subcutaneous fat. This highly aggressive tumor appears with a latency interval of several years after surgery and adjuvant radiation therapy. The clinical presentation is varied. In some patients, the lesion is preceded by the appearance of atypical vascular changes while in others single or multiple nodular subcutaneous lesions arise de novo and simulate a cancer relapse close to the surgical scar. Sampling by FNB of these lesions yields a highly cellular harvest mainly consisting of epithelioid cells that tend to aggregate in three-dimensional clusters, or are loosely cohesive, or completely non-cohesive. Spindle cells may also be present. The cells tend to cluster around prominent capillary vessels, which are visible inside the aggregates (Fig. 2.35) [59]. The differential diagnosis encompasses poorly differentiated adenocarcinoma, metaplastic carcinoma, or epithelioid-cell melanoma. A definitive diagnosis relies upon immunocytochemical demonstration of endothelial differentiation of the tumor cells.

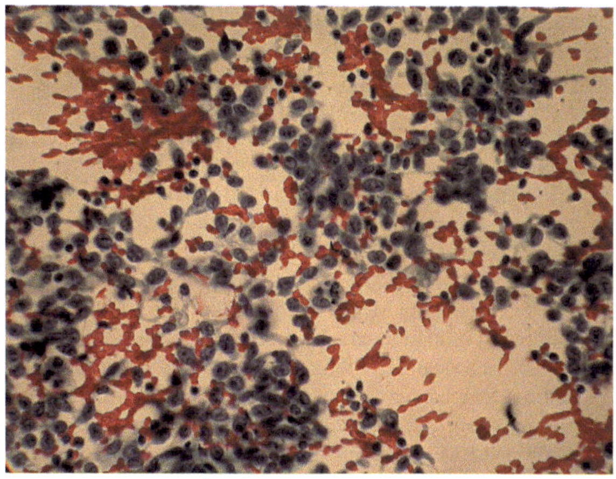

Fig. 2.35 Variably clustered or non-cohesive spindle and epithelioid cells with round nuclei and prominent nucleoli are characteristically found in FNB samples of angiosarcoma developing after breast conservative surgery. P stain, ×400

References

1. Silverstein MJ (2000) The Van Nuys Breast Center: the first free-standing multidisciplinary breast center. Surg Oncol Clin North Am 9:159–175.
2. Tubiana M, Koscielny S (1999) The rationale for early diagnosis of cancer-the example of breast cancer. Acta Oncol 38:295–303.
3. Abner AL, Collins L, Peiro G et al (1998) Correlation of tumor size and axillary lymph node involvement with prognosis in patients with T1 breast carcinoma. Cancer 83:2502–2508.
4. Zarbo RJ, Howanitz PJ, Bachner P (1991) Interinstitutional comparison of performance in breast fine-needle aspiration cytology. A Q-probe quality indicator study. Arch Pathol Lab Med 115:743–750.
5. Ciatto S, Bonardi R, Cariaggi MP (1995) Performance of fine-needle aspiration cytology of the breast-multicenter study of 23,063 aspirates in ten Italian laboratories. Tumori 81:13–17.
6. Arisio R, Cuccorese C, Accinelli G et al (1998) Role of fine-needle aspiration biopsy in breast lesions: analysis of a series of 4,110 cases. Diagn Cytopathol 18:462–467.
7. Ingram DM, Sterrett GF, Sheiner HJ, Shilkin KB (1998) Fine-needle aspiration cytology in the management of breast disease. Med J Aust 2:170–173.
8. Patel JJ, Gartell PC, Smallwood J et al (1987) Fine needle aspiration cytology of breast masses: an evaluation of its accuracy and reasons for diagnostic failure. Ann R Coll Surg Engl 69:156–159.
9. Elston CW, Cotton RE, Davies CJ, Blamey RW (1978) A comparison of the use of the "Tru-Cut" needle and fine needle aspiration cytology in the pre-operative diagnosis of carcinoma of the breast. Histopathology 2:239–254.
10. Ballo MS, Sneige N (1996) Can core needle biopsy replace fine-needle aspiration cytology in the diagnosis of palpable breast carcinoma. A comparative study of 124 women. Cancer 78:773–777.
11. Sun W, Li A, Abreo F, Turbat-Herrera E, Grafton WD (2001) Comparison of fine-needle aspiration cytology and core biopsy for diagnosis of breast cancer. Diagn Cytopathol 24:421–425.
12. Westenend PJ, Sever AR, Beekman-De Volder HJ, Liem SJ (2001) A comparison of aspiration cytology and core needle biopsy in the evaluation of breast lesions. Cancer 93:146–150.
13. Houssami N, Ciatto S, Ellis I, Ambrogetti D (2007) Underestimation of malignancy of breast core-needle biopsy: concepts and precise overall and category-specific estimates. Cancer 109:487–495.
14. Kumaroswamy V, Liston J, Shaaban AM (2008) Vacuum assisted stereotactic guided mammotome biopsies in the management of screen detected microcalcifications: experience of a large breast screening centre. J Clin Pathol 61:766–769.
15. Kikuchi M, Tsunoda-Shimizu H, Kawasaki T et al (2007) Indications for stereotactically-guided vacuum-assisted breast biopsy for patients with category 3 microcalcifications. Breast Cancer 14:285–291.
16. Cobb CJ, Raza AS Obituary (2005) Alas poor FNA of breast-we knew thee well!. Diagn Cytopathol 32:1–4.

17. Levine T (2004) Breast cytology–is there still a role? Cytopathology 15:293–296.
18. Dray M, Mayall F, Darlington A (2000) Improved fine needle aspiration (FNA) cytology results with a near patient diagnosis service for breast lesions. Cytopathology 11:32–37.
19. Brown LA, Coghill SB (1992) Cost effectiveness of a fine needle aspiration clinic. Cytopathology 3:275–280.
20. Masood S, Frykberg ER, McLellan GL et al (1991) Cytologic differentiation between proliferative and nonproliferative breast disease in mammographically guided fine-needle aspirates. Diagn Cytopathol 7:581–590.
21. Sneige N, Staerkel GA, Caraway NP et al (1994) A plea for uniform terminology and reporting of breast fine needle aspirates. M.D. Anderson Cancer Center proposal. Acta Cytol 38:971–972.
22. Perry N, Broeders M, de Wolf C, Törnberg S (eds) (2001) Pathology in mammography screening-non-operative diagnosis. European Guidelines for Quality Assurance in Mammographic Screening, 3rd Ed. Luxembourg: European Commission, pp 162–172.
23. Wilson ARM, Asbury D, Cooke J et al (2001) Clinical Guidelines For Breast Cancer Screening Assessment. Sheffield, NHS Breast Screening Programme (NHSBSP Publication No 49).
24. Ellis IO, Humphreys S, Michell M et al (2001) Cytology Sub-group of the National Coordinating Group for Breast Screening Pathology. Guidelines for Non-operative Diagnostic Procedures and Reporting in Breast Cancer Screening. Sheffield, NHS Cancer Screening Programmes 2001 (NHSBSP Publication No 50).
25. Brancato B, Bonardi R, Crocetti E et al (2004) Clinical significance and optimal management of patients with an "atypia, probably benign" (C3) report at FNAC of the breast. Breast J 10:458–489.
26. Zhao C, Raza A, Martin SE et al (2009) Breast fine-needle aspiration samples reported as "proliferative breast lesion": clinical utility of the subcategory "proliferative breast lesion with atypia". Cancer Cytopathol 117:137–147.
27. Martelli G, Pilotti S, Coopmans de Yoldi G et al (1990). Diagnostic efficacy of physical examination, mammography, fine needle aspiration cytology (triple-test) in solid breast lumps: an analysis of 1708 consecutive cases Tumori 76:476–479.
28. Irwig L, Macaskill P, Houssami N (2002) Evidence relevant to the investigation of breast symptoms: the triple test. Breast 11:215–220.
29. Rosai J (2004). Breast. In: Rosai and Ackerman's Surgical Pathology. 9th Ed, Vol 2. Mosby, Edinburgh, pp. 1787–1838.
30. Foxcroft LM, Evans EB, Porter AJ (2007) Difficulties in the pre-operative diagnosis of phyllodes tumours of the breast: a study of 84 cases. Breast 16:27–37.
31. Ibarra JA (2006) Papillary Lesions of the Breast. The Breast Journal 12:237–251.
32. Dawson AE, Mulford DK(1994) Benign versus malignant papillary neoplasms of the breast. Diagnostic clues in fine needle aspiration cytology. Acta Cytol 38:23–28.
33. Tavassoli FA, Hoefler H. Rosai J et al (2003) Intraductal proliferative lesions. In: Tavassoli FA, Devilee P (eds) Pathology and Genetics of Tumours of the Breast and Female Genital Organs. World Health Organization Classification of Tumours. IARC Press, Lyon, pp 60–75.
34. Burstein HJ, Polyak K, Wong JS et al (2004) Ductal carcinoma in situ of the breast. N Engl J Med 350:1430–1441.
35. Gherardi G, Marveggio C (1999) Cytologic score and DNA-image analysis in the classification of borderline breast lesions: a prospective study on 47 fine-needle aspirates. Diagn Cytopathol 20:212–218.
36. Haji BE, Das DK, Al-Ayadhy B et al (2007) Fine-needle aspiration cytologic features of four special types of breast cancers: mucinous, medullary, apocrine, and papillary. Diagn Cytopathol 35:408–416.
37. Cheng L, Lee WY, Chang TW (2004) Benign mucocele-like lesion of the breast: how to differentiate from mucinous carcinoma before surgery. Cytopathology 15:104–108.
38. Carder PJ, Murphy CE, Liston JC (2004) Surgical excision is warranted following a core biopsy diagnosis of mucocoele-like lesion of the breast. Histopathology 45:148–154.
39. de la Torre M, Lindholm K, Lindgren A (1994) Fine needle aspiration cytology of tubular breast carcinoma and radial scar. Acta Cytol 38:884–890.
40. Lamb J, McGoogan E (1994) Fine needle aspiration cytology of breast in invasive carcinoma of tubular type and in radial scar/complex sclerosing lesions. Cytopathology 5:17–26.
41. Fadare O, Tavassoli FA (2008) Clinical and pathologic aspects of basal-like breast cancers. Nat Clin Pract Oncol 5:149–159.
42. Chen L, Fan Y, Lang RG et al (2008) Breast carcinoma with micropapillary features: clinicopathologic study and long-term follow-up of 100 cases. Int J Surg Pathol 16:155–163.
43. Lui PC, Lau PP, Tse GM et al (2007) Fine needle aspiration cytology of invasive micropapillary carcinoma of the breast. Pathology 39:401–405.
44. Ng WK, Poon CS, Kong JH (2001) Fine needle aspiration cytology of invasive micropapillary carcinoma of the breast: review of cases in a three-year period. Acta Cytol 45:973–979.
45. Tanaka K, Imoto S, Wada N et al (2008). Invasive apocrine carcinoma of the breast: clinicopathologic features of 57 patients. Breast J 14:164–168.
46. Soon SR, Yong WS, Ho GH et al (2008) Adenoid cystic breast carcinoma: a salivary gland-type tumour with excellent prognosis and implications for management. Pathology 40:413–415.
47. Tse GM, Tan PH, Lui PC, Putti TC (2008) Spindle cell lesions of the breast–the pathologic differential diagnosis. Breast Cancer Res Treat 109:199–207.
48. Malberger E, Yerushalmi R, Tamir A, Keren R (1997) Diagnosis of fibroadenoma in breast fine needle aspirates devoid of typical stroma. Acta Cytol 41:1483–1438.
49. Ventura K, Cangiarella J, Lee I et al (2003) Aspiration biopsy of mammary lesions with abundant extracellular mucinous material. Review of 43 cases with surgical follow-up. Am J Clin Pathol 120:194–202.
50. Simsir A, Tsang P, Greenebaum E (1998) Additional mimics of mucinous mammary carcinoma: fibroepithelial lesions. Am J Clin Pathol 109:169–172.
51. Dusenbery D, Frable WJ (1992) Fine needle aspiration cytology of phyllodes tumor. Potential diagnostic pitfalls. Acta Cytol 36:215–221.

52. Simsir A, Waisman J, Thorner K, Cangiarella J (2003) Mammary lesions diagnosed as "papillary" by aspiration biopsy: 70 cases with follow-up. Cancer 99:156–165.
53. Kobayashi TK, Ueda M, Nishino T et al (1992) Spontaneous infarction of an intraductal papilloma of the breast: cytological presentation on fine needle aspiration. Cytopathology 3:379–384.
54. Shihara A, Kobayashi TK (2006). Infarcted intraductal papilloma of the breast: cytologic features with stage of infarction. Diagn Cytopathol 34:373–376.
55. Ng WK, Kong JH (2003) Significance of squamous cells in fine needle aspiration cytology of the breast. A review of cases in a seven-year period. Acta Cytol 47:27–35.
56. Wong NL, Wan SK (2000) Comparative cytology of mucocele-like lesion and mucinous carcinoma of the breast in fine needle aspiration. Acta Cytol 44:765–770.
57. Yeoh GP, Cheung PS, Chan KW (1999) Fine-needle aspiration cytology of mucocele-like tumors of the breast. Am J Surg Pathol 23:552–559.
58. Guadagni M, Nazzari G (2008) Zuska's disease. G Ital Dermatol Venereol 143:157–160.
59. Gherardi G, Rossi S, Perrone S, Scanni A (2005) Angiosarcoma after breast-conserving therapy: fine-needle aspiration biopsy, immunocytochemistry, and clinicopathologic correlates. Cancer 105:145–151.

Thyroid

3

3.1 Introduction

Fine-needle biopsy (FNB) is the most effective and efficient diagnostic procedure to study thyroid nodular lesions [1–9]. It is inexpensive, rapidly performed, very well-tolerated by the patient in any context, and immediately repeatable. In experienced hands, FNB is highly reliable in the diagnosis of benign lesions and in the identification and typing of a significant number of malignant tumors. Since the predictive value of a negative diagnosis is very high, the patient can be confidently assured and followed up unless other clinical conditions or risk factors warrant a more aggressive approach. The positive predictive value of the procedure is similarly high and the most appropriate oncological therapy can be started immediately after a FNB diagnosis of malignancy. There are, however, a few cases in which the diagnosis remains inevitably indeterminate in terms of possible malignancy [2,10]. These fall into the diagnostic category "follicular proliferation" and account for about 10–30% of cases in most series [2,10,11–14] . In such patients, the thyroid lesion should be surgically excised to obtain a definitive histopathological diagnosis. The category "follicular proliferation" is the real gray zone of FNB because no more than one third of these cases correspond to malignant lesions; in the remaining cases, patients undergo a major surgical procedure for diagnostic purposes only.

3.2 Indications for FNB

3.2.1 *Palpable Nodule*

The palpable thyroid nodule is a frequent clinical finding in the general population. These nodules are generally ≥1 cm in diameter, and their diagnostic work-up requires a thorough patient history and physical examination [14]. Access to previous investigations, laboratory tests, and relevant surgical documentation is very important. The patient should be asked about a family history of thyroid carcinoma (especially medullary carcinoma and papillary carcinoma), a possible history of radiation exposure to the neck, thyroiditis, and symptoms potentially indicative of vocal cord paralysis (hoarseness of voice, dysphagia, odynophagia, etc.) or tracheal deviation or infiltration (coughing, shortness of breath, stridor, etc.). Physical examination should focus on the size of the nodule, its consistency, its mobility during swallowing, possible fixation of the mass to surrounding structures, possible tracheal deviation, enlarged cervical lymph nodes, etc.

If the lesion was noted by the patient, then the growth behavior of the nodule should be discussed. Finally, a possible history of malignancy in other organs should be ruled out, especially in elderly patients, as the thyroid lesion might represent a metastatic tumor.

As a basic diagnostic step, thyroid function should be assessed with a set of tests, including thyroid stimulating hormone (TSH), and the lesion should be evaluated ultrasonographically [14]. This imaging technique is effective at distinguishing cystic from solid lesions, delineating the architecture and measuring the size of the lesion, determining whether the nodule is solitary or part of a multinodular gland, and accurately demonstrating any regional lymph node enlargement. Sonographic findings suggesting a higher risk of malignancy include hypoechogenicity of the nodule, the detection of microcalcifications and irregular margins, and central blood flow. TSH titers above normal are an immediate indication for FNB, while patients with normal or depressed TSH should have a radionuclide thyroid scan, the results of which should be correlated with the sonographic findings [1,3,6,7,11]. The incidence of malignancy in a functioning thyroid nodule in the absence of significant clinical findings is very low, such that FNB investigation is not required in these cases [14].

There are no significant contraindications to performing FNB, except in the uncooperative patient and in patients with a severe bleeding diathesis. The most significant complication of thyroid FNA is intrathyroidal hemorrhage, but it has been reported very rarely [14].

3.2.2 Non-Palpable Nodule Discovered via Imaging

Thyroid nodular lesions can be discovered incidentally via imaging; for example, during an ultrasonographic investigation of the neck that is carried out to evaluate enlarged lymph nodes or a mass in the salivary glands, during a carotid Doppler scan or scans done for parathyroid disease, or during ^{18}FDG-PET, CT, or MRI scans. These lesions are generally of small size (<1 cm in diameter). The assessment of TSH has a limited role in the decision whether the lesion should be investigated by FNB. The procedure is indicated if a dedicated ultrasonographic study demonstrates the nodule to be abnormal in echogenicity and echotexture. In addition, all lesions detected by ^{18}FDG-PET scan should be considered for FNB sampling, irrespective of their ultrasonographic features. The diagnostic work-up of nodular lesions >1 cm that are not clinically detectable due to various reasons should follow the same scheme as used for palpable lesions [14].

3.3 FNB Sampling Technique

Needles to be used for FNB should have a caliber ranging between 22G and 27G. On occasion, larger needles can be employed, e.g., for evacuating a cyst containing a viscous fluid. Prior to puncture, the skin is rapidly cleansed but a sterile drape is not required and in most cases neither is local anesthesia. The patient lies supine while hyperextending the neck; this position is obtained by placing a pillow directly under his or her neck. The patient is then asked to swallow two to three times. During swallowing, the palpable nodule will increase in consistency, which facilitates its immobilization by the examining physician using two fingers. The patient is then asked not to speak or swallow and the needle is quickly introduced into the nodule. For palpable nodules, this is done under visual guidance; for those that are non-palpable, the needle is inserted under ultrasound guidance [15]. Sampling is performed with a series of advance-withdraw motions; the maneuver should last no more than 3–4 s. The first pass can be done using the non-aspiration technique and a very thin needle (27G or 25G) followed by the use of a larger needle under forced aspiration, depending on the type of harvest obtained. The non-aspiration procedure is effective for sampling hypervascular nodules [15]. The immediate appearance of blood in the needle hub is indicative of a suboptimal sampling due to bloody dilution and obscuration and/or an insufficient cellular component in the diagnostic yield. Three to four passes constitute the minimal requirement for representative FNB sampling. The use of core-needle biopsy is advocated by some clinicians to examine certain solid thyroid nodules but in practice this is very rarely required. Following the procedure, the biopsy site is gently compressed with manual pressure for about 1 min, then a bandage is applied and an ice pack is maintained on the puncture site under slight compression for about 10 min. For most patients, normal activities can be resumed after a 20- to 30-min observation period, which is required to rule out possible rapid progressive swelling and ecchymoses. If a cystic fluid is evacuated, the patient should be asked to present again within the following 2–3 days if the cyst swells; in this case, re-aspiration provides a much more abundant cellular yield.

3.4 The Cold Nodule: Histopathological Findings and Clinicopathological Correlates

3.4.1 Nodular Hyperplasia

Nodular hyperplasia (or nodular sporadic goiter) is by far the most frequent disease of the thyroid, with an incidence reaching 40–45% of the population in endemic areas. Clinical onset is characterized by a single nodular swelling in an otherwise normal or

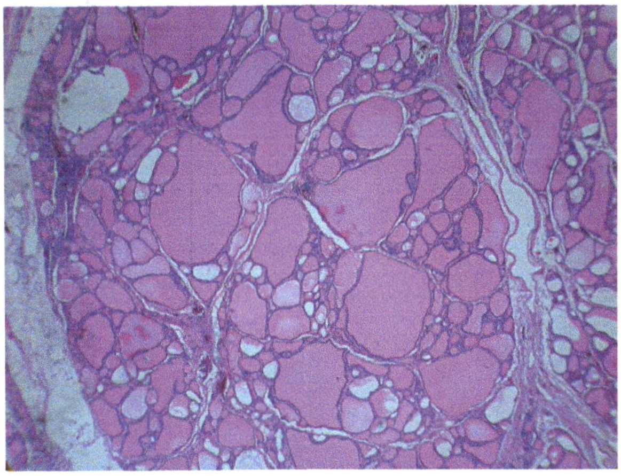

Fig. 3.1 Histology of macrofollicular nodular hyperplastic nodule. Hematoxylin & eosin (H&E) stain, ×40

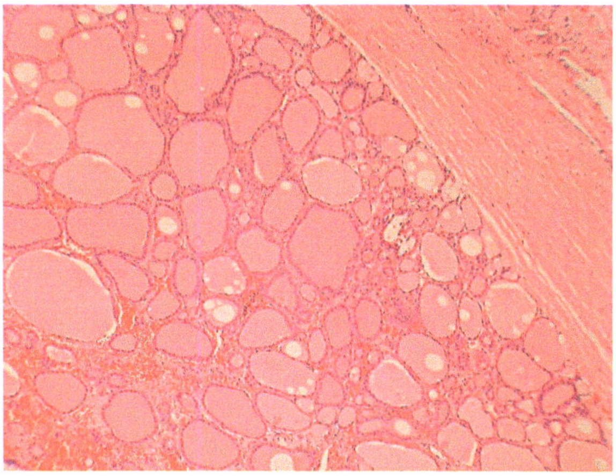

Fig. 3.2 Histology of a follicular adenoma, showing a delimiting fibrous capsule. H&E stain, ×100

diffusely enlarged thyroid. The patient often reports a recent size increase of the lesion, perhaps in association with pain. In some cases, the thyroid appears to expand retrosternally into the superior mediastinum. Histologically, the lesion consists of a nodular pseudotumor composed of follicles of varying size and surrounded by a thin, incomplete fibrous capsule [16]. Follicular size may vary from very small, with little colloid (microfollicular pattern), to very large, with abundant colloid (macrofollicular pattern) (Fig. 3.1). Cells delimiting follicular structures consist of cuboid thyrocytes or as large eosinophilic oncocytoid cells (Hürthle or Ashkenazy cells). Degenerative changes within follicles, including hemorrhagic necrosis, pseudocystic transformation, dystrophic calcification, and bone deposition, are variably but constantly detected. Collections of histiocytes with foamy cytoplasm containing hemosiderin granules are always present within colloid. Cholesterol crystals, hemosiderin, and possibly oxalate crystals are often seen.

3.4.2 Follicular Adenoma

Follicular adenoma comprises a monoclonal proliferation of well-differentiated thyrocytes or Hürthle cells [16,17]. The lesion is more often solitary and the surrounding parenchyma is either normal or appears to develop in the context of multinodular hyperplasia or thyroiditis. The tumor is most frequently detected in middle-aged euthyroid adults, with a higher prevalence in females. It is rarely responsible for increased hormone secretion ("hot" or hyperfunctioning adenoma). Clinical onset is characterized by a slowly growing mass that may compress surrounding structures. Tumor size at onset ranges between 1 and 3 cm. Histologically, the tumor has a follicular pattern of growth and is delimited by a continuous and thin fibrous capsule (Fig. 3.2). Follicle size is only slightly variable throughout the tumor. The pattern of growth may be microfollicular or macrofollicular. In some variants, the follicular content is barely discernible and the tumor assumes a solid or trabecular growth pattern. Thyrocytes delimiting follicular cavities are polygonal or cuboid cells of small size displaying a round to oval nucleus with small nucleoli. When the Hürthle cell component of the tumor is >75%, it is defined as a Hürthle cell adenoma. Follicular adenoma frequently undergoes involutive changes, such as hemorrhagic necrosis, fibrosis, calcium deposition, and pseudocystic transformation. Foamy histiocytes containing hemosiderin granules and cholesterol crystals within colloid are common findings.

3.4.3 Hyaline Trabecular Adenoma

This tumor of the follicular epithelium is of uncertain malignant potential and can develop in association with lymphocytic thyroiditis [16,17]. It is entirely characterized by elongated cells that are assembled in parallel and form long and tortuous trabecular structures (Fig. 3.3a). The longer axis of the cells is generally orthogonal to the axis of the trabecular structure.

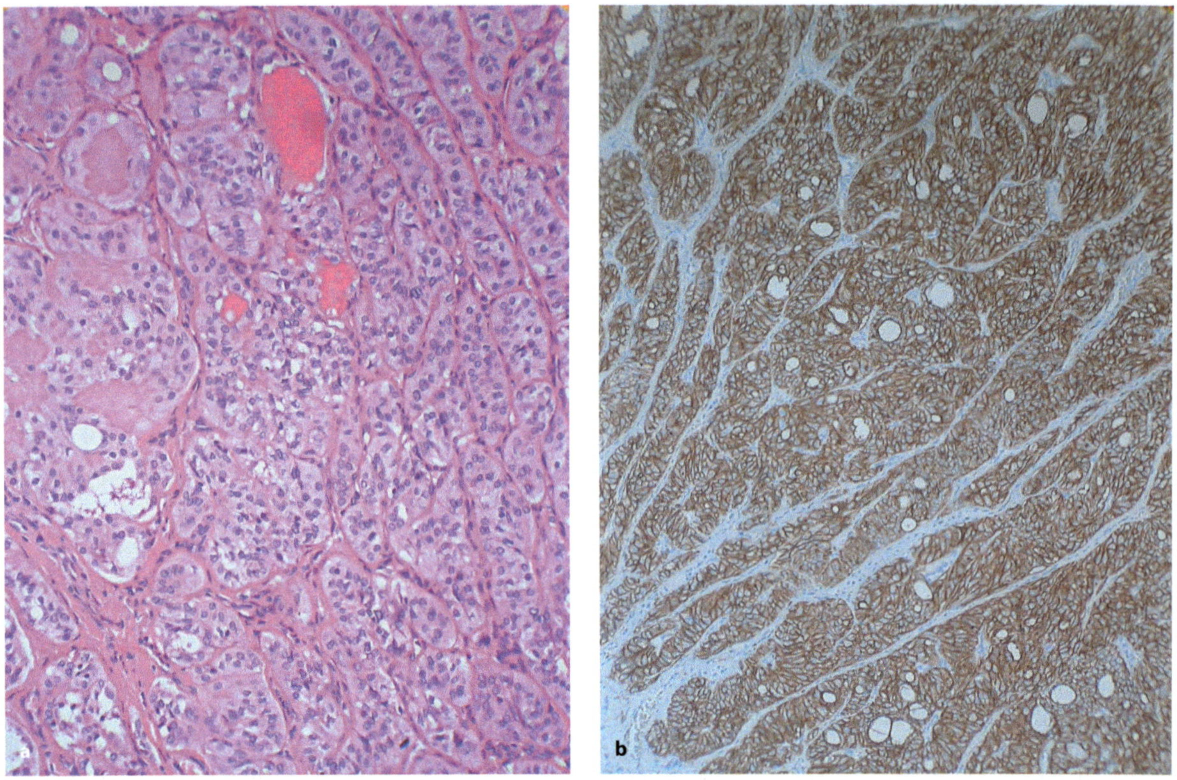

Fig. 3.3 **a** Histology of hyaline follicular adenoma; the lesion is composed of elongated cells that are assembled in parallel and form long and tortuous trabecular structures. H&E stain, ×200. **b** Same case as in **a**. Immunostaining for Ki-67/MIB1 decorates the cytoplasm of cells. Counterstained with hematoxylin, ×100

Tumor growth is associated with the deposition of an interstitial hyaline matrix. The nuclei of tumor cells are oval or elongated and often appear to contain grooves and nuclear inclusions identical to those of papillary carcinoma cells. The cytoplasm is eosinophilic and contains characteristic inclusion bodies that consist of giant lysosomes [16,17].

3.4.4 Thyroiditis

3.4.4.1 Autoimmune Thyroiditis

The definition of autoimmune thyroiditis encompasses both lymphocytic throiditis and Hashimoto's thyroiditis [16]. The former affects younger individuals and is rarely responsible for the development of a nodular lesion. The latter, by contrast, is seen in adults 40 years of age and older and its course may be characterized by the development of a nodular lesion. Autoimmune thyroiditis is associated with significant disturbance of thyroid function and the presence of autoantibodies in the serum. The clinical onset is typically a syndrome of pain and the sensation of constraint in the neck, accompanied by a sore throat and low fever, followed by the development of thyroid enlargement and hypothyroidism. The thyroid is massively infiltrated by inflammatory cells, mostly small lymphocytes and plasma cells with sparse granulocytes and multinucleated cells. Residual follicles are delimited by oxyphilic cells (Hürthle cells) (Fig. 3.4), often showing a clear chromatin with nuclear grooves and possible pseudoinclusions, thus simulating the nuclear changes seen in papillary carcinoma. In later phases, the oxyphilic cells may undergo squamous metaplasia and the inflammatory infiltrate is replaced by a fibrosing process. Hashimoto's thyroiditis can produce a pseudonodular tumefaction due to asymmetric involvement of the gland by the inflammatory process or it may harbor a nodular

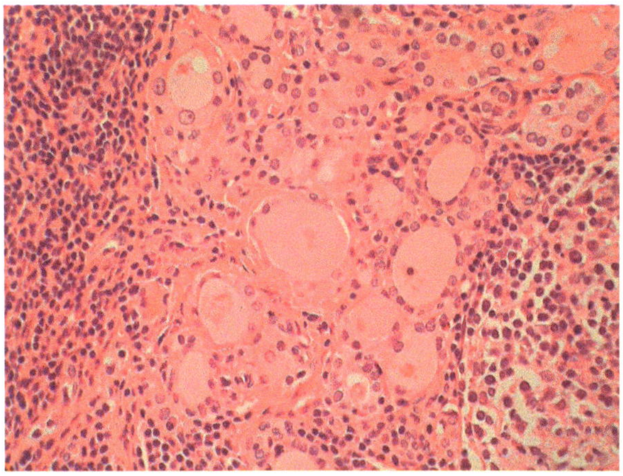

Fig. 3.4 Histology of lymphocytic thyroiditis; residual follicles are found in between lymphoid follicles and are delimited by oxyphilic cells. H&E stain, ×200

hyperplasia composed of Hürthle cells or even a Hürthle cell adenoma. Papillary carcinoma can also develop in the context of Hashimoto's thyroiditis. In some cases, finally, the lymphoid proliferation is so florid as to simulate a malignant lymphoma [16,17].

3.4.4.2 De Quervain's Thyroiditis

This peculiar inflammatory process of the thyroid mainly affects middle-aged adults or the elderly. It is characterized by an acute clinical onset, with fever and pharyngodynia, which is followed by a rapidly progressive glandular enlargement and a tendency to hypothyroidism. In this phase, patients with the disease may present with a nodular swelling simulating a malignancy. Histologically, the gland is effaced by a non-necrotic granulomatous inflammatory infiltrate with a significant component of foreign-body-type multinucleated cells, a minor component of small lymphocytes, and a marked tendency to fibrosis [16].

3.4.4.3 Riedel's Thyroiditis

Riedel's thyroiditis is quite rare and almost exclusively seen in elderly patients. Its main clinical feature consists of a diffuse or nodular swelling of the gland, which has a very hard consistency and is responsible for tracheal constriction. This clinical picture closely simulates that of anaplastic carcinoma. Histologically, the thyroid parenchyma is massively substituted by a fibrosing process that includes chronic inflammatory cells with occasional eosinophils and which leads to heavy collagen deposition [16].

3.4.5 Papillary Carcinoma

Papillary carcinoma is by far the most frequent malignancy of the thyroid and its incidence is continuously increasing [16–19]. It is seen at any age group, including in pediatric patients, but is markedly frequent in women between 20 and 50 years of age. By definition, papillary carcinoma is a neoplasia derived from the follicular epithelium. These cells show a peculiar set of nuclear changes that are pathognomonic and a group of additional features that are variably present and/or particularly expressed in selected variants. The set of nuclear changes consists of: (a) large size (up to 3–5×RBC); (b) an oval to elongated shape; (c) an irregular profile, marked by the presence of incomplete or complete grooves; (d) a clear or finely granular chromatin, with small nucleoli; (e) intranuclear inclusions of the cytoplasm, which is of variable shape and size due to invagination of the nuclear membrane (Fig. 3.5a,b) [16–19]. The tumor is particularly prone to the invasion of lymphatic vessels; in fact, the detection of a lymph node metastasis in the neck from an occult primary is rather commonly seen (up to 20% of cases, especially in young patients) [19]. Several variants of the tumor have been described, the most common being the follicular, the oxyphil cell, the clear cell, the columnar cell, and the tall cell variants. The *follicular variant* is characterized by a follicular (macro- and microfollicular) pattern of growth such that the tumor closely simulates a follicular adenoma or carcinoma (Fig. 3.5a). This resemblance is also reinforced by the reduced presence of the characteristic nuclear changes, compared to the other variants. Cells in the *tall cell variant* have a long axis that is at least three times their width; in addition, they show an eosinophilic cytoplasm and prominent nuclear changes. In the *columnar cell variant*, the tumor cell nuclei are elongated and pseudostratified; the cytoplasm contains clear vacuoles resembling those seen in endometrial cells, with secretory changes. These latter two variants bear a more aggressive biological course and show an early involvement of the lymph nodes [17].

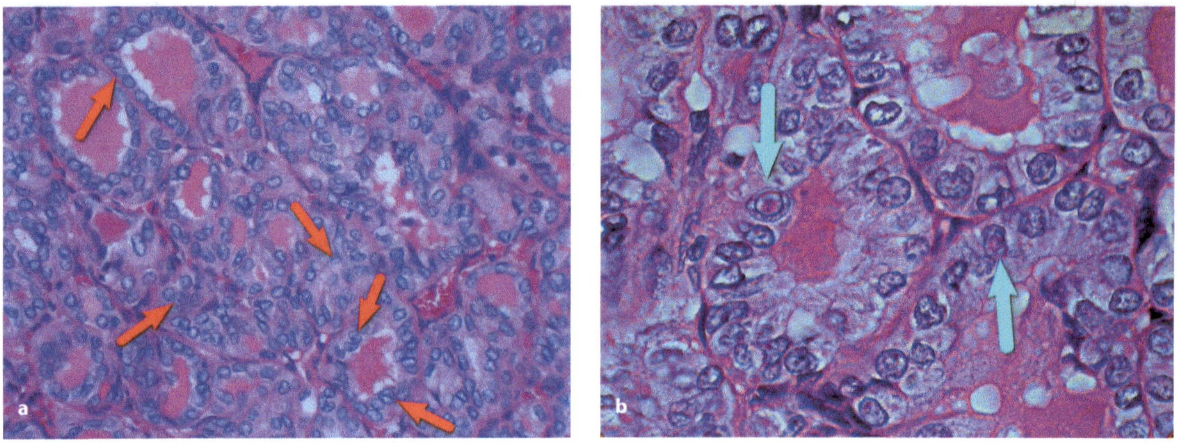

Fig. 3.5 **a** Histology of papillary carcinoma, follicular variant. The nuclei have an irregular outline due to nuclear grooves (*arrows*) and the chromatin is clear or finely granular with small nucleoli. H&E stain, ×400. **b** Histology of papillary carcinoma, usual variant; high-power view discloses intranuclear cytoplasmic inclusions (*arrows*). H&E stain, ×1000

3.4.6 Follicular Carcinoma

Follicular carcinoma represents only 10–15% of malignant tumors of the thyroid [16,20–23]. It mainly occurs in adults in the 6th and 7th decade, without a sex predilection. The neoplastic cells recapitulate the morphology of normal thyrocytes or Hürthle cells [24,25]. The clinical onset is typically characterized by the appearance of a slowly growing nodular swelling of the thyroid. Distant metastases are present in about 20% of patients, even in this early phase. The preferred sites for metastatic involvement are the lung, bone, subcutis, and brain. The two variants differ with respect to local tumor aggressiveness and malignant potential. In the capsulated and minimally invasive variant, the tumor is surrounded by a thick and continuous fibrous capsule and closely resembles an otherwise typical follicular adenoma. The detection of capsular permeation by tumor growth (Fig. 3.6) and/or foci of invasion of capsular vessels (Fig. 3.7) provides evidence of the malignant behavior of the lesion. The implications of the former vs. the latter are different in terms of risk of distant metastasis. In practice, tumors with only capsular invasion are locally aggressive but the risk of distant metastasis is close to zero [21,22]. By contrast, tumors showing invasion of less than four capsular vessels are associated with distant metastasis in about 5% of cases, and those showing four or more foci of vascular invasion are associated with distant metastases in up to 18% of the cases [23]. Based on these facts, total thyroidectomy for tumor excision is not totally justified [21–23]. The risk of metastasis is higher if the tumor is composed of Hürthle cells [24,25]. In summary, the factors predicting an aggressive course of this variant are the number of foci of vascular invasion and a prevailing Hürthle cell morphology of the tumor cells. The massively infiltrating variant of follicular carcinoma is a much more aggressive malignancy [26]. The tumor cells may resemble normal thyrocytes but more commonly have

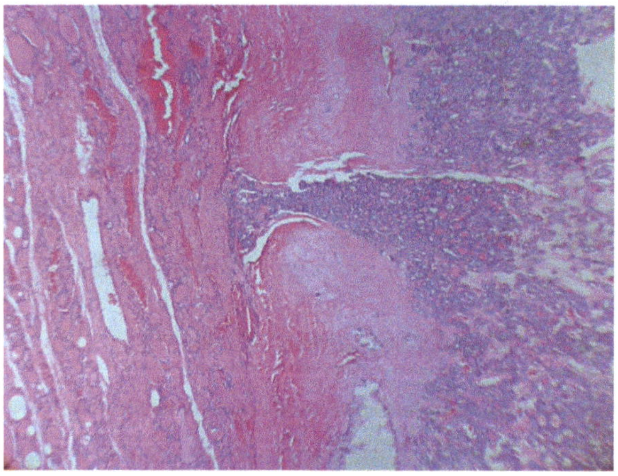

Fig. 3.6 Histology of encapsulated follicular carcinoma; the image shows a focus of capsular violation by the tumor. H&E stain, ×40

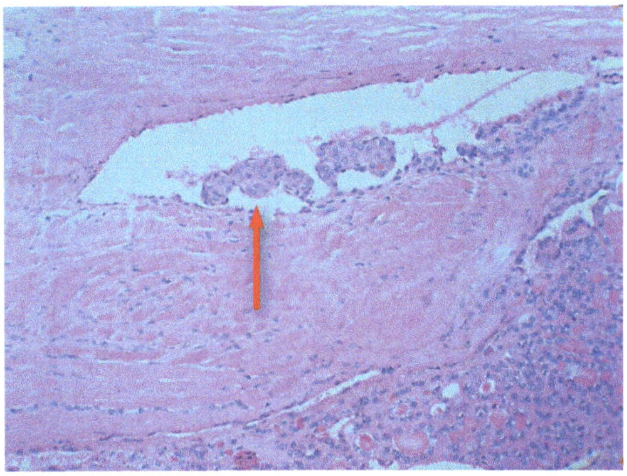

Fig. 3.7 Histology of encapsulated follicular carcinoma; the image shows a capsular vessel containing neoplastic thrombi (*arrow*). H&E stain, ×400

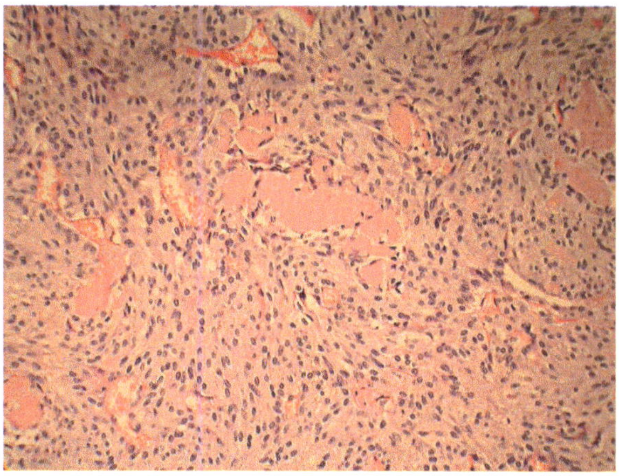

Fig. 3.8 Histology of medullary carcinoma showing cords of spindle cells admixed with amyloid extracellular deposits. H&E stain, ×400

enlarged nuclei with a higher nuclear/cytoplasmic ratio. The tumor may be partially capsulated and shows a massive infiltration of the surrounding parenchyma as well as multiple sites of blood vessel invasion [26].

3.4.7 Medullary Carcinoma

Medullary carcinoma is a rare malignancy that can present as either a sporadic or a familiar form. The former is more common, accounting for 70–80% of the cases. The tumor starts as a rapidly growing thyroid mass that is frequently associated with pain, dysphagia, and enlarged lymph nodes in the neck [16,27,28]. In about one third of cases, patients experience a concomitant chronic diarrhea. An elevation of serum CEA occurs early in the course of the disease and can represent the only manifestation of the tumor. The familiar form develops in young individuals and is frequently multicentric and bilateral. Histologically, medullary carcinoma is characterized by a greatly variable appearance. In general, the tumor cells are of intermediate size, with a polygonal or elongated and epithelioid appearance (Fig. 3.8); alternatively, they may have a plasmacytoid appearance. The pattern of tumor growth is in solid nests and cords, or it may assume a trabecular, pseudopapillary, tubular, microglandular, or cribriform pattern. The interstitium may contain amyloid substance in variable amounts (Fig. 3.8).

3.4.8 Poorly Differentiated Follicular ("Insular") Carcinoma

Insular carcinoma characteristically occurs in middle aged and elderly subjects, is more prevalent in females, and belongs to the category of poorly differentiated follicular tumors of the thyroid [29,30]. The tumor presents as a rapidly growing mass in patients with a history of a solitary thyroid nodule of long duration. Wide metastatic involvement of regional lymph nodes is generally present at clinical onset. Histologically, the tumor consists of solid nests and cords ("insulae") of small to intermediate-sized cells with a large nucleus and scant cytoplasm. Nuclei are round to oval and monomorphous in appearance (Fig. 3.9a). They are densely hyperchromatic or may be characterized by vesicular chromatin and contain multiple small nucleoli [31,32]. Necrotic changes are obvious and the tumor cells appear to be mitotically active. Multiple foci of lymphatic and blood vessel invasion by the tumor are characteristically seen. The morphological features of this tumor may partially overlap those of the widely invasive variant of follicular carcinoma; in fact, abortive follicular structures are frequently detected.

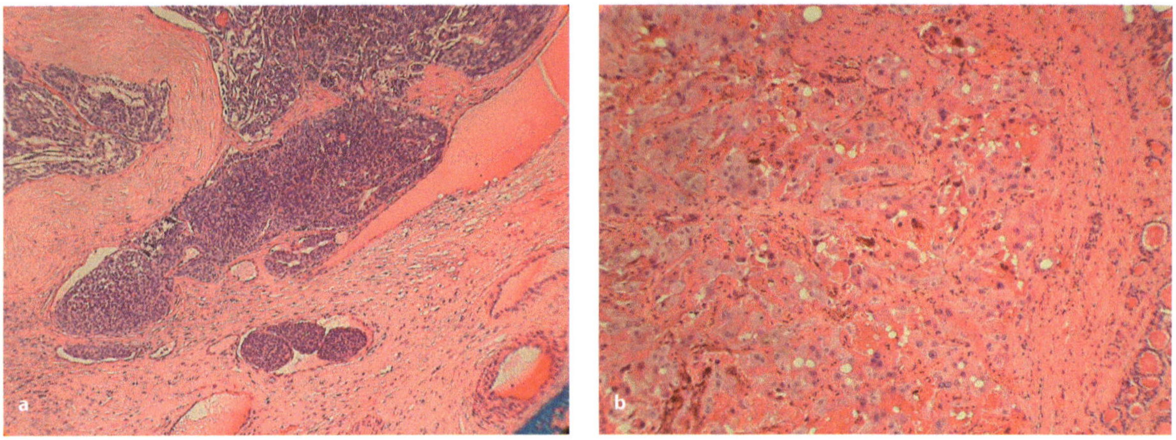

Fig. 3.9 **a** Histology of poorly differentiated follicular carcinoma; the image shows massive vascular invasion by tumor cells. H&E stain, ×250. **b** Histology of a poorly differentiated Hürthle cell carcinoma. The tumor cells are pleomorphic and display prominent nucleoli. H&E stain, ×400

3.4.9 Poorly Differentiated Carcinomas with Papillary, Hürthle Cell, or Medullary Carcinoma Cell Features

It is worth noting that otherwise "usual" forms of papillary, Hürthle cell, or medullary carcinoma can harbor a secondary component characterized by a loss of cellular differentiation and significant changes in the pattern of tumor growth. The latter features are consistent with a more aggressive course. Indeed, since the biological behavior of these tumors resembles that of anaplastic carcinoma they are classified under the heading of "poorly differentiated" tumors of the thyroid. In Hürthle cell carcinoma, this phenomenon is manifested by the appearance of a highly pleomorphic cellular component, displaying large and bizarre nuclei and prominent nucleoli, that shows prominent infiltration of the surrounding parenchyma (Fig. 3.9b) [31].

3.4.10 Undifferentiated (Anaplastic) Carcinoma

Anaplastic carcinoma is typically detected in middle-aged adults and the elderly, with a geographic incidence paralleling that of endemic goiter [16,32]. It is characterized by a rapidly progressive disease course, with the appearance of a mass in the thyroid that is very hard in consistency and compresses the surrounding structures. The tumor may develop in a patient with a history of a long-standing thyroid nodule or it may appear ex novo in an otherwise normal thyroid. Moreover, it can develop in a patient who has already undergone thyroid surgery for the treatment of a papillary carcinoma or a follicular tumor. The wide ranging histopathological morphologies of the tumor include a spindle and giant cell sarcomatoid appearance, mostly spindle cells in fibrosarcoma-like or malignant fibrous-histiocytoma-like patterns, epithelioid cells with an angiosarcoma-like or hemangiopericytoma-like pattern, or a pattern reminiscent of squamous cell carcinoma [32–34]. The differential diagnosis includes sarcoma, large-cell lymphoma, metastatic carcinoma, parathyroid carcinoma, and Riedel's thyroiditis [33,34].

3.4.11 Intrathyroid Parathyroid Tumors

Parathyroid glands can occur within the thyroid parenchyma or capsule [35] and can be affected by primary or secondary hyperplasia, adenoma, and carcinoma. Parathyroid neoplasms are solid or cystic lesions, easily misinterpreted clinically and on imaging as thyroid primary lesions, especially if clinical or biochemical signs of hyperparathyroidism are not evident [36]. Histologically, intrathyroid parathyroid adenoma and well-differentiated carcinoma are characterized by a follicular, solid and multinodular, or

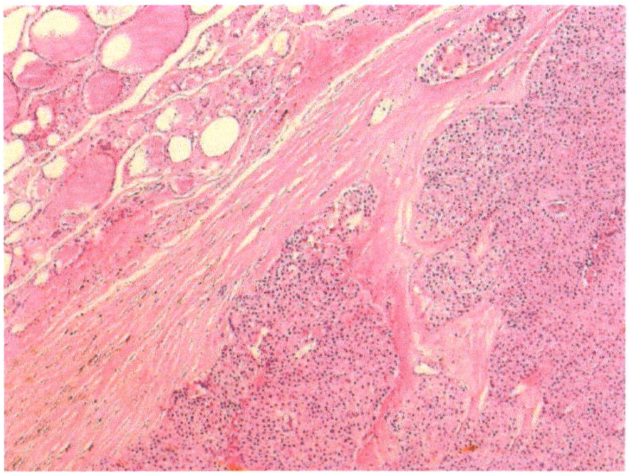

Fig. 3.10 Histology of intrathyroid parathyroid carcinoma. The tumor is encapsulated and contains intratumoral fibrous trabeculae; normal thyroid tissue is evident in the upper left part of the figure. H&E stain, ×250

trabecular pattern of growth (Fig. 3.10). Follicles containing colloid-like material can closely simulate thyroid follicular neoplasms. In addition, tumor cells may appear as clear cells or oncocytic cells. The distinction between adenoma and well-differentiated carcinoma may be difficult or impossible. Highly predictive signs of malignancy are capsular invasion and disruption in addition to intravascular tumor growth, but these findings may be very subtle or completely lacking in parathyroid carcinoma.

3.5 Immunohistochemistry of Thyroid Lesions

Immunohistochemical diagnostic markers consist of thyroid secretion products, such as thyroglobulin (TG), calcitonin (CT), and CEA, as well as different types of cytokeratins, adhesion molecules (galectin 3), receptors (RET and EGFR), gene transcription factors (TTF-1), and membrane products (HBME-1) [37,38]. TG is expressed in tumors of follicular derivation whereas CT and CEA are associated only with tumors of parafollicular derivation. TTF-1 is expressed both in tumors of follicular and parafollicular derivation. Galectin 3 and HBME are mainly expressed in malignant tumors of follicular derivation (papillary and follicular carcinomas) but also in a significant percentage of follicular adenomas. Cytokeratin 19 expression is diffusely prominent in papillary carcinoma, less so in medullary carcinoma, and sparse and focal in follicular adenoma. Cytokeratin 7 is focally expressed in anaplastic carcinoma, which is of help in the distinction of this tumor from a sarcoma or malignant melanoma. Hyaline trabecular adenoma cells show a strong cytoplasmic immunoreactivity for cytokeratin 19 and Ki-67/MIB1 (Fig. 3.3b) [35]. Anaplastic carcinoma cells express vimentin and the epidermal growth factor receptor (EGFR) in most cases while cytokeratins are coexpressed in about 50% of cases [38].

3.6 Analytical Approach to the Cytological Sample

The systematic approach to a thyroid smear requires evaluation of the background and the ancillary cellular components first, followed by the thyroid cellular yield.

3.6.1 Background

The background may contain the following components.

3.6.1.1 Blood

The amount of blood in the smear may be rather abundant in a thyroid sample due to the density of capillaries at the sampling site. The thyroid is perfused by an abundant microcirculation network whose density per volume is inversely proportional to the size of the thyroid follicles. Thus, microfollicular nodules are hypervascularized while macrofollicular nodules contain fewer vessels but a larger amount of colloid. In general, the larger the size of the follicle within the sampled area, the less the amount of blood contamination in the smear.

3.6.1.2 Colloid

Colloid is a proteinaceous amorphous substance that stains pink, orange, or yellow in ethanol-fixed and Papanicolaou-stained smears, or grayish to green in air-dried preparations stained with May Grünwald

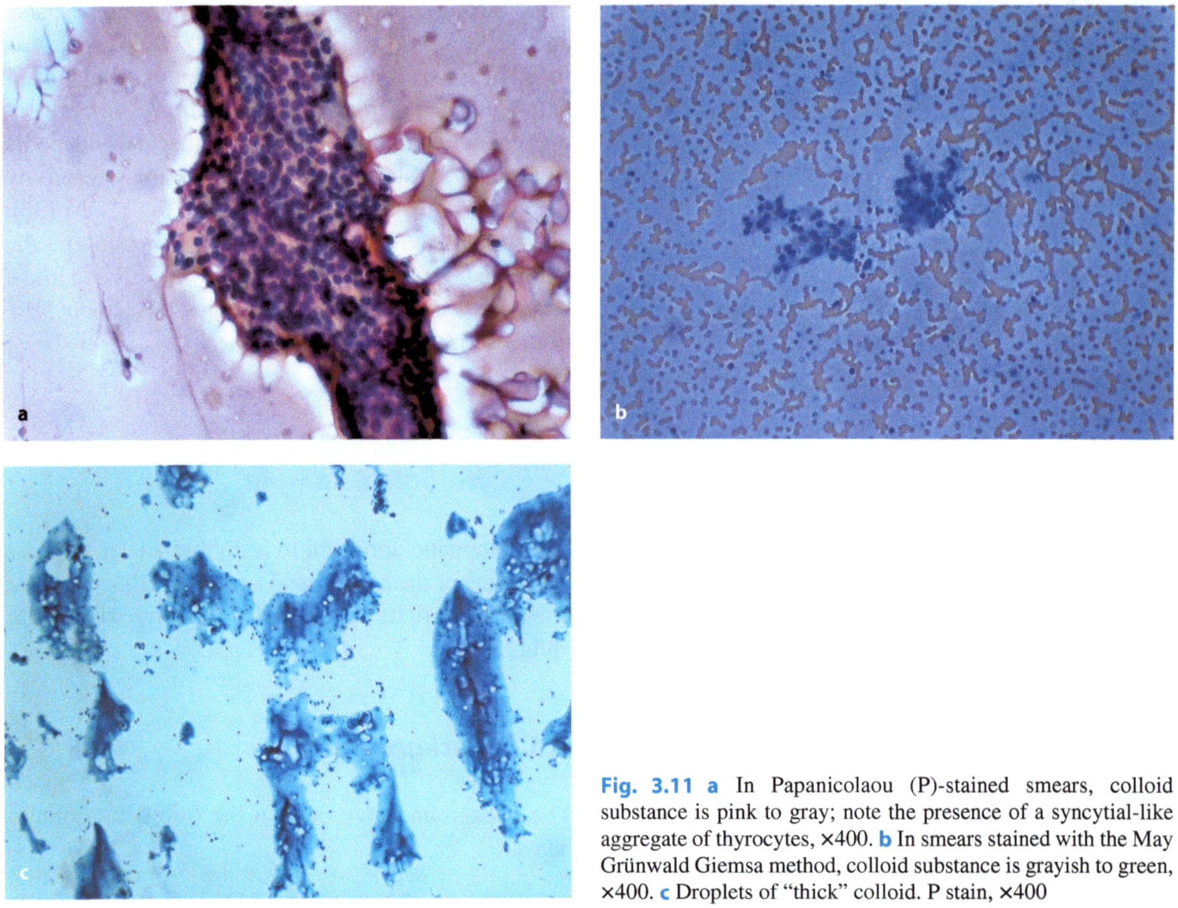

Fig. 3.11 **a** In Papanicolaou (P)-stained smears, colloid substance is pink to gray; note the presence of a syncytial-like aggregate of thyrocytes, ×400. **b** In smears stained with the May Grünwald Giemsa method, colloid substance is grayish to green, ×400. **c** Droplets of "thick" colloid. P stain, ×400

Giemsa stain. It can appear either as a transparent patina all over the slide, in large globules, or as discrete, rounded, or irregularly shaped droplets. These latter accumulations may be slightly basophilic and non-transparent (Fig. 3.11). The amount of colloid in a FNB sample is proportional to the wideness of the follicular cavities at the puncture site. When colloid is abundant, the amount of blood contaminating the smear is reduced and vice versa.

3.6.1.3 Stromal Fragments

Stromal fragments may consist of loose to dense fibrous tissue containing a variable amount of capillaries and entrapped thyrocytes or inflammatory cells; they may also comprise aggregates of adipocytes (a rare finding) or amyloid substance.

Papanicolaou-stained smears evidence the presence of hyaline collagen, which appears homogeneously pink (Fig. 3.12), while May Grünwald Giemsa-stained preparations are metachromatic. Calcified material may be present as well. The capillary vessel

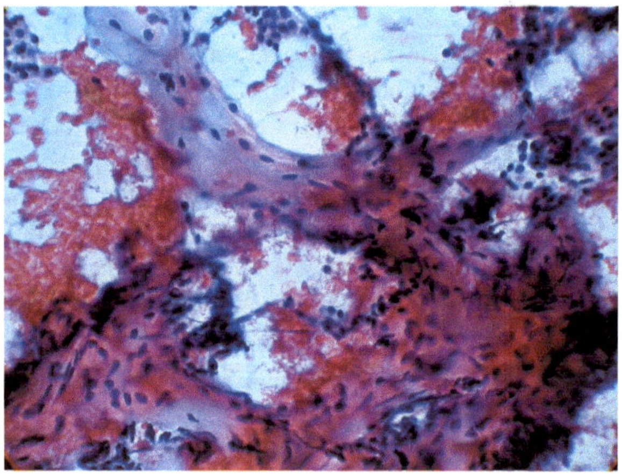

Fig. 3.12 Stromal fragments containing fibrocytes in an amorphous collagen background containing capillary vessels. P stain, ×400

component is variable but may be very abundant. Capillaries may show prominent endothelial cells containing vesicular nuclei and well-evident nucleoli. Amyloid or pseudoamyloid accumulations are homogeneous, fibrillary, and of various shape and size.

3.6.1.4 Inflammatory Cells and Crystals

The most commonly found inflammatory cells in FNB smears are small lymphocytes, plasma cells, and histiocytes. Histiocytes may be mononucleated or multinucleated. In the former case, the cells are generally of intermediate size with an abundant foamy cytoplasm. Their nucleus is centrally or eccentrically located and contains vesicular chromatin as well as a small nucleolus (Fig. 3.13a). The cytoplasm includes lipids, cholesterol crystals, or hemosiderin, all of which are better seen in smears stained according to the May Grünwald Giemsa method (Fig. 3.13b). Other examples of mononucleated macrophages are the epithelioid histiocytes seen in various granulomatous processes; these cells possess a dense cytoplasm and are elongated in shape. Multinucleated histiocytes can be very large and may assume the morphology of foreign-body macrophages, which contain numerous randomly distributed nuclei and a vacuolated or granular cytoplasm (Fig. 3.13c). A peculiar variant of multi-nucleated histiocytes is seen in papillary and medullary carcinomas; it represents an integral component of the neoplastic population of these tumors (see below). The number of nuclei rarely exceeds 10–20 and they are characterized by an irregular profile due to the presence of clefts. Finally, inorganic crystals, mostly cholesterol (Fig. 3.13b), or deposits of various types, usually calcium (Fig. 3.14), can be seen extracellularly in the background.

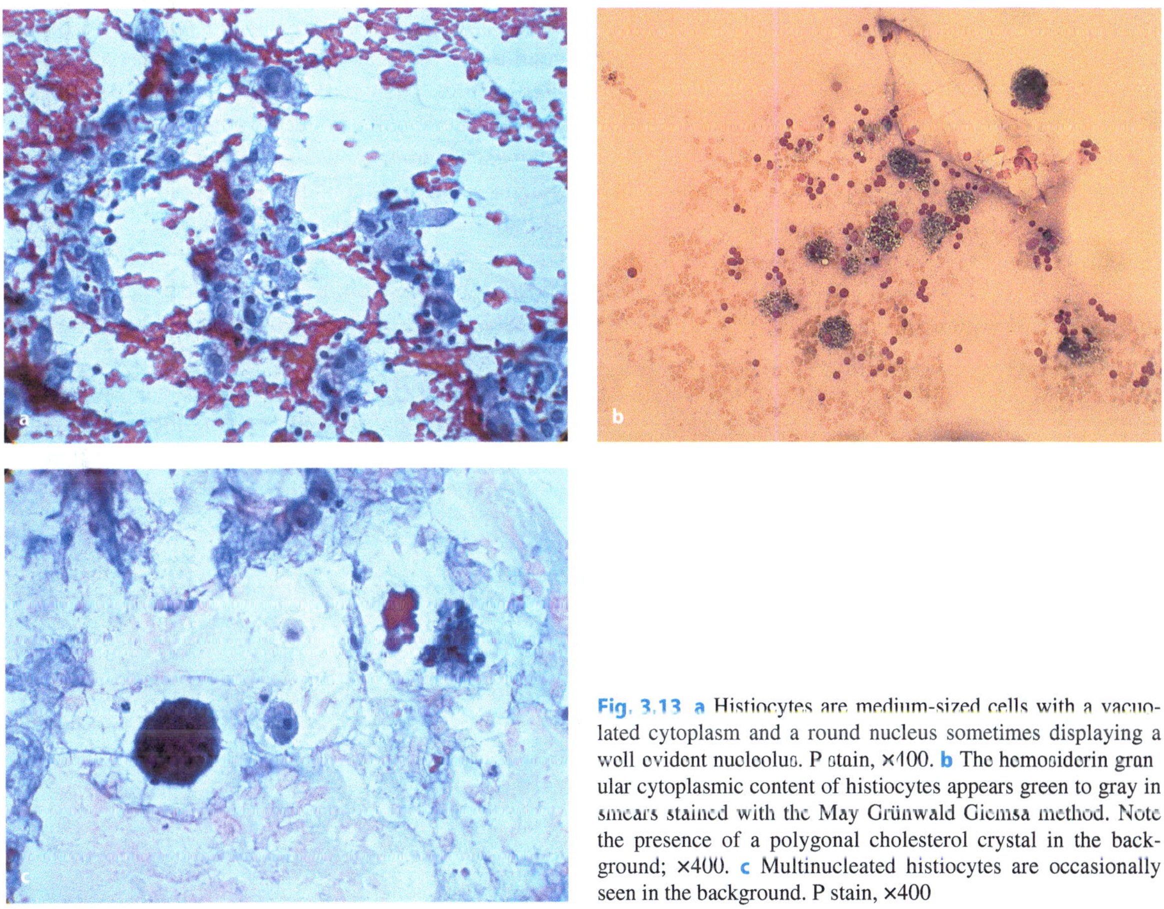

Fig. 3.13 **a** Histiocytes are medium-sized cells with a vacuolated cytoplasm and a round nucleus sometimes displaying a well evident nucleolus. P stain, ×100. **b** The hemosiderin granular cytoplasmic content of histiocytes appears green to gray in smears stained with the May Grünwald Giemsa method. Note the presence of a polygonal cholesterol crystal in the background; ×400. **c** Multinucleated histiocytes are occasionally seen in the background. P stain, ×400

3.6.2 Proper Thyroid Cell Types

3.6.2.1 Follicular Thyrocytes

Follicular thyrocytes are found in two-dimensional sheets (Figs. 3.14, 3.15a), syncytium-like aggregates (Fig. 3.11a), or three-dimensional aggregates (Fig. 3.15b). In the latter, they are assembled in follicular clusters of variable size. Follicular cells are small to intermediate in size and contain a variable amount of cytoplasm. Their nuclei have a round to oval shape, a smooth border, and are rarely larger than 2×RBC (Fig. 3.15c). The chromatin is finely granular with small chromocenters and sometimes small nucleoli (Fig. 3.15d). The cytoplasm is amphophilic or eosinophilic. Follicular cells may also be found as non-cohesive elements dispersed in the background (Fig. 3.15e). Their nuclei are small and darkly stained, resembling those in apoptotic cells. The cytoplasm of dispersed cells is generally very scant or even unapparent. These cells, even in completely benign conditions, may show variable degrees of anisonucleosis but they always retain a round to oval regular contour.

3.6.2.2 Oxyphil Cells

Oxyphil cells (also known as oncocytes, Hürthle cells, or Ashkenazy cells) are intermediate to large in size and differ from follicular cells with respect to their cytoplasmic and nuclear features. The cytoplasm is abundant and homogeneous or finely granular and eosinophilic (Fig. 3.15f). The nucleus is round, larger than 2×RBC, and, most importantly, often contains a well-evident nucleolus. By definition, the nuclear contour is round to oval with a smooth border. Oxyphil cells are seen as single isolated elements dispersed in the background, or in syncytium-like sheets, in two-dimensional sheets, or in three-dimensional follicular aggregates.

3.6.2.3 Miscellaneous Cell Types

Several additional cell types can be detected in FNB smears in various pathological conditions. In particular, thyroid cells may assume an *epithelioid* or elongated and *spindle-like* configuration, as is observed in thyroiditis and various types of primary carcinoma.

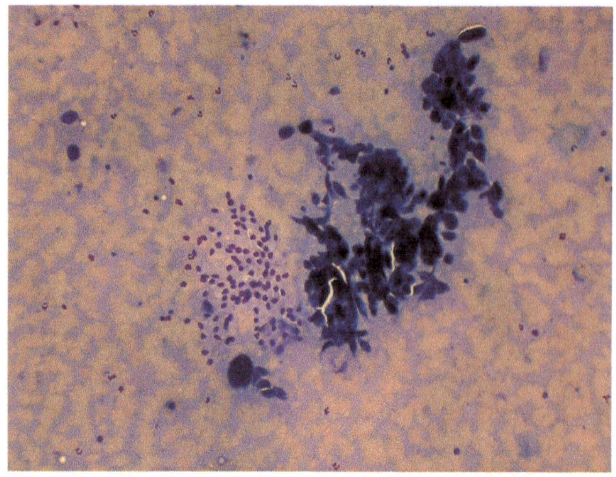

Fig. 3.14 Extracellular calcium deposits are stained intensely blue in smears stained with the May Grünwald Giemsa method. Note the presence of a two-dimensional aggregate of thyrocytes; ×400

These cells should be differentiated from epithelioid histiocytes, fibroblasts, and fibrocytes. Cells assuming a *squamoid* or definitely squamous cell morphology are seen in FNB smears obtained from various benign conditions, such as thyroditis, and represent metaplastic cells. Their morphology is identical to that of the squamous cells found in other normal epithelia. Atypical squamoid cells resembling those of non-keratinizing squamous cells may appear in some variants of papillary carcinoma and anaplastic carcinoma. *Giant cells,* which contain one or multiple nuclei showing bizarre features (large size, hyperchromasia, irregular shape, prominent nucleoli, etc.), are the hallmark of several primary and metastatic malignancies of the thyroid. The cytoplasm of these cells is generally abundant and densely amphiphilic or basophilic but may also be vacuolated. They should be differentiated from multinucleated histiocytes.

3.6.3 Specimen Adequacy

The minimal requirements for the adequacy of a thyroid nodule specimen obtained by FNB have been the subject of several debates [39–45]. Consequently, the lack of uniform criteria for adequacy assessment has created diagnostic discrepancies between pathologists and thus significantly compromised the clinical applicability of the cytological diagnosis. It is difficult to state any general rules because the cellular yield

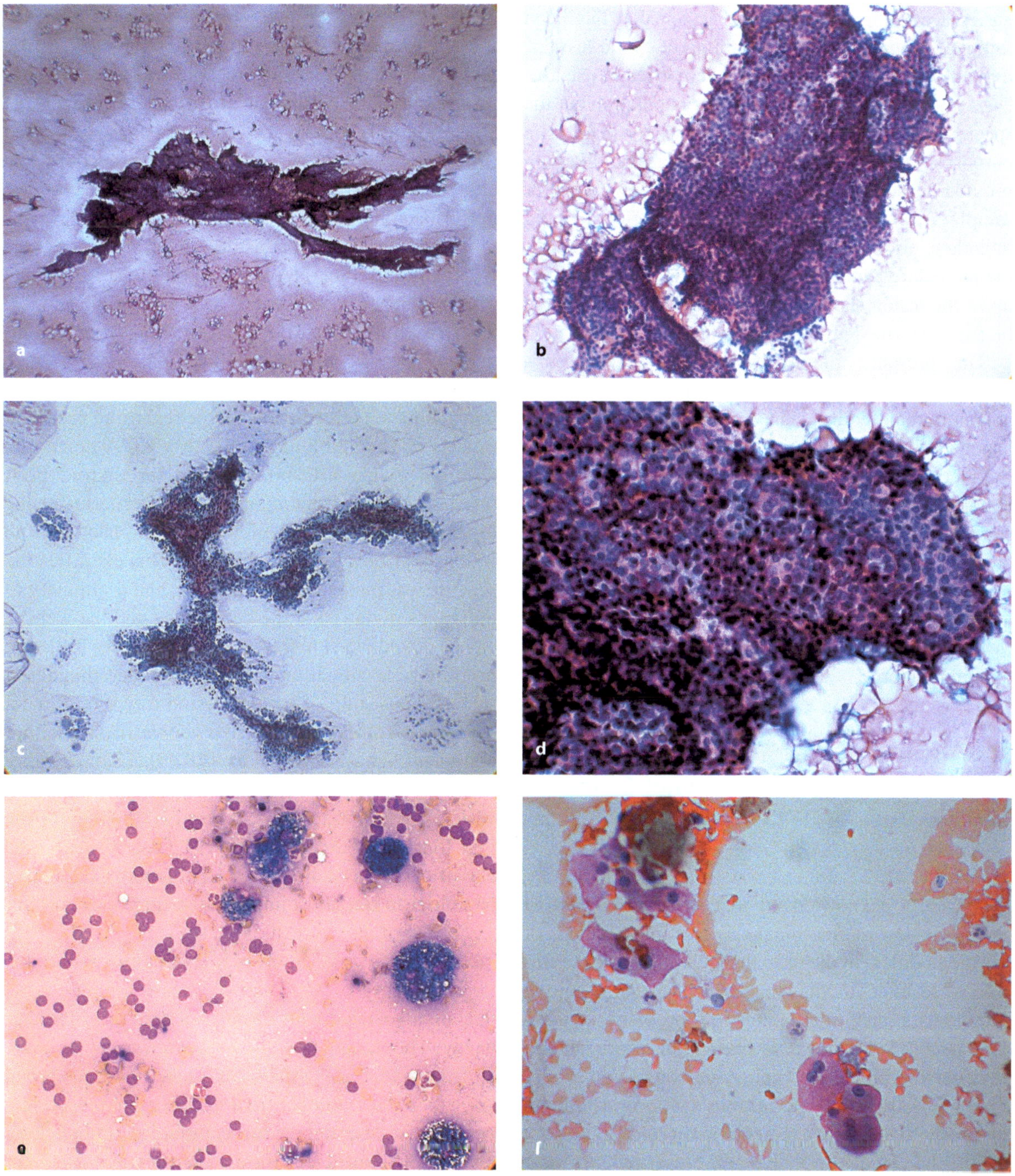

Fig. 3.15 a A two-dimensional and irregularly shaped aggregate of thyrocytes is seen against a background rich in colloid. P stain, ×200. b A three-dimensional aggregate of thyrocytes. P stain, ×400. c A three-dimensional aggregate with a definite follicular configuration. P stain, ×200. d At high magnification, thyrocytes within aggregates appear to have round nuclei with little or no variation in size and shape. Their chromatin is finely granular. P stain, ×1000. e Dispersed thyrocytes practically devoid of cytoplasm and showing a finely granular chromatin. May Grünwald Giemsa stain, ×1000. f Hürthle cells appear as medium-sized and polygonal elements with a granular eosinophilic cytoplasm and a centrally located nucleus containing a well-evident nucleolus. P stain, ×1000

varies according to the thyroid lesion that has been sampled. In practice, FNB sampling of cystic lesions, hypocellular colloid nodules, or hemorrhagic pseudocysts may yield a very scant cellular population but the specimen is not necessarily inadequate for diagnostic purposes. In these cases, a repeat biopsy is not likely to provide an additional or more representative cellular sample; thus, the diagnostic formulation should include a brief comment outlining the limitations of the procedure and all possible implications. A follow-up of the lesion should be recommended and a repeat biopsy performed after 3–6 months.

The presence of at least six cellular groups containing at least ten cells each represents a reasonable minimal requirement for diagnosing follicular lesions [45] but this does not constitute a general rule. In fact, when such a sparse amount of cells consists of abnormal or atypical cells, any definitive diagnosis should be discouraged and adequate sampling should be obtained by repeat biopsy. In conclusion, the most important rule in assessing specimen adequacy is to acknowledge the possible nature of the thyroid lesion by judicious correlation with clinical findings and imaging features.

3.7 Towards a Uniform Diagnostic Terminology: The National Cancer Institute (NCI) Classification Scheme, 2008

It is widely acknowledged that FNB is the test of choice for the routine diagnosis and management of thyroid nodules. In the past, the lack of uniform terminology resulted in diagnostic inconsistency among pathologists and communication problems among clinicians [45–47]. For this reason, all efforts should be made to promote the implementation of universally accepted diagnostic criteria, thus favoring a rational approach to the management of thyroid lesions. It should be recognized that the scrutiny of most morphological parameters in thyroid cytology is greatly open to subjective interpretation, which negatively impacts the diagnostic reproducibility of the procedure. Attempts to reduce subjectivity as much as possible are therefore of paramount importance as this will increase the clinical applicability of the procedure. The aim of a consensus-based terminology is also to clearly define the most proper context justifying the diagnosis of "indeterminate for malignancy," which is inevitably rendered in as many as one third of the thyroid follicular lesions recognized as "follicular proliferation" or "follicular neoplasm." However, the abuse of this diagnostic category has decreased the positive predictive value of the procedure and caused unnecessary and unjustified thyroidectomies, performed only for diagnostic purposes [46,47].

The National Cancer Institute (NCI) sponsored the NCI Thyroid Fine-Needle Aspiration (FNA) State of the Science Conference, on October 22 and 23, 2007, in Bethesda, MD. This meeting was accompanied by a permanent informational website (http://thyroidfna.cancer.gov) that serves as an unprecedented information source regarding nearly all aspects of needle biopsy of the thyroid. A diagnostic terminology/classification scheme for thyroid FNA interpretation and cytomorphological criteria for the diagnosis of various benign and malignant thyroid lesions was developed (Table 3.1). This classification scheme was published in 2008 [48], and a summary of the topics reviewed at the conference and the website can be downloaded free from several sources [49]. The proposed classification is a six-category diagnostic scheme consisting of benign, lesion (atypia) of undetermined significance, follicular neoplasm, suspicious, malignant, and unsatisfactory [48,49]. Each category identifies a different ''risk of malignancy,'' which varies from <1% to a maximum of 70–80% for the first four categories in the list. The use of this tiered classification system favors reproducibility among pathologists and, most importantly, improves the clinical utility of the cytopathological diagnosis. The main merit of the classification is to distinguish within the large category of follicular-patterned samples those that are associated with a low vs. a high risk of malignancy. The designation "*follicular lesions of undetermined significance*" represents a heterogeneous group "in which the cytologic findings are not convincingly benign, yet the degree of cellular or architectural atypia is not sufficient for an interpretation of follicular neoplasm or suspicious for malignancy" [48]. The category should represent ideally less than 7% of all thyroid FNB interpretations; the risk of malignancy for such lesions is 5–10%. Further management of these patients is based on proper correlation with clinical findings and imaging data. Generally, the patient should be followed up and a repeat FNB performed after a short time, as it can help differentiate benign

Table 3.1 The National Cancer Institute (NCI) Classification Scheme (2008)

Suggested categories	Alternate category(ies) terms	Risk of malignancy
Benign		<1%
Follicular lesion of undetermined significance	Atypia of undetermined significance R/O neoplasm Atypical follicular lesion Cellular follicular lesion	5–10%
Follicular neoplasm	Suspicious for follicular neoplasm	20–30%
Suspicious for malignancy		50–75%
Malignant		100%
Non-diagnostic	Unsatisfactory	

from potentially malignant tumors. The category of "*follicular neoplasm/suspicious for follicular neoplasm*" applies to non-papillary follicular-patterned lesions/neoplasms and Hürthle cell lesions/neoplasms. The risk of malignancy is higher (20–30%) and varies depending on the size of the lesion or the relative prevalence of Hürthle cells. Most patients with this diagnosis will undergo lobectomy/hemithyroidectomy and a definite diagnosis (adenomatoid nodule vs. adenoma vs. carcinoma) is rendered on surgical pathology examination. Finally, the category "*suspicious for malignancy*" includes lesions suspicious for the follicular variant of papillary carcinoma, medullary carcinoma, anaplastic carcinoma, or other primary (for example, malignant lymphoma) or metastatic tumors in which cytological findings are not totally diagnostic due to several reasons, including poor cellularity, artifacts, necrosis, and specimens inadequate to perform confirmatory immunostains (for medullary carcinoma). A repeat biopsy is generally of help to better define the lesion and the patient should be referred for thyroid lobectomy.

3.8 Pattern Profiling of FNB Samples

Pattern profiling and the cytomorphological classification tree of thyroid FNB samples is based on the evaluation of the following features: (a) background; (b) extent of cellularity and the nature of the cell types present, including ancillary elements; (c) the structure of cellular aggregates; and (d) the fine morphology of the nuclei and cytoplasm of each cellular component. Examination of the samples according to these criteria requires accurate observation and orderly classification. The end result is that the cytological expressions can be conveniently divided into three large groups indicating benign, indeterminate, and malignant lesions. Once the major pattern has been identified, the diagnostic possibilities are dramatically reduced and the next step is to home in on the exact diagnosis by using the NCI classification scheme, 2008.

3.8.1 Benign and Non-Neoplastic Follicular Lesions

3.8.1.1 Colloid Nodule

- *Background:* abundant colloid, with possible stromal fragments and sparse red blood cells.
- *Cellularity:* poor (slightly above adequacy requirements).
- *Cell types present:* follicular thyrocytes (Fig. 3.11a,b), histiocytes with hemosiderin granules (Fig. 3.13), lymphocytes (optional), Hürthle cells (occasional elements).
- *Aggregation pattern:* two-dimensional aggregates (Fig. 3.11a) with well-defined follicular spaces and equidistant nuclei; sparse non-cohesive cells.
- *Fine cellular morphology:* small, round, monomorphous and mostly hyperchromatic nuclei; sparse or barely evident cytoplasm.

3.8.1.2 Hypercellular Colloid Nodule

- *Background:* moderate amount of colloid that stains clear or appears transparent, together with a significant component of red blood cells and stromal fragments.
- *Cellularity:* moderate to abundant.
- *Cell types present:* mostly follicular thyrocytes, histiocytes with hemosiderin granules, lymphocytes

(sparse), Hürthle cells (no more than occasional elements).

- *Aggregation:* two-dimensional aggregates (Fig. 3.15a) with well-defined follicular spaces and equidistant nuclei, microfollicular aggregates (Fig. 3.15b) with minor degree of nuclear overlap (Fig. 3.15d); a significant component of non-cohesive cells (Fig. 3.15e).
- *Fine cellular morphology:* small, round, monomorphous and mostly hyperchromatic nuclei; sparse or practically absent cytoplasm (Fig. 3.15c).

The above descriptions differ with respect to the amount of follicular cells detected in the smear but they share the following features: (a) abundant colloid in the background, (b) easily detected histiocytes with hemosiderin granules, (c) prevalence of two-dimensional aggregates of follicular cells with an ordered distribution of nuclei, (d) monomorphous round nuclei showing a smooth external contour and dense chromatin. By definition, follicular cells in this group of lesions show a typical nuclear morphology and any irregularity of the nuclear profile, even in occasional elements, excludes the case from this category [3,6,9,41,43]. The presence of occasional Hürthle cells is not influential (Fig. 3.15f). Additional findings include the presence of cholesterol crystals, lipid material accumulation, calcium deposits, and oxalate crystals and serve as evidence of intralesional regressive changes. Lymphocytes and plasma cells are constantly found, at least in minor amounts. Histiocytes are always present and they are seen as dispersed elements in the background. Sometimes, however, they can occur as large tissue fragments and may display nuclear atypia (nuclear grooves, elongated shape, membrane thickening, chromatin clearing) mimicking the cytological changes characteristic of papillary carcinoma [50].

3.8.1.3 Chronic Lymphocytic Thyroiditis

- *Background:* red blood cells, stromal fragments, absence of colloid, with lymphoglandular bodies.
- *Cellularity:* scant to moderate.
- *Cell types present:* Hürthle cells, i.e., cells larger than follicle cells, of variable shape (rounded to polygonal), and having an abundant gray to eosinophilic cytoplasm and a round nucleus, plus a polymorphous lymphoid population consisting of small lymphocytes, centrocytes, and some centroblasts, with plasma cells, neutrophils, histiocytes; and possibly multinucleated histiocytes (Fig. 3.16a).
- *Aggregation:* Hürthle cells present in monolayered sheets (Fig. 3.16b) but also in small groups, or non-cohesive.
- *Fine cellular morphology:* possible significant anisonucleosis (variable shape and size of nuclei) of Hürthle cells, with prominent nucleoli (Fig. 3.16c) and/or nuclear clearing and occasional grooving phenomena; lymphocytes frequently adhering to or infiltrating the cytoplasm of Hürthle cells.

If the FNB smear shows a dual population of Hürthle cells and activated lymphocytes, the diagnosis of chronic lymphocytis is generally straightforward [51]. The detection, however, of extensive Hürthle cell pleomorphism is a major cause of false-positive diagnoses, including poorly differentiated follicular and anaplastic carcinomas. In addition, nuclear clearing may suggest papillary carcinoma, and prominent nucleoli a Hürthle cell tumor [52]. In general, in these cases the detection of even scattered lymphocytes should suggest thyroiditis and necessitates antibody titers, if not already available. Moreover, taking into proper account the clinical presentation of the nodular lesion is of paramount importance to avoid a misdiagnosis of malignancy.

3.8.2 Potentially Neoplastic Lesions

The group of indeterminate cases includes categories 2–4 of the NCI classification scheme, 2008. The cytological picture is similar that seen for benign lesions but the detection of additional findings dealing with the cellular aggregation pattern and fine morphology dictates a more cautious approach. In this setting, cytological data are to be considered inconclusive and indeterminate for possible malignancy but a clear-cut distinction between low- and high-risk lesions should be reached. Additional actions should be taken, ranging from strict clinical follow-up of the patient and/or repeat biopsy to immediate surgical excision of the nodule for thorough histological evaluation.

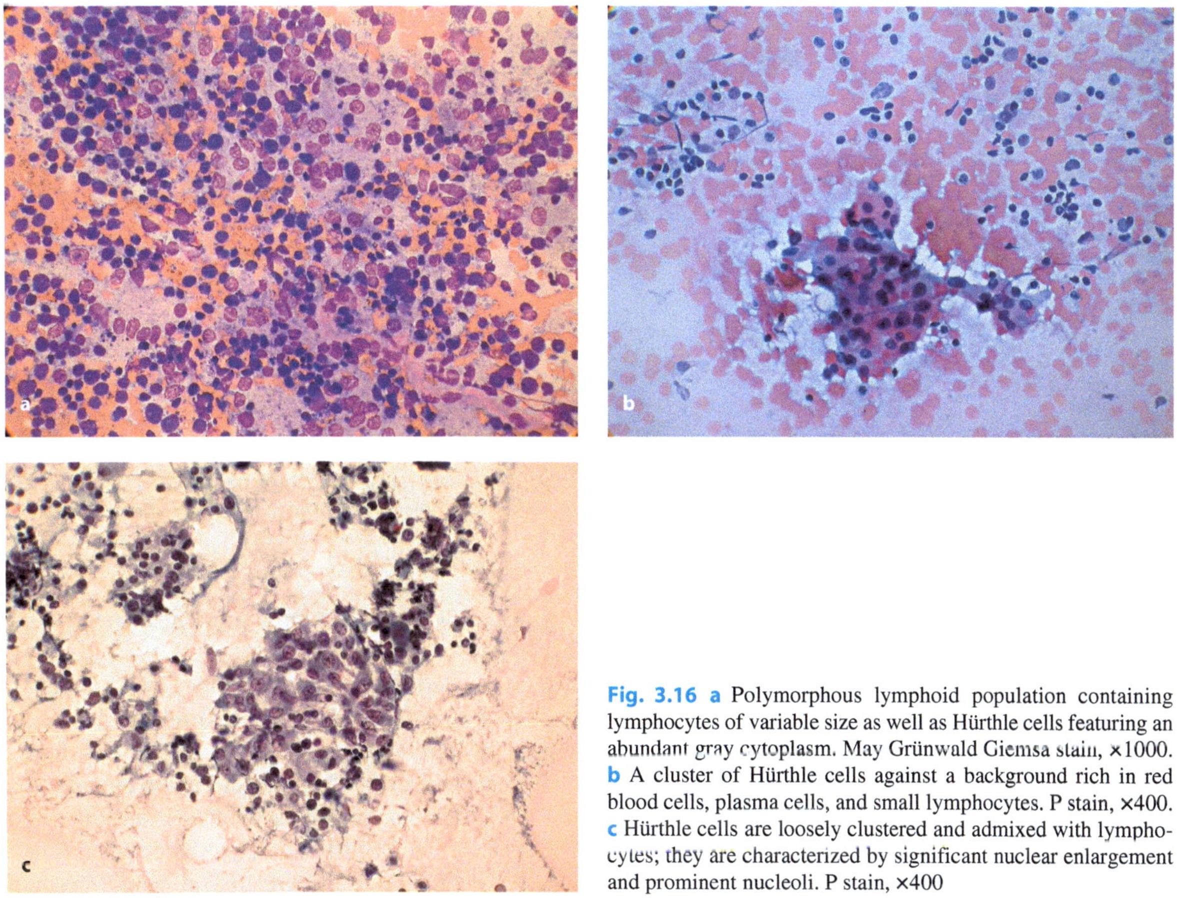

Fig. 3.16 **a** Polymorphous lymphoid population containing lymphocytes of variable size as well as Hürthle cells featuring an abundant gray cytoplasm. May Grünwald Giemsa stain, ×1000. **b** A cluster of Hürthle cells against a background rich in red blood cells, plasma cells, and small lymphocytes. P stain, ×400. **c** Hürthle cells are loosely clustered and admixed with lymphocytes; they are characterized by significant nuclear enlargement and prominent nucleoli. P stain, ×400

3.8.2.1 Follicular Lesion of Undetermined Significance

- *Background:* moderate to sparse colloid, blood and stromal fragments.
- *Cellularity:* poor to moderate.
- *Cell types present:* mostly follicular thyrocytes, sparse or any histiocytes with hemosiderin granules, lymphocytes (sparse), Hürthle cells (no more than occasional elements).
- *Aggregation:* two-dimensional aggregates with well-defined follicular spaces and equidistant nuclei, minor degree of nuclear overlap; a significant component of non-cohesive cells.
- *Fine cellular morphology:* follicular thyrocytes with typical morphology (see above) plus a minor component (<10%) of cells with large nuclei (diameter >2×RBC) with chromatin clearing, and occasional nuclear clefts (Fig. 3.17).

Cytological findings in this pattern are essentially similar to those of the previous category; however, based on the sparsity of colloid and histiocytes with hemosiderin pigment granules as well as the detection of occasional nuclear clearing or an irregular nuclear profile, the possibility of a follicular variant of papillary carcinoma cannot be ruled out. Colloid scarcity can be attributed to incomplete sampling of an otherwise typical colloid nodule, and some cases are placed in this category because of a compromised specimen (e.g., low cellularity, poor fixation, obscuring blood). The detection of a partially deviant nuclear morphology of follicular cells suggests that a more cautious approach to the case is needed. In general, patients should undergo repeat biopsy to disclose possible additional findings that may be of help in better defining the case. A closer re-evaluation of imaging data and clinical findings often leads to a definitive decision.

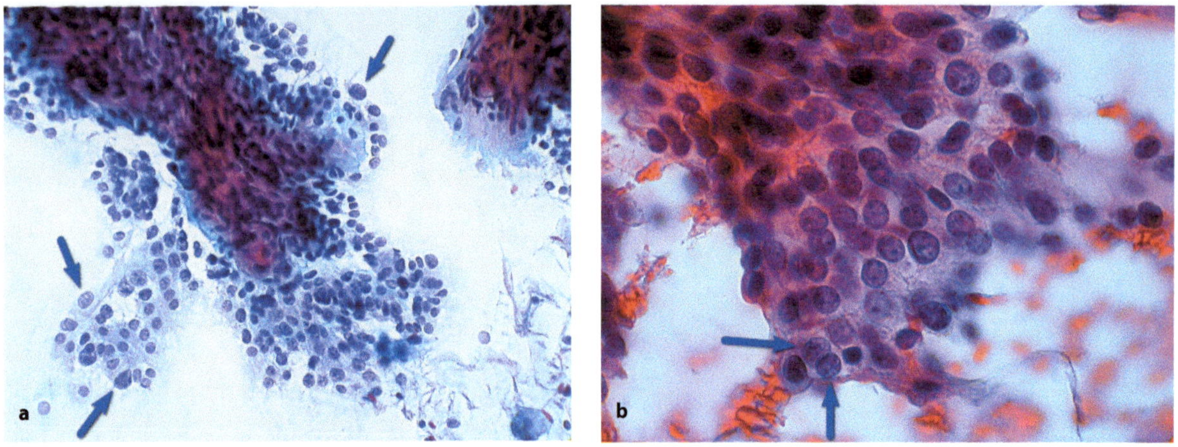

Fig. 3.17 a Occasional nuclear enlargement (*arrows*) is seen in this aggregate of thyrocytes. P stain, ×1000. b Occasional nuclear grooving in two cells (*arrows*) coexists in an aggregate with thyrocytes having an otherwise typical morphology. P stain, ×1000

3.8.2.2 Follicular Proliferation/Neoplasm

- *Background:* blood and stromal fragments, no colloid.
- *Cellularity:* moderate to abundant (Fig. 3.18a,b).
- *Cell types present:* follicular thyrocytes (Fig. 3.18c) or Hürthle cells (Fig. 3.18d), sparse lymphocytes, no histiocytes with hemosiderin granules.
- *Aggregation:* three-dimensional aggregates composed of overlapping microfollicular structures (Fig. 3.18a), microfollicles occurring as single and isolated structures, a significant component of non-cohesive cells (Fig. 3.18c).
- *Fine cellular morphology:* follicular thyrocytes with typical morphology (round to oval shape and a smooth border, finely granular chromatin with small chromocenters, no nucleoli) and the absence of: nuclei of larger size, chromatin clearing, and nuclear clefts; enlarged nuclei with centrally located nucleoli in Hürthle cells, but no nuclear clearing or clefts.

This category invokes a cytological picture marked by a high cellularity, a microfollicular pattern of aggregation, and a decidedly monomorphous appearance of the nuclei [10–12,53]. Samples containing Hürthle cells may show prominent cellular dissociation and a more pronounced nuclear pleomorphism but they are similarly included in this category. By definition, the colloid in the background is absent or very sparse and transparent. In addition, histiocytes with pigment granules are not seen. The exclusion criteria for the diagnosis of follicular proliferation are listed in Table 3.2.

The above-described picture does not identify a particular disease entity of the thyroid but a *specific cytological pattern* that is observed in the FNB smears collected from distinct variants of benign hyperplastic nodules, follicular adenoma, and well-differentiated follicular carcinoma [10,12]. These share a microfollicular pattern of growth and a relative monomorphism of proliferating cells. The differential diagnosis of these lesions is solely based on the histological evaluation of additional morphological features, which mainly include the presence of a well-defined and continuous capsule, the detection of capsular infiltration to a significant extent, and the presence of capsular angioinvasiveness. In summary, the thyrocyte population shares exactly the same morphological features, whether comprising benign hyperplastic nodules, adenoma, or carcinoma. The only morphological markers of malignancy are possibly detected at the interface of the nodule with the surrounding parenchyma. These markers thus represent histological and *not* cytological findings. The follicular variant of papillary carcinoma can have the same microfollicular pattern of growth as the above lesions, but neoplastic cells should be characterized by a markedly different nuclear morphology (see below). In a significant proportion of FNB samples of this tumor variant, however, the characteristic nuclear changes may be completely lacking such that the cytological picture inevitably falls into the category of follicular proliferation.

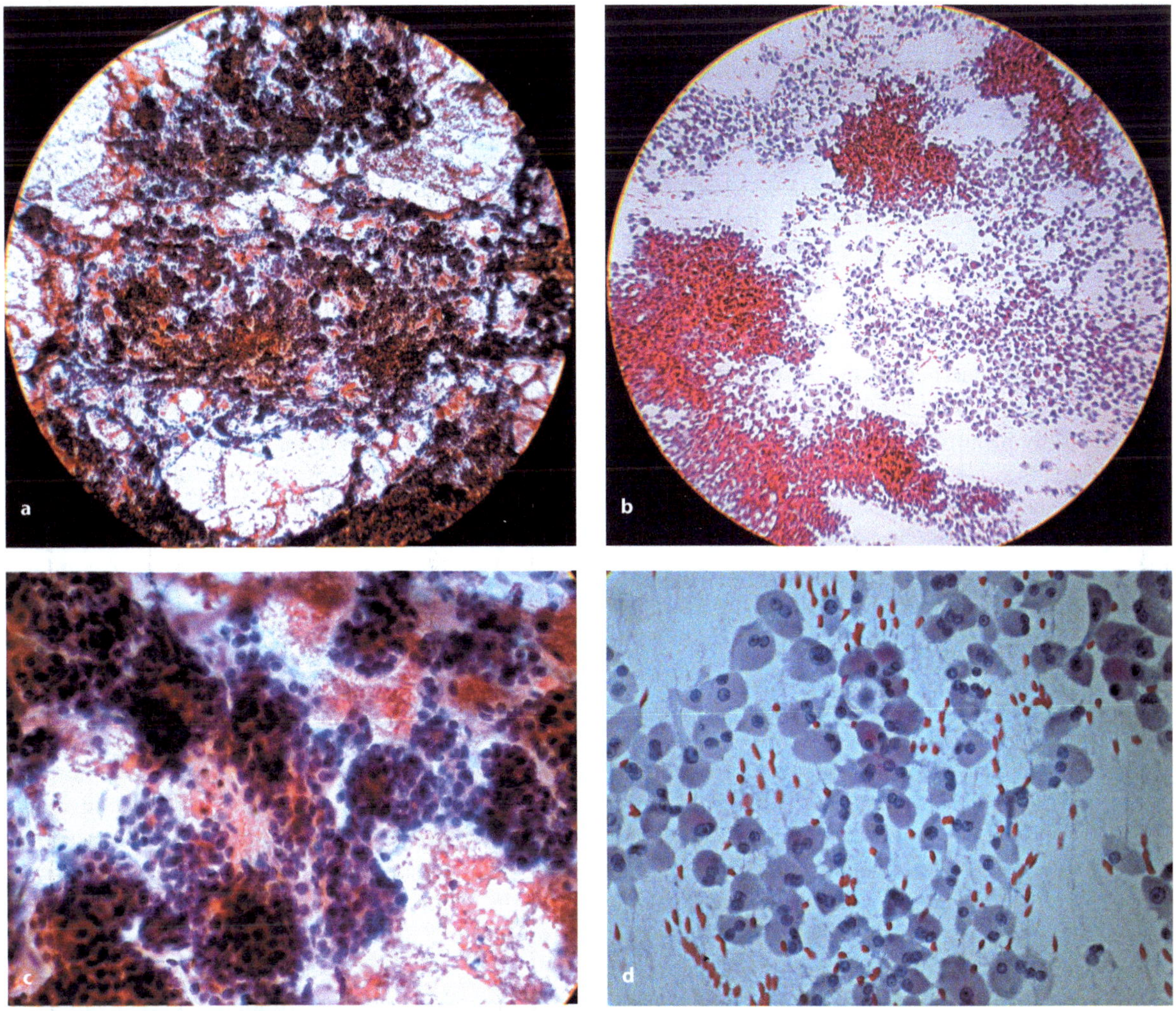

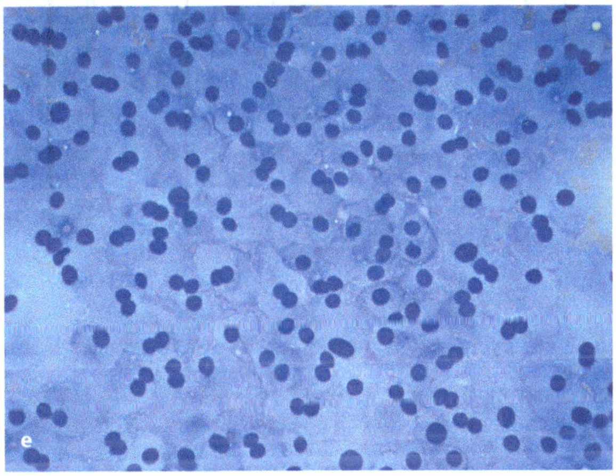

Fig. 3.18 **a** Low-magnification view of a smear containing abundant microfollicular aggregates. P stain, ×40. **b** Low-magnification view of a smear containing an abundant population of cohesive and non-cohesive Hürthle cells. P stain, ×40. **c** High-power view of three-dimensional microfollicular aggregates. P stain, ×400. **d** Hürthle cells may occasionally appear binucleated, with medium-sized nuclei and prominent nucleoli. P stain, ×400. **e** Appearance of Hürthle cells in May Grünwald Giemsa-stained smears, ×600

Table 3.2 Criteria to exclude the diagnosis of follicular proliferation/neoplasm

Nuclear polymorphism, with a significant component (>10%) of enlarged nuclei
Nuclear inclusions (pseudonucleoli) and nuclear clefts (even if only occasionally detected)
Polygonal or spindle cell morphology
Sparse cellularity

Loewagen et al. [54,55] first gave form to the definition of "follicular neoplasm" in the early 1960s, when the nuclear changes of papillary carcinoma had not been fully identified and follicular carcinoma was considered the most frequent malignancy of the thyroid. In the following decades, the follicular variant of papillary carcinoma became increasingly recognized and the incidence of follicular carcinoma dramatically decreased [56]. In addition, the minimally invasive and the widely invasive variants of follicular carcinoma were fully characterized and Hürthle cell neoplasms were included in the group of follicular neoplasms [21,22,53]. Despite these revolutionary changes, the concept of "follicular proliferation/neoplasm" still retains its validity in the practice of cytology because it identifies a group of lesions that should be considered as indeterminate for possible malignancy and inevitably require excisional biopsy for a conclusive diagnosis [8,10]. As already mentioned, the definition is also used for samples that are mostly or totally characterized by Hürthle cells, provided that no significant nuclear alteration is detected (nuclear clefts, chromatin clearing, nuclear inclusions, etc.), which would suggest papillary or medullary carcinoma. Finally, the term "follicular proliferation" should not be used for samples with a poor cellularity; instead, it is better to resort to the diagnosis of follicular lesion of indeterminate significance.

The positive predictive value of this diagnostic category is no higher than about 30%, i.e., only roughly one third of these lesions turn to be malignant upon histological evaluation of the surgically excised thyroid (Table 3.3) [10,57–63]. As noted in the Introduction, this represents the real gray zone of FNB of the thyroid and many efforts have been focused on the identification of possible concomitant ancillary criteria that decrease the level of indeterminacy. Surveys of large series have shown that, when the lesion is solitary and especially when abnormal echogenicity and echotexture are detected, the risk of malignancy in lesions diagnosed as follicular proliferation is higher in males and in adults older than 40 years of age [59,64]. Repeat biopsy in these patients is useful to better disclose a significant proportion of cases that actually are "suspicious for carcinoma" or even "diagnostic for carcinoma" [65]. Intraoperative frozen section examination of the nodule does not provide a significant increase in the positive predictive value unless a cytological examination of imprint smears is done [66]. Testing for cellular expression of galectin-3 has contributed to the detection of lesions at increased risk of being malignant. In histological specimens, positive galectin 3 immunostaining is found in 27–100% of cases but it is also detected in up to 45% of follicular adenomas and, albeit rarely, in nodular hyperplasia [67]. Immunostaining of cytological smears, however, is associated with a significant number of false-positive results and thus should be done only in cell-block material of needle-rinse samples or in paraffin sections from core biopsies [68,69]. Testing for the co-expression of CD44 is of help in identifying samples

Table 3.3 Cytohistological correlation for cases diagnosed as "follicular proliferation/neoplasm"

Bibliographic reference	Number of cases	Malignant (%)	Follicular carcinoma	Follicular variant/papillary carcinoma
[10]	122	36 (29.5)	11	25
[58]	219	26 (11.9)	19	7
[59]	888	103 (11.6)	76	27
[60]	84	19 (22.6)	8	11
[61]	96	28 (29.1)	6	22
[62]	120	21 (17.5)	9	12
[63]	147	23 (15.6)	15	8
[64]	201	51(25)	31	11

indicating truly malignant disease, thus increasing the specificity of the procedure [67]. Nowadays, molecular genetics offers a very promising tool to identify the malignant cases among the group diagnosed as follicular proliferation [70], but its application in the routine clinical context is not yet feasible.

3.8.3 Malignant Lesions

3.8.3.1 Papillary Carcinoma

The diagnosis of papillary carcinoma is based on the detection of several "major" and "minor" cytological features, listed in Table 3.4. The major features are pathognomonic criteria for papillary carcinoma and their detection is essential to the diagnosis, while the minor cytological features lack any diagnostic specificity but their detection can reinforce a diagnostic suspicion. All major criteria should be present together for a reliable diagnosis of papillary carcinoma but when one or more of them is lacking the detection of some minor criteria can help support the diagnosis of "suspicious for malignancy" (category 4 of the NCI, 2008 classification scheme).

Incomplete or complete *nuclear grooving* [71–75] is found in nuclei that have an ovoid shape and perhaps a thick nuclear membrane (Fig. 3.19a). The latter shows an irregular profile, being angulated or sometimes convoluted. Nuclei are >2×RBC in diameter. The chromatin is finely granular in texture, and nuclei contain multiple and eccentrically placed small nucleoli (best seen in Papanicolaou-stained smears) (Fig. 3.19b). *Pseudonucleoli* consist of intranuclear cytoplasmic inclusions delimited by a sharp, well-defined membrane [75–77]; they contain a cytoplasmic matrix that should look the same as that of the rest of the cytoplasm (Figs. 3.19a, 3.20). *Papillary fragments* are

Table 3.4 Major and minor diagnostic criteria for papillary carcinoma

Major criteria	Minor criteria
Incomplete or complete nuclear grooving in diffusely enlarged nuclei	Variability of cellular aggregation pattern
	Papillary fragments
Finely granular ("powdery") chromatin texture with multiple and eccentrically placed small nucleoli	Psammoma bodies
	Multinucleated cells
Pseudonucleoli	Squamoid appearance of cells
	Occasional "giant" nuclei
	Thick colloid

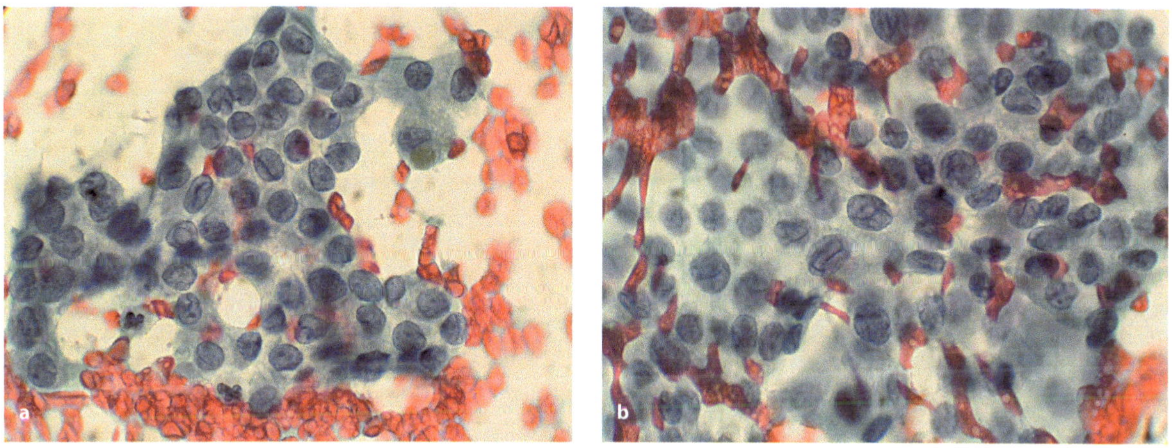

Fig. 3.19 a Complete and incomplete nuclear grooves are seen in the majority of cells as well as a single nuclear inclusion (pseudonucleolus). P stain, ×400. **b** At closer view, the irregular outlines of the nuclei are evident, and nuclei contain single or even double clefts. P stain, ×1000

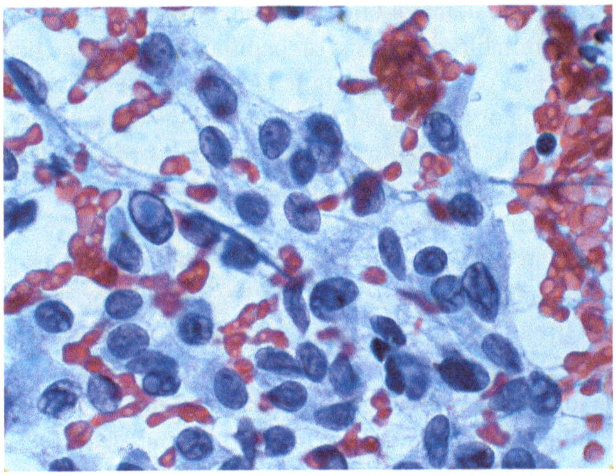

Fig. 3.20 Prominent nuclear inclusions are seen in several cells. P stain, ×1000

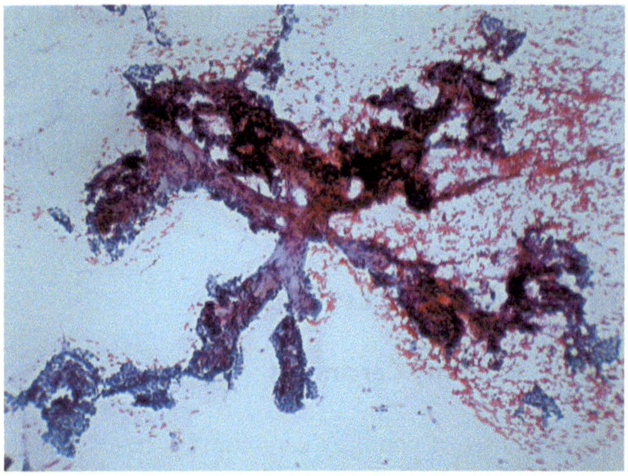

Fig. 3.21 A complex papillary aggregate with a connective-tissue stalk. P stain, ×100

detected in a minor proportion of cases [75,78] and they are pathognomonic of papillary carcinoma only if cells of the covering epithelium show the characteristic and above-described nuclear changes (Fig. 3.21). *Two-dimensional aggregates* are characteristic although not pathognomonic of papillary carcinoma and occur much more frequently than papillary fragments; due to their structure, they represent the site of choice for initially searching for the subtle nuclear changes of the tumor (Fig. 3.22) [71,75,78]. *Psammoma bodies* are not commonly encountered and by no means can be considered a specific feature of papillary carcinoma. Additional findings are occasional *giant nuclei* (their size reaching 3–5×RBC) within epithelial aggregates or in isolated elements (Fig. 3.23) and peculiar *multinucleated cells* (Fig. 3.24) similar to those found in some cases of active thyroiditis and in FNB samples of medullary carcinoma. Finally, a *squamoid appearance*, in which the cells have a peculiar polygonal or spindle-like shape, a densely hyperchromatic nucleus, as well as a homogeneous and eosinophilic cytoplasm with sharp cellular borders, is especially evident in two-dimensional aggregates (Fig. 3.25) [75].

The cytological picture is highly variable in terms of background features, cellularity, cellular aggregation pattern, and type of ancillary cell components. This variability reflects the diversity of histological variants of papillary carcinoma. Basically, two main variants are encountered in common daily practice, namely, the “usual” and the “follicular” variant.

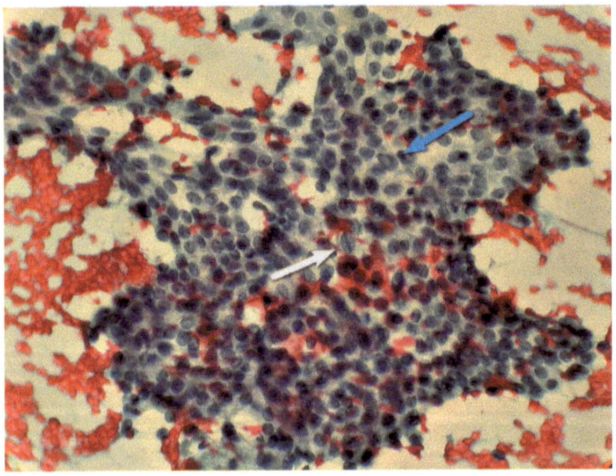

Fig. 3.22 A characteristic two-dimensional cellular aggregate containing nuclear grooves (*blue arrow*) and a nuclear inclusion (*white arrow*). P stain, ×400

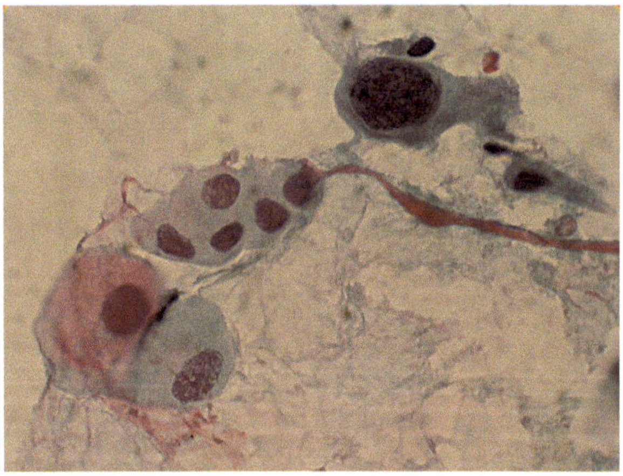

Fig. 3.23 Giant nuclei are found in some cells. P stain, ×1000

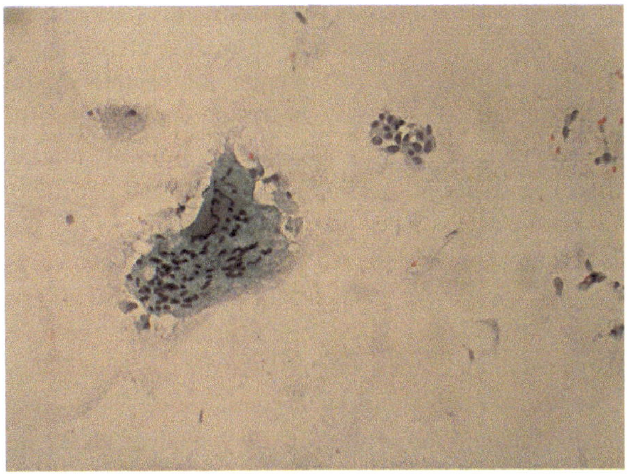

Fig. 3.24 A large multinucleated cell and an aggregate of elongated epithelioid cells are seen. P stain, ×400

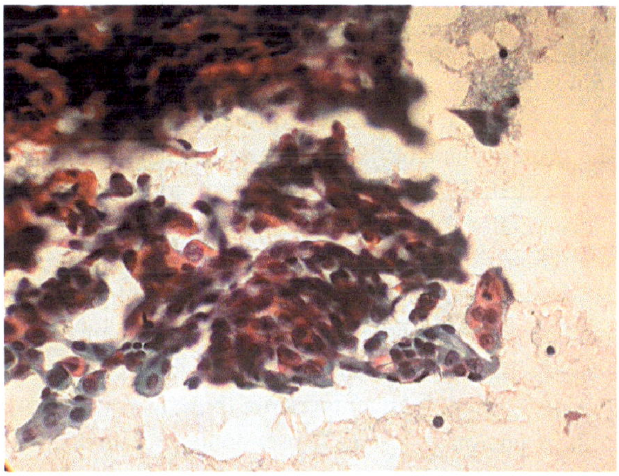

Fig. 3.25 Tumor cells sometimes appear elongated and with an eosinophilic cytoplasm, thus resembling squamous cells. P stain, ×400

Papillary Carcinoma, "Usual" Variant

- *Background:* blood and stromal fragments, sparse colloid, and deposits of "thick" colloid in the background, moderate to abundant cellularity.
- *Aggregation pattern:* variable (two-dimensional, follicular, three-dimensional) in different fields (Fig. 3.26).
- *Cells morphology:* polygonal to oval to round cells (best observed within two-dimensional aggregates) with pinkish (in smears stained using the May Grünwald Giemsa method) or gray-green (in Papanicolaou-stained smears) cytoplasm having a distinct external outline (Fig. 3.22).
- *Nuclear morphology:* enlarged nuclei (size >2×RBC), with a round to elongated shape and external-membrane thickening; also, partial or complete clefts, finely granular ("powdery") chromatin with small chromocenters, small and eccentrically placed nucleoli, single or multiple nuclear inclusions of variable size containing a matrix that shows the same tinctorial features as the cytoplasm (Figs. 3.19, 3.20).
- *Inconsistent features:* papillary aggregates (Fig. 3.21), psammoma bodies within the background or embedded within cellular aggregates, squamoid appearance of the cells (Fig. 3.25), multinucleated cells (Fig. 3.24), histiocytes containing hemosiderin pigment granules.

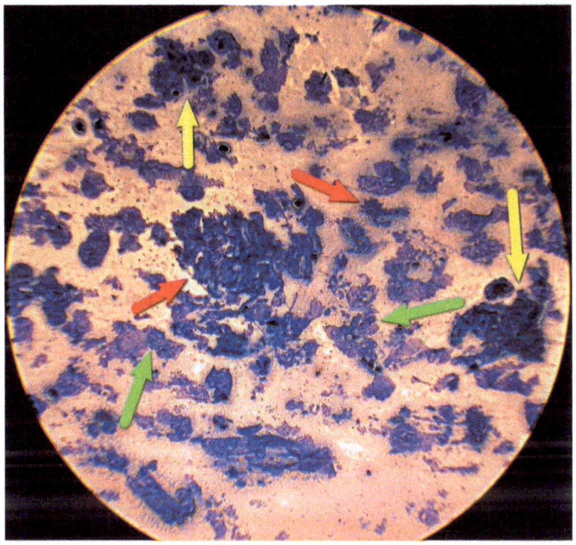

Fig. 3.26 A variable aggregation pattern is a characteristic and peculiar finding in FNB smears of papillary carcinoma. Some aggregates are three-dimensional and follicularly patterned (*yellow arrows*), while others have a papillary (*red arrows*) or two-dimensional (*green arrows*) configuration

The cytological diagnosis of the classical variant of papillary carcinoma is easily accomplished if the specific nuclear changes can be detected in a significant proportion of cells in adjunct to other features, including abundant cellularity with a significant component of two-dimensional cellular aggregates, the frequent squamoid appearance of the cells, as well as multinucleated cells and "thick" colloid in the background. The variability of the cytological picture reflects the intrinsic variability of the tumor itself in each case, since in the "usual" variant areas of classical papillary growth alternate with areas having either a solid, syncytial, or trabecular appearance or a minor component with a follicular pattern of growth.

An essential diagnostic requirement is detection of the nuclear changes that are specific to papillary carcinoma, listed in Table 3.3. These alterations can occasionally be seen also in benign conditions including diffuse hyperplasia (Graves' disease) and Hashimoto's thyroiditis [79,80]. A somewhat similar nuclear clearing can also result from a technical artifact, due to improper smearing, excessive dehydration before fixation, high temperature (bullous transformation of nuclei or "pseudo"-pseudonuclear inclusions) [79]. If technical artifacts can be ruled out, the detection of nuclear clefts and pseudoinclusions should be evaluated using a semi-quantitative approach. Yang and Demirci, 2003 [81], provided several key suggestions regarding the reading of these changes in FNB smears that have contributed significantly to increasing the reproducibility of interpretation among observers. The diagnostic algorithm is illustrated in Figure 3.27. Samples should be evaluated at high microscopic power in at least five representative fields, focusing attention on those areas where nuclear changes occur most frequently. Nuclear clefts are classified as occurring in >20%, in 10–19%, and in <10% of cells. In the first case, a concomitant detection of nuclear inclusions provides a reliable basis for a conclusive diagnosis of papillary carcinoma; the absence of inclusions justifies a more prudent diagnosis of "suspicious for carcinoma" (category 4, NCI, 2008). If the incidence of nuclear clefts ranges between 10 and 19% of the cells, the sample should be evaluated for the possible concomitant presence of nuclear inclusions and/or an extent of nuclear enlargement >2×RBC. Detection of the former definitely favors the diagnosis of papillary carcinoma. If nuclear inclusions are not detected but nuclear enlargement is evident, a clear-cut suspicion of carcinoma should be recorded (category 4, NCI, 2008). The lack of both these ancillary criteria supports the diagnosis of follicular lesion of indeterminate significance. This diagnostic formulation is to be used if nuclear clefts are detected in <10% of cells. Finally, nuclear inclusions may happen to be detected in the absence of nuclear clefts: this may reflect incomplete sampling of a papillary carcinoma, or a diagnosis of either hyalinizing trabecular adenoma or medullary carcinoma. Basically, if no other hints to a specific diagnosis are available, then the cytological picture is inconclusive and should prompt a repeat biopsy. Yang and Demirci, 2003 [81], showed that the detection of nuclear clefts in amounts >20% and between 10 and 19% occurred, respectively, in 65 and 35% of their cases of papillary carcinoma. No malignant case fell into the category of samples showing nuclear clefts in a proportion <10% of cells. It was therefore concluded that the detection of nuclear clefts in a proportion of cells >20% bears a 65% positive predictive value for papillary carcinoma.

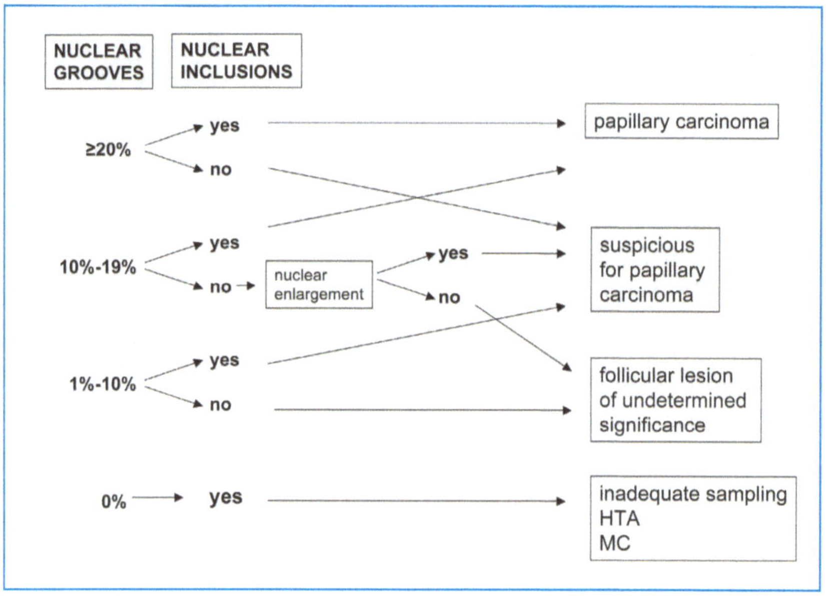

Fig. 3.27 Suggested decision tree based on the amount of nuclear grooves and the presence nuclear inclusions in FNB smears of papillary carcinoma. Adapted from Yang and Demirci, 2003 [81]. *HTA*, hyalinizing trabecular adenoma; *MC*, medullary carcinoma

Follicular Variant of Papillary Carcinoma

- *Background:* blood and stromal fragments, with no colloid (or accumulations of "thick" colloid inconsistently found).
- *Cellularity:* moderate to abundant.
- *Aggregation pattern:* branching two-to three-dimensional microfollicular aggregates (Fig. 3.28a,b) possibly containing a basophilic "colloid ball" (Fig. 3.28c), three-dimensional follicularly patterned clusters highly similar to what is seen in follicular proliferation/neoplasm, or dissociated microfollicles (Fig. 3.28d).
- *Cellular features:* cell size larger than that of normal follicular cells, with a round to oval shape and a small amount of cytoplasm.
- *Nuclear features:* enlarged and elongated nuclei (>2×RBC), with clear chromatin and a thick nuclear membrane as a common but inconsistent feature (Fig. 3.29a); nuclear clefts and nuclear inclusions only in about two-thirds and one-third of cases, respectively (Fig. 3.29b).

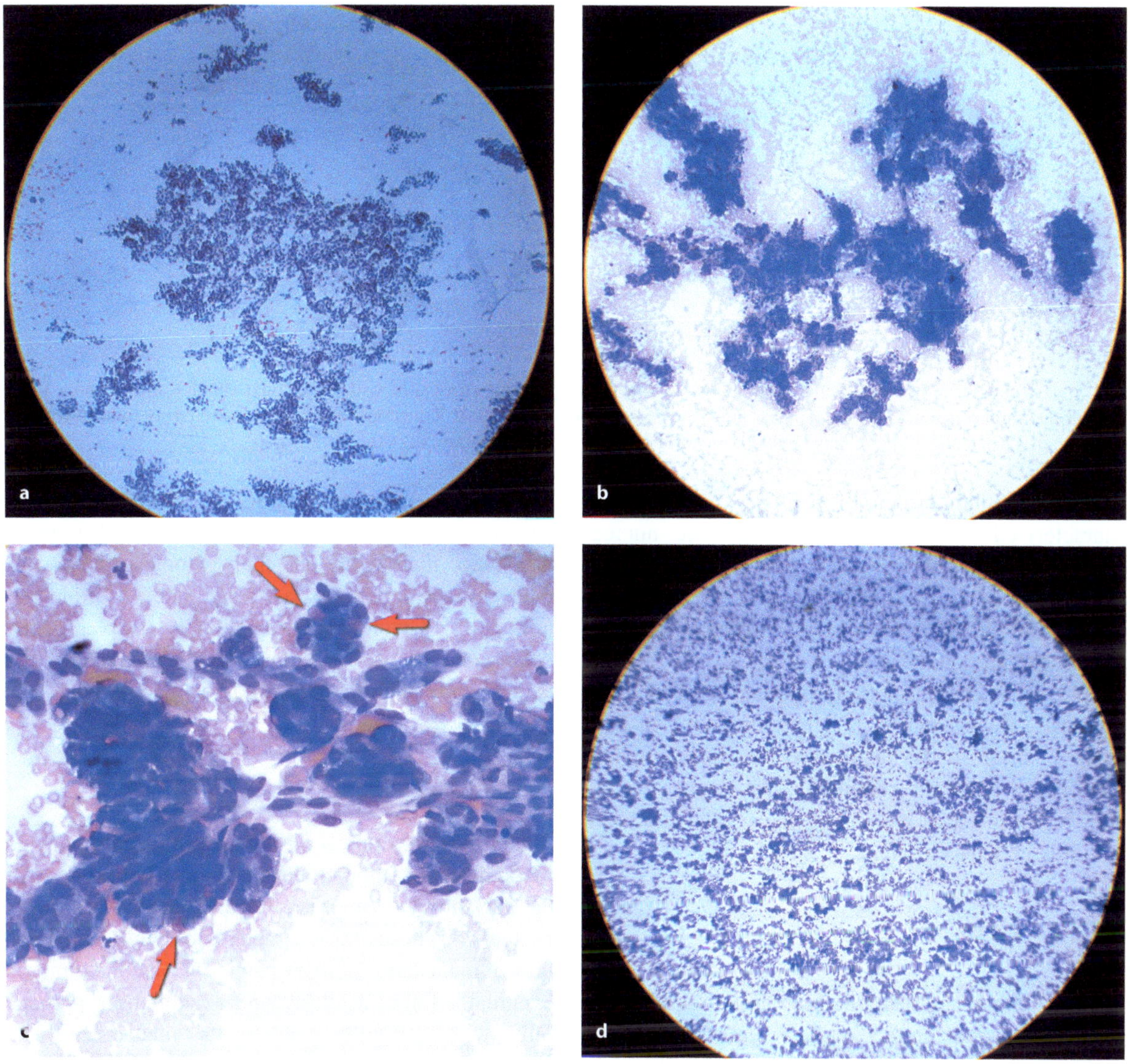

Fig. 3.28 **a** Aggregate with a two-dimensional follicular configuration. May Grünwald Giemsa stain, ×200. **b** Aggregate with a three-dimensional follicular configuration. May Grünwald Giemsa stain, ×200. **c** Some microfollicular structures contain basophilic colloid "balls" (*arrows*). May Grünwald Giemsa stain, ×480. **d** Low-power view of a FNB smear showing a myriad of dissociated microfollicular structures or single cells, ×200. May Grünwald Giemsa stain, ×40

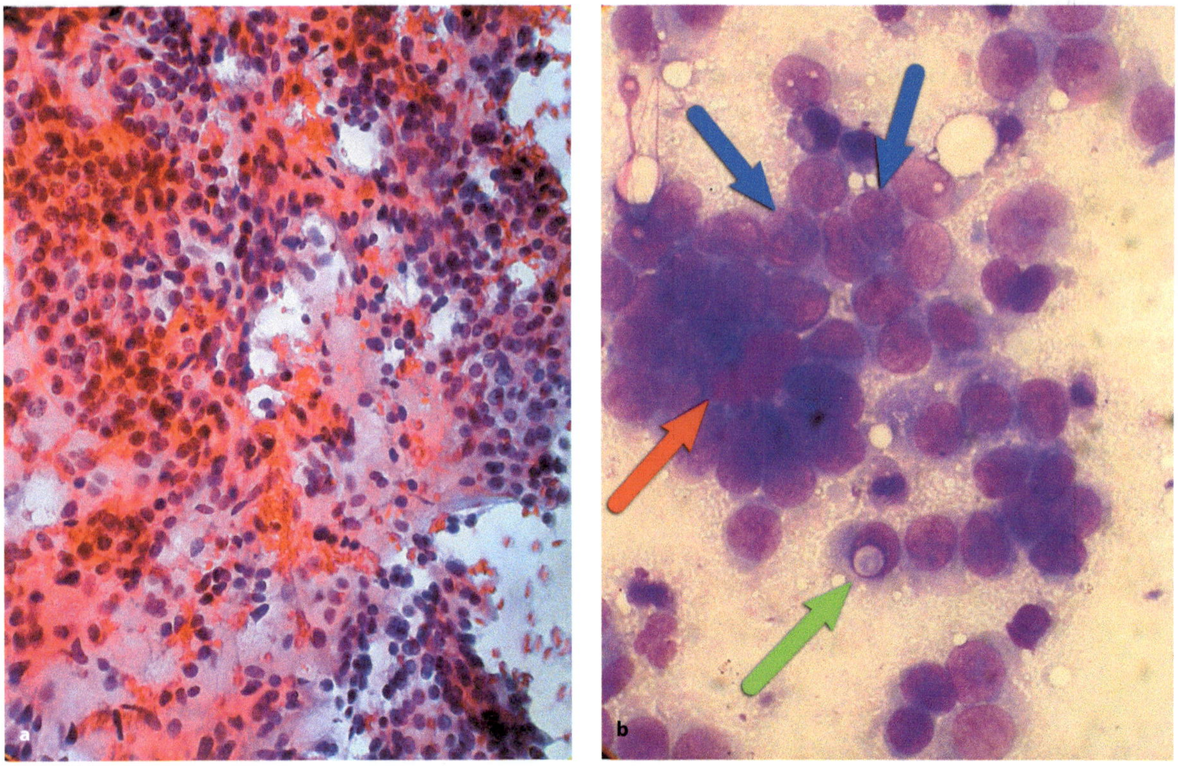

Fig. 3.29 **a** Nuclei in microfollicular aggregates show a finely granular chromatin with occasional small nucleoli and a thick nuclear membrane. P stain, ×800. **b** Nuclear grooves (*blue arrows*) and nuclear inclusions (*green arrow*) are rarely found. Note the presence of a basophilic colloid "ball" (*red arrow*). May Grünwald Giemsa stain, ×2000

The follicular variant of papillary carcinoma is characterized by a scarcity of diagnostic nuclear changes and a particular cell pattern of follicular aggregation of the cells [82–87]. Both these features can prevent the tumor from being correctly diagnosed and instead interpreted as a follicular lesion of indeterminate significance or as a follicular proliferation/neoplasm. Repeat biopsy is generally useful in these cases to disclose the distinctive diagnostic nuclear features of papillary carcinoma, which are usually unevenly distributed within the smear and better seen in highly cellular samples.

Rare Variants

Papillary carcinoma has a highly variable histopathological appearance; in fact, while several variants have been reported their cytopathological appearance is poorly described in the medical literature due to the rarity of the cases and the correspondingly limited number of reports. The only two variants that need to be mentioned here are the tall cell and the columnar cell types. FNB samples from tumors of the *tall cell variant* comprise a population of cells whose length is more than twice their width and their cytoplasm may stain intensely eosinophilic so as to simulate a Hürthle cell tumor [88]. Cytological evaluation of samples of the *columnar cell variant* shows highly elongated cells lacking any oxyphilic changes of the cytoplasm [89].

The Clinically Occult Papillary Carcinoma

Sometimes, the clinical onset of papillary carcinoma is marked by the enlargement of a single lymph node in the neck and the tumor is clinically occult. FNB unexpectedly discloses the characteristic cytological findings of metastatic papillary carcinoma and the tumor is eventually found at ultrasound examination, perhaps only with difficulty due to its small size. The metastatic lymph node can also appear as a cystic lesion and the patient generally reports a rapid enlargement of the lesion [90,91]. These "cysts" are often located in sites that would be atypical for lateral branchial cleft cysts and should raise a high index of clinical suspicion. It is important to remember that cytological evaluation of the cystic content may often show only a meager cellular content consisting of histiocytes and cytoplasmic debris. The patient should be asked to present for a repeat aspiration if the lesion reappears, which generally occurs within hours to a few days after the first evacuation of the cyst. The second aspiration inevitably provides an abundant cellular sample and the definitive diagnosis of cystic metastasis of papillary carcinoma is easily obtained.

3.8.3.2 Poorly Differentiated Follicular ("Insular") Carcinoma

- *Background:* blood and stromal fragments, no colloid, with possible necrotic debris.
- *Cellularity:* moderate to abundant (Fig. 3.30a).
- *Cell types present:* follicular thyrocytes with enlarged nuclei, a coarsely granular chromatin with occasional prominent nucleoli, no clefts or pseudonucleoli, and sparse or barely discernible cytoplasm (Fig. 3.30b), and possibly histiocytes with hemosiderin granules or a foamy cytoplasm.
- *Aggregation pattern:* microfollicular structures with a great tendency to cellular non-cohesion.

Poorly differentiated follicular carcinoma can occur as a single nodular tumefaction or as a diffuse enlargement of an entire thyroid lobe. Patients tend to be elderly and they report a rapid enlargement of the lesion. The diagnosis of malignancy is straightforward due to the lesion's high cellularity and cellular atypia. The most prominent finding is the great tendency of cells to non-cohesion [92].

3.8.3.3 Poorly Differentiated Hürthle Cell Carcinoma

- *Background:* blood and stromal fragments, no colloid with possible necrotic debris.
- *Cellularity:* moderate to abundant.

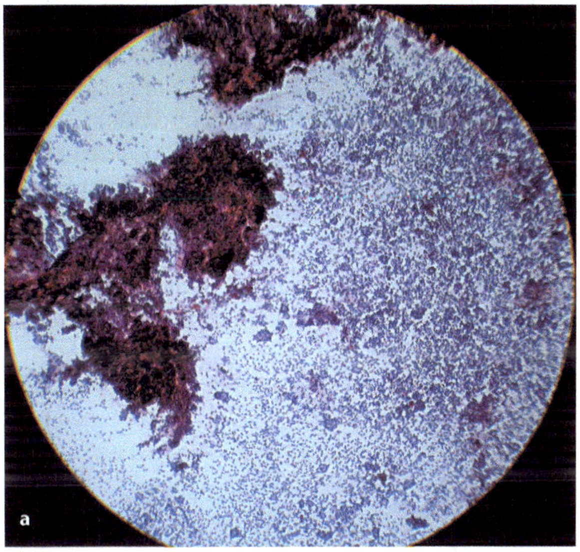
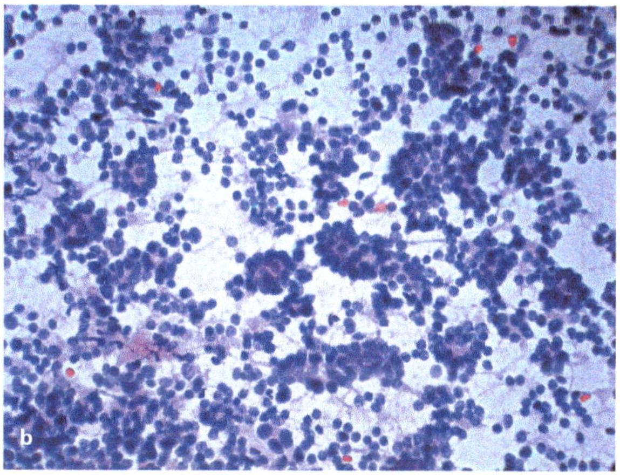
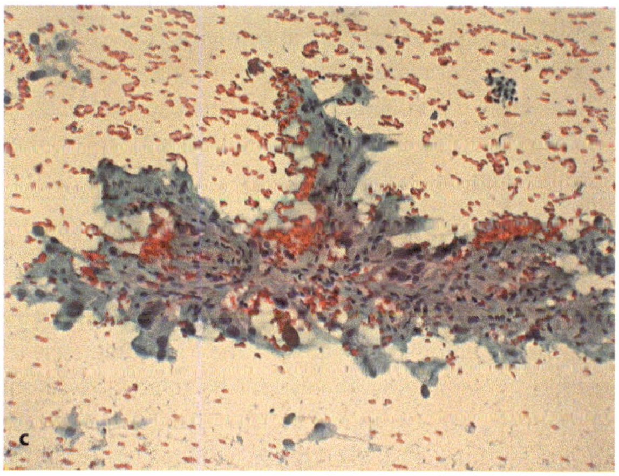

Fig. 3.30 **a** Low-power view showing abundant cellularity in the FNB sample; cells are detected in follicular aggregates or as isolated single elements. P stain, ×200. **b** High power view showing medium-sized cells characterized by round nuclei containing a coarsely granular chromatin and little or barely discernible cytoplasm. P stain, ×400. **c** A stromal fragment with entrapped large and pleomorphic Hürthle cells characterized by abundant cytoplasm, a large nucleus, and sometimes a large prominent nucleolus. Compare the size of these cells with that of normal thyrocytes seen in the upper right portion of the image. P stain, ×400

- *Cell types present:* large and pleomorphic Hürthle cells with abundant cytoplasm, a large nucleus with a coarsely granular cytoplasm, and a large prominent nucleolus (Fig. 3.30c).
- *Aggregation pattern:* syncytial-like three-dimensional aggregates or non-cohesive cells.

Poorly differentiated Hürthle cell carcinoma is a rare and rather aggressive malignancy occurring in adults in middle age and in the elderly [31]. The most prominent finding in FNB smears is a great pleomorphism of tumor cells [93]. The differential diagnosis includes medullary carcinoma and anaplastic cell carcinoma (see below).

3.8.3.4 Medullary Carcinoma

- *Background features:* blood with no colloid and few if any histiocytes; occasionally with eosinophilic ground substance (amyloid).
- *Cellularity:* moderate to abundant.
- *Aggregation pattern:* great tendency to cellular dissociation, with the detection of clusters of few cells.
- *Cell features:* intermediate to large size, round, oval, or elongated to spindled shape with marked cellular pleomorphism (Fig. 3.31a); green or grayish, granular cytoplasm in Papanicolaou-stained preparations (Fig. 3.31b), blue to metachromatic in smears stained with the May Grünwald Giemsa method (Fig. 3.31c) with possible detection of intensely red ("magenta") granules (Fig. 3.31d).
- *Nuclei:* round (Fig. 3.31c,e) to elongated (Fig. 3.31a), centrally or eccentrically placed, in the latter case giving the cell a plasmacytoid appearance (Fig. 3.31a, arrow); finely granular chromatin with a "salt and pepper" appearance (Fig. 3.31e) or coarsely granular with occasional prominent nucleoli; pseudonucleoli (i.e., nuclear cytoplasmic inclusions) as a frequent finding (Fig. 3.31c) but rare or absent nuclear grooves.

The cytomorphology of medullary carcinoma in FNB smears is variable [94–96] and reflects the diverse histopathological appearance of this tumor in surgical pathology. As a caveat, the FNB diagnosis of medullary carcinoma should not be released without laboratory confirmation of an increased calcitonin titer in the serum. The differential diagnosis includes Hürthle cell tumors (which show a higher degree of atypia and a homogeneous, not granular, cytoplasm), some papillary carcinoma variants (which show abundant nuclear grooves and few or any nuclear inclusions), metastatic neuroendocrine carcinoma, and intrathyroid parathyroid tumors. Since the latter may be indistinguishable from medullary carcinoma (see below), the distinction is based on proper correlation with clinical findings as well as imaging and laboratory data.

3.8.3.5 Anaplastic Carcinoma

- *Background:* necrotic cellular debris, with inflammatory cells (possibility of an "abscess-like" sample), and stromal fragments.
- *Cellularity:* variable in amount, with possible acellular samples.
- *Cell features:* intermediate to large size, epithelioid, spindled, or bizarre shape (Fig. 3.32a,b) and bright eosinophilic squamoid cytoplasm (squamous-cell-like variant, Fig. 3.32c) or clear cytoplasm with possible lymphophagocytosis ("emperipolesis"), possibility of a biphasic population of spindle cells and giant multinucleated cells (Fig. 3.32d).
- *Nuclei:* large size with possible bizarre shape, large and prominent nucleoli, multinucleation (Fig. 3.32a–d).

The diagnosis of anaplastic carcinoma is easy when highly pleomorphic and bizarre cells are observed in the smear [41–97], but in about half the cases the sample can be completely acellular or necrotic, with sparse inflammatory cells, thus preventing a conclusive diagnosis. Such samples are due to the extensive fibrosis or the necrosis and inflammation that can occur within the tumor as a consequence of its active growth. The patient frequently reports a rapidly enlarging tumor mass, and a stone-hard neck mass is palpated. If the sample is indeed necrotic or "abscess-like," the differential diagnosis should include suppurative thyroiditis or necrotic de Quervain's thyroiditis. However, since these disease entities are not likely to cause the dramatic symptomatology, then, especially when the clinical evidence is contradictory, a repeat FNB sampling of the tumor should be done to acquire a more representative cellular yield. A repeat biopsy commonly allows proper documentation of the

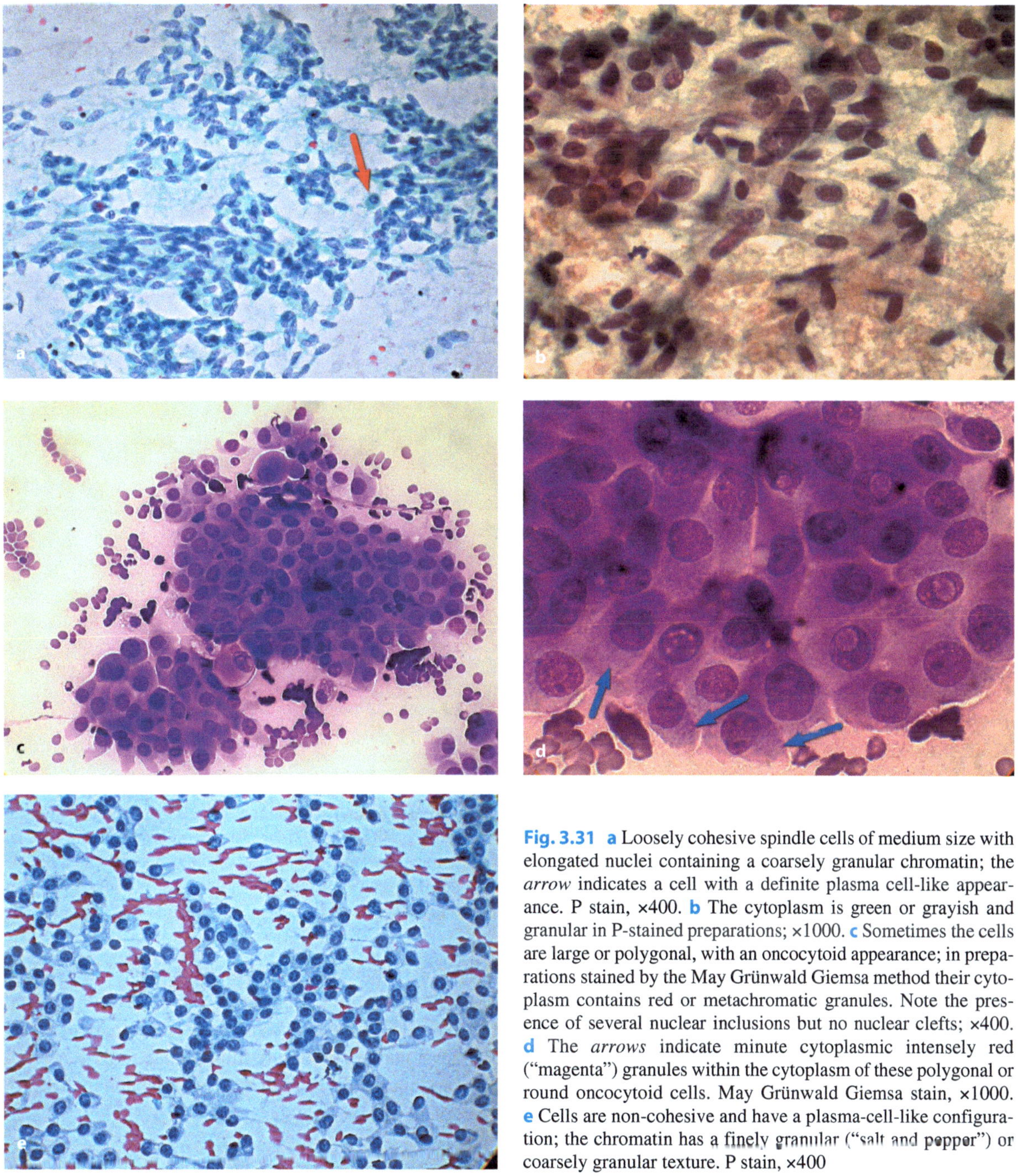

Fig. 3.31 a Loosely cohesive spindle cells of medium size with elongated nuclei containing a coarsely granular chromatin; the *arrow* indicates a cell with a definite plasma cell-like appearance. P stain, ×400. b The cytoplasm is green or grayish and granular in P-stained preparations; ×1000. c Sometimes the cells are large or polygonal, with an oncocytoid appearance; in preparations stained by the May Grünwald Giemsa method their cytoplasm contains red or metachromatic granules. Note the presence of several nuclear inclusions but no nuclear clefts; ×400. d The *arrows* indicate minute cytoplasmic intensely red ("magenta") granules within the cytoplasm of these polygonal or round oncocytoid cells. May Grünwald Giemsa stain, ×1000. e Cells are non-cohesive and have a plasma-cell-like configuration; the chromatin has a finely granular ("salt and pepper") or coarsely granular texture. P stain, ×400

diagnosis, which is of paramount importance in these patients to permit palliative treatment without surgical intervention. The differential diagnosis of anaplastic carcinoma from the FNB sample should always include intrathyroid metastatic malignancies, i.e., carcinomas primary in the lung and pancreas (large-cell anaplastic variants), the kidney (clear-cell variants), or the aerodigestive tract (squamous-cell-like variants), and amelanotic malignant melanoma. The clinical onset of anaplastic carcinoma of the thyroid can be also characterized by the appearance of a metastatic tumor mass in the viscera (especially lung and liver) or bone, thus simulating a tumor primary in these sites.

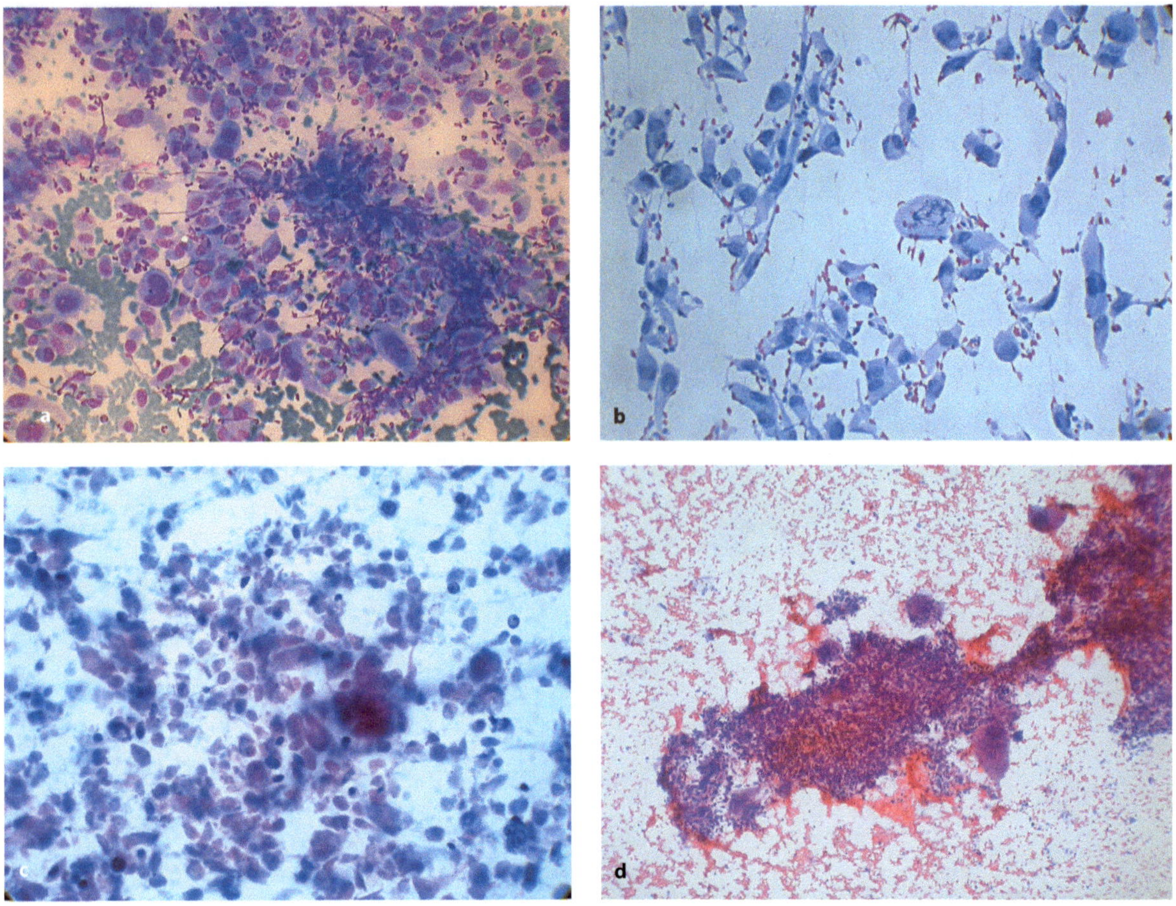

Fig. 3.32 **a** Large polygonal or elongated cells with pleomorphic nuclei are a characteristic finding in FNB samples of anaplastic thyroid carcinoma. May Grünwald Giemsa stain, ×400. **b** Large elongated to spindle cells with occasional multinucleation; note an atypical mitotic figure in one of the elements. P stain, ×400. **c** Cells sometimes have an eosinophilic cytoplasm and contain hyperchromatic nuclei, thus resembling atypical squamous cells. Coagulative necrosis is also prominent in this field. P stain, ×400. **d** A biphasic population of spindle cells and giant multinucleated cells. P stain, ×200

3.8.3.6 Intrathyroid Parathyroid Tumors

- *Background features:* blood with an amorphous proteinaceous ground substance (no colloid and few, if any, histiocytes).
- *Cellularity:* moderate to abundant (Fig. 3.33a).
- *Aggregation pattern:* variable, with large, tight three-dimensional clusters, sheets, and syncytia, trabeculae, rare microfollicles (Fig. 3.33a,b), and a strong tendency to cellular dissociation, resulting in bare nuclei (Fig. 3.33b).
- *Cell features:* mostly medium sized cells, round to oval to polygonal in shape; occasionally elongated and somewhat spindle-shaped; abundant eosinophilic but also amphophilic and clear cytoplasm (Fig. 3.33b).
- *Nuclei:* generally round in shape with slight pleomorphism; sometimes eccentrically placed (Fig. 3.33b), finely granular chromatin with small occasional nucleoli, rare multinucleation, occasional pseudonucleoli (intranuclear cytoplasmic inclusion), nuclear grooves always absent (Fig. 3.33c).

On FNB cytology, intrathyroid parathyroid lesions may be confused with several cytomorphological look-alikes of thyroid neoplasms [98–101], thus posing true diagnostic challenges especially in the absence of overt hyperparathyroidism. The differential diagnosis includes medullary carcinoma, and Hürthle cell or follicular cell tumors. Careful evaluation of the cell size, the complexity of the cellular arrangement, with a rich capillary component and abundant monomorphic

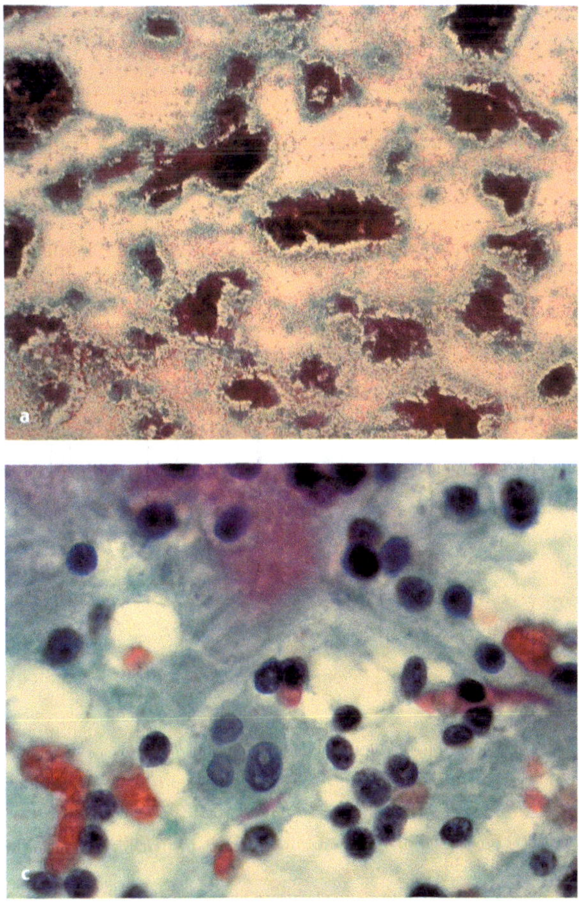

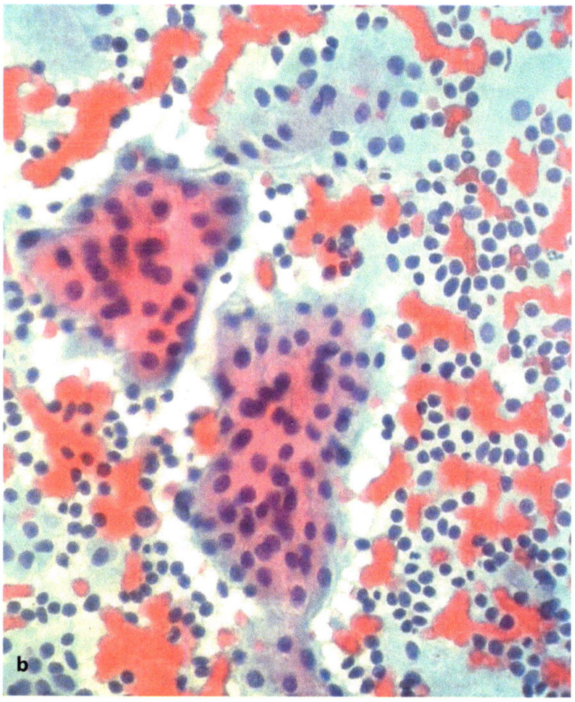

Fig. 3.33 **a** Abundant cellularity consisting of cohesive cells in three-dimensional clusters or non-cohesive cells. P stain, ×100. **b** Cells are medium-sized and round to polygonal in shape. They have an abundant cytoplasm which may look eosinophilic or clear; round bare nuclei are abundant in the background. P stain, ×450. **c** Distinct nuclear vacuoles are sometimes seen in parathyroid tumor cells. P stain, ×1000

bare nuclei, and the concomitant presence of oncocytoid and clear cells can help exclude the possibility of the above-listed tumor entities. Nonetheless, a prudent correlation with clinical findings, in particular increased titers of parathyroid hormone in the serum and hypercalcemia, is sometimes the only basis for a conclusive diagnosis. FNB cytological findings cannot provide any conclusive preoperative data regarding the lesion's malignant behavior since the distinction of benign lesions of the parathyroid from those that are well-differentiated carcinoma is practically impossible.

3.8.3.7 Metastatic Malignancies and Malignant Lymphoma

The thyroid, as already mentioned, may be the site of involvement of epithelial malignancies that originate in various primary sites (mainly the lower respiratory tract and kidney); this generally happens in the setting of widespread metastatic dissemination. Indeed, the tumor that most commonly involves the thyroid even at an early stage of the disease is malignant melanoma [31], including of the uveal tract [102]. The main differential diagnoses in FNB thyroid samples are medullary carcinoma and anaplastic carcinoma, especially the spindle and epithelioid cell variants. Due to the protean morphology of melanoma cells, the correct diagnosis can be difficult to achieve, especially when careful inspection of the FNB sample fails to demonstrate melanin granules in the cytoplasm. Malignant lymphoma primarily involving the thyroid generally manifests as a high-grade tumor composed of large cells. The FNB sample is characterized by the presence of lymphoglandular bodies in the background and the lack of thyroid follicular cells.

References

1. Mazeh H, Beglaibter N, Prus D et al (2007) Cytohistologic correlation of thyroid nodules. Am J Surg 194:161–163.
2. Ogilvie JB, Piatigorsky EJ, Clark OH (2006) Current status of fine needle aspiration for thyroid nodules. Adv Surg 40:223–238.
3. Smith J, Cheifetz RE, Schneidereit N et al (2005) Can cytology accurately predict benign follicular nodules? Am J Surg 189:592–595.
4. Morgan JL, Serpell JW, Cheng MS (2003) Fine-needle aspiration cytology of thyroid nodules: how useful is it? ANZ J Surg 73:480–483.
5. Cheung YS, Poon CM, Mak SM et al (2007) Fine-needle aspiration cytology of thyroid nodules—how well are we doing? Hong Kong Med J 13:12–15.
6. Bajaj Y, De M, Thompson A (2006) Fine needle aspiration cytology in diagnosis and management of thyroid disease. J Laryngol Otol 120:467–479.
7. Cáp J, Ryska A, Rehorková P et al (1999) Sensitivity and specificity of the fine needle aspiration biopsy of the thyroid: clinical point of view. Clin Endocrinol (Oxf) 51:509–515.
8. Leonard N, Melcher DH (1997) To operate or not to operate? The value of fine needle aspiration cytology in the assessment of thyroid swellings. J Clin Pathol 50:941–943.
9. Sclabas GM, Staerkel GA, Shapiro Seet al (2003) Fine-needle aspiration of the thyroid and correlation with histopathology in a contemporary series of 240 patients. Am J Surg 186:702–709.
10. Baloch ZW, Fleisher S, LiVolsi VA, Gupta PK (2002) Diagnosis of "follicular neoplasm": a gray zone in thyroid fine-needle aspiration cytology. Diagn Cytopathol 26:41–44.
11. Kim ES, Nam-Goong IS, Gong G et al (2003) Postoperative findings and risk for malignancy in thyroid nodules with cytological diagnosis of the so-called "follicular neoplasm". Korean J Intern Med 18:94–97.
12. Sahin M, Gursoy A, Tutuncu NB, Guvener DN (2006) Prevalence and prediction of malignancy in cytologically indeterminate thyroid nodules. Clin Endocrinol (Oxf) 65:514–518.
13. Miller B, Burkey S, Lindberg G et al (2004) Prevalence of malignancy within cytologically indeterminate thyroid nodules. Am J Surg 188:459–462.
14. Cibas ES, Alexander EK, Benson CB et al (2008) Indications for thyroid FNA and pre-FNA requirements: a synopsis of the National Cancer Institute Thyroid Fine-Needle Aspiration State of the Science Conference. Diagn Cytopathol 36:390–399.
15. Pitman MB, Abele J, Ali SZ et al (2008) Techniques for thyroid FNA: a synopsis of the National Cancer Institute Thyroid Fine-Needle Aspiration State of the Science Conference. Diagn Cytopathol 36:407–424.
16. Rosai J (2004) Thyroid gland. In: Rosai and Ackerman's Surgical Pathology. Mosby, Edinburgh, pp 515–594.
17. Hedinger C, Williams ED, Sobin LH (1988) Histological typing of thyroid tumors. WHO international histological classification of tumors, 2nd Ed. Springer-Verlag, Berlin.
18. Carcangiu ML, Zampi G, Pupi A et al (1985) Papillary carcinoma of the thyroid. A clinicopathologic study of 241 cases treated at the University of Florence, Italy. Cancer 55:805–828.
19. Chan JK (1990). Papillary carcinoma of thyroid: classical and variants. Histol Histopathol 5:241–257.
20. Shaha AR, Shah JP, Loree TR (1997) Differentiated thyroid cancer presenting initially with distant metastasis. Am J Surg 174:474–476.
21. van Heerden JA, Hay ID, Goellner JR et al (1992) Follicular thyroid carcinoma with capsular invasion alone: a nonthreatening malignancy. Surgery 112:1130–1136.
22. Thompson LD, Wieneke JA, Paal E et al (2001) A clinicopathologic study of minimally invasive follicular carcinoma of the thyroid gland with a review of the English literature. Cancer 91:505–524.
23. Lang W, Choritz H, Hundeshagen H (1986) Risk factors in follicular thyroid carcinomas. A retrospective follow-up study covering a 14-year period with emphasis on morphological findings. Am J Surg Pathol 10:246–255.
24. Gosain AK, Clark OH (1984) Hürthle cell neoplasms. Malignant potential. Arch Surg 119:515–519.
25. Bronner MP, LiVolsi VA (1988) Oxyphilic (Askanazy/Hürthle cell) tumors of the thyroid: microscopic features predict biologic behavior. Surg Pathol 1:137–150.
26. Collini P, Sampietro G, Pilotti S (2004) Extensive vascular invasion is a marker of risk of relapse in encapsulated non-Hürthle cell follicular carcinoma of the thyroid gland: a clinicopathological study of 18 consecutive cases from a single institution with a 11-year median follow-up. Histopathology 44:35–39.
27. Williams ED (1966) Histogenesis of medullary carcinoma of the thyroid. J Clin Pathol 19:114–118.
28. Saad MF, Ordonez NG, Rashid RK et al (1984) Medullary carcinoma of the thyroid. A study of the clinical features and prognostic factors in 161 patients. Medicine (Baltimore) 63:319–342.
29. Pilotti S, Collini P, Mariani L et al (1997). Insular carcinoma: a distinct de novo entity among follicular carcinomas of the thyroid gland. Am J Surg Pathol 21:1466–1473.
30. Volante M, Collini P, Nikiforov YE et al (2007) Poorly differentiated thyroid carcinoma: the Turin proposal for the use of uniform diagnostic criteria and an algorithmic diagnostic approach. Am J Surg Pathol 31:1256–1264.
31. Baloch ZW, LiVolsi VA (2008) Unusual tumors of the thyroid gland. Endocrinol Metab Clin North Am 37:297–310.
32. Rosai J, Saxén EA, Woolner L (1985) Undifferentiated and poorly differentiated carcinoma. Semin Diagn Pathol 2:123–136.
33. Tan RK, Finley RK 3rd (1995). Anaplastic carcinoma of the thyroid: a 24-year experience. Head Neck 17:41–47.
34. Aldinger KA, Samaan NA, Ibanez M, Hill CS Jr (1978) Anaplastic carcinoma of the thyroid: a review of 84 cases of spindle and giant cell carcinoma of the thyroid. Cancer 41:2267–2275.
35. Rosai J (1996) Parathyroid glands. In: Ackerman's Surgical Pathology. Mosby, St Louis, pp 577–578.
36. Kirsten LJ, Ghosh BL (2001) Intrathyroidal parathyroid carcinoma. J Surg Oncol 77:136–138.
37. Rosai J (2003) Immunohistochemical markers of thyroid tumors: significance and diagnostic applications. Tumori 89:517–519.
38. Fischer S, Asa SL (2008) Application of immunohistochemistry to thyroid neoplasms. Arch Pathol Lab Med 132:359–372.

39. Redman R, Zalaznick H, Mazzaferri EL, Massoll NA (2006). The impact of assessing specimen adequacy and number of needle passes for fine-needle aspiration biopsy of thyroid nodules. Thyroid 16:55–60.
40. Goellner JR, Gharib H, Grant CS, Johnson DA (1987) Fine needle aspiration cytology of the thyroid, 1980 to 1986. Acta Cytol 31:587–590.
41. Kini SR (1987) Guides to clinical aspiration biopsy – Thyroid. Igaku Shoin, New York, pp 307–314.
42. Kelly NP, Lim JC, DeJong S et al (2006). Specimen adequacy and diagnostic specificity of ultrasound-guided fine needle aspirations of nonpalpable thyroid nodules. Diagn Cytopathol 34:188–190.
43. Nguyen GK, Ginsberg J, Crockford PM (1991) Fine-needle aspiration biopsy cytology of the thyroid. Its value and limitations in the diagnosis and management of solitary thyroid nodules. Pathol Annu 26 Pt 1:63–91.
44. Guidelines of the Papanicolaou Society of Cytopathology for the Examination of Fine-Needle Aspiration Specimens from Thyroid Nodules (1996). The Papanicolaou Society of Cytopathology Task Force on Standards of Practice. Mod Pathol 9:710–715.
45. Jing X, Michael CW, Pu RT (2008) The clinical and diagnostic impact of using standard criteria of adequacy assessment and diagnostic terminology on thyroid nodule fine needle aspiration. Diagn Cytopathol 36:161–166.
46. Wang HH (2006) Reporting thyroid fine-needle aspiration: literature review and a proposal. Diagn Cytopathol 34:67–76.
47. Redman R, Yoder BJ, Massoll NA (2006) Perceptions of diagnostic terminology and cytopathologic reporting of fine-needle aspiration biopsies of thyroid nodules: a survey of clinicians and pathologists. Thyroid 16: 1003–1008.
48. Baloch ZW, LiVolsi VA, Asa SL et al (2008) Diagnostic terminology and morphologic criteria for cytologic diagnosis of thyroid lesions: a synopsis of the National Cancer Institute Thyroid Fine-Needle Aspiration State of the Science Conference. Diagn Cytopathol 36: 425–437.
49. Baloch ZW, Cibas ES, Clark DP et al (2008) The National Cancer Institute Thyroid fine needle aspiration state of the science conference: A summation. CytoJournal 5:6.
50. Nassar A, Gupta P, LiVolsi VA, Baloch Z (2003) Histiocytic aggregates in benign nodular goiters mimicking cytologic features of papillary thyroid carcinoma. Diagn Cytopathol 29:243–245.
51. Kumar N, Ray C, Jain S (2002) Aspiration cytology of Hashimoto's thyroiditis in an endemic area. Cytopathology 13:31–39.
52. Montone KT, Baloch ZW, LiVolsi VA (2008) The thyroid Hürthle (oncocytic) cell and its associated pathologic conditions: a surgical pathology and cytopathology review. Arch Pathol Lab Med 132:1241–1250.
53. Renshaw A (2001) Follicular lesions of the thyroid. Am J Clin Pathol 115:782–785.
54. Lowhagen T (1974) Thyroid. In: Zajicek J (ed) Aspiration Biopsy Cytology, Part 1, Cytology of supradiaphragmatic organs, Monographs in Clinical Cytology, vol 4. Karger, Basel, pp 67–89.
55. Lowhagen T, Willems J-S (1981) Aspiration biopsy cytology in diseases of the thyroid. Adv Clin Cytol 201–231.
56. LiVolsi VA, Asa SL (1994) The demise of follicular carcinoma of the thyroid gland. Thyroid 4:233–236.
57. Schlinkert RT, van Heerden JA, Goellner JR et al (1997) Factors that predict malignant thyroid lesions when fine-needle aspiration is "suspicious for follicular neoplasm". Mayo Clin Proc 72:913–916.
58. Ravetto C, Colombo L, Dottorini ME (2000) Usefulness of fine-needle aspiration in the diagnosis of thyroid carcinoma: a retrospective study in 37,895 patients. Cancer 90:357–363.
59. Lin JD, Hsueh C, Chao TC et al (1997) Thyroid follicular neoplasms diagnosed by high-resolution ultrasonography with fine needle aspiration cytology. Acta Cytol 41:687–691.
60. Greaves TS, Olvera M, Florentine BD et al (2000). Follicular lesions of thyroid: a 5-year fine-needle aspiration experience. Cancer 90:335–341.
61. Raber W, Kaserer K, Niederle B, Vierhapper H (2000) Risk factors for malignancy of thyroid nodules initially identified as follicular neoplasia by fine-needle aspiration: results of a prospective study of one hundred twenty patients. Thyroid 10:709–712.
62. Yang GC, Liebeskind D, Messina AV (2003) Should cytopathologists stop reporting follicular neoplasms on fine-needle aspiration of the thyroid? Cancer 99:69–74.
63. Mihai R, Parker AJ, Roskell D, Sadler GP (2009) One in four patients with follicular thyroid cytology (THY3) has a thyroid carcinoma. Thyroid 19:33–37.
64. Frates MC, Benson CB, Doubilet PM et al (2006) Prevalence and distribution of carcinoma in patients with solitary and multiple thyroid nodules on sonography. J Clin Endocrinol Metab 91:3411–3417.
65. Baloch Z, LiVolsi VA, Jain P et al (2003) Role of repeat fine-needle aspiration biopsy (FNAB) in the management of thyroid nodules. Diagn Cytopathol 29:203–206.
66. Miller MC, Rubin CJ, Cunnane M et al (2007) Intraoperative pathologic examination: cost effectiveness and clinical value in patients with cytologic diagnosis of cellular follicular thyroid lesion. Thyroid 17:557–565.
67. Maruta J, Hashimoto H, Yamashita H et al (2004) Immunostaining of galectin-3 and CD44v6 using fine-needle aspiration for distinguishing follicular carcinoma from adenoma. Diagn Cytopathol 31:392–396.
68. Bartolazzi A, Orlandi F, Saggiorato E et al (2008) Galectin-3-expression analysis in the surgical selection of follicular thyroid nodules with indeterminate fine-needle aspiration cytology: a prospective multicentre study. Lancet Oncol 9:543–549.
69. Carpi A, Naccarato AG, Iervasi G et al (2006) Large needle aspiration biopsy and galectin-3 determination in selected thyroid nodules with indeterminate FNA-cytology. Br J Cancer 95:204–209.
70. DeLellis RA (2006) Pathology and genetics of thyroid carcinoma. J Surg Oncol 94:662–669.
71. Kaur A, Jayaram G (1991) Thyroid tumors: cytomorphology of papillary carcinoma. Diagn Cytopathol 7:462–468.
72. Gould E, Watzak L, Chamizo W, Albores-Saavedra J (1999) Nuclear grooves in cytologic preparations. A study of the utility of this feature in the diagnosis of papillary carcinoma. Acta Cytol 33:16–20.

73. Deligeorgi-Politi H (1987) Nuclear crease as a cytodiagnostic feature of papillary thyroid carcinoma in fine-needle aspiration biopsies. Diagn Cytopathol 3:307–310.
74. Rupp M, Ehya H (1998) Nuclear grooves in the aspiration cytology of papillary carcinoma of the thyroid. Acta Cytol 33:21–26.
75. Akhtar M, Ali MA, Huq M, Bakry M (1991) Fine-needle aspiration biopsy of papillary thyroid carcinoma: cytologic, histologic, and ultrastructural correlations. Diagn Cytopathol 7:373–379.
76. Das DK, Sharma PN (2005) Intranuclear cytoplasmic inclusions and nuclear grooves in fine needle aspiration smears of papillary thyroid carcinoma and its variants: advantage of the count under an oil-immersion objective over a high-power objective. Anal Quant Cytol Histol 27:83–94.
77. Christ ML, Haja J (1979) Intranuclear cytoplasmic inclusions (invaginations) in thyroid aspirations. Frequency and specificity. Acta Cytol 23:327–331.
78. Gupta S, Sodhani P, Jain S, Kumar N (2004) Morphologic spectrum of papillary carcinoma of the thyroid: role of cytology in identifying the variants. Acta Cytol 48:795–800.
79. Rosai J, Kuhn E, Carcangiu ML (2006) Pitfalls in thyroid tumour pathology. Histopathology 49:107–120.
80. Tahlan A, Dey P (2001) Nuclear grooves. How specific are they? Acta Cytol 45:48–50.
81. Yang YJ, Demirci SS (2003) Evaluating the diagnostic significance of nuclear grooves in thyroid fine needle aspirates with a semiquantitative approach. Acta Cytol 47:563–570.
82. Logani S, Gupta PK, LiVolsi VA et al (2000) Thyroid nodules with FNA cytology suspicious for follicular variant of papillary thyroid carcinoma: follow-up and management. Diagn Cytopathol 23:380–385.
83. Aron M, Mallik A, Verma K (2006). Fine needle aspiration cytology of follicular variant of papillary carcinoma of the thyroid: Morphologic pointers to its diagnosis. Acta Cytol 50:663–668.
84. Shih SR, Shun CT, Su DH et al (2005) Follicular variant of papillary thyroid carcinoma: diagnostic limitations of fine needle aspiration cytology. Acta Cytol 49:383–386.
85. El Hag IA, Kollur SM (2004) Benign follicular thyroid lesions versus follicular variant of papillary carcinoma: differentiation by architectural pattern. Cytopathology 15:200–205.
86. Wu HH, Jones JN, Grzybicki DM, Elsheikh TM (2003) Sensitive cytologic criteria for the identification of follicular variant of papillary thyroid carcinoma in fine-needle aspiration biopsy. Diagn Cytopathol 29:262–266.
87. Powari M, Dey P, Saikia UN (2003) Fine needle aspiration cytology of follicular variant of papillary carcinoma of thyroid. Cytopathology 14:212–215.
88. Das DK, Mallik MK, Sharma P et al (2004) Papillary thyroid carcinoma and its variants in fine needle aspiration smears. A cytomorphologic study with special reference to tall cell variant. Acta Cytol 48:325–336.
89. Jayaram G (2000) Cytology of columnar-cell variant of papillary thyroid carcinoma. Diagn Cytopathol 22:227–229.
90. Lin JD, Hsuen C, Chen JY et al (2007) Cystic change in thyroid cancer. ANZ J Surg 77:450–454.
91. Ustün M, Risberg B, Davidson B, Berner A (2002) Cystic change in metastatic lymph nodes: a common diagnostic pitfall in fine-needle aspiration cytology. Diagn Cytopathol 27:387–392.
92. Nguyen GK, Akin MR (2001) Cytopathology of insular carcinoma of the thyroid. Diagn Cytopathol 25:325–330.
93. Ghofrani M, Sosa JA, Ocal IT, Angeletti C (2006) Fine needle aspiration of poorly differentiated oxyphilic (Hürthle cell) thyroid carcinoma: a case report. Acta Cytol 50:560–562.
94. Schaffer R, Muller HA, Pfeifer U et al (1984) Cytological findings in medullary carcinoma of the thyroid. Path Res Pract 178:461–466.
95. Mendonca ME, Ramos SM, Soares J (1991) Medullary carcinoma of thyroid: a re-evaluation of the cytological criteria of diagnosis. Cytopathol 2:93–102.
96. Bhanot P, Yang J, Schnadig VJ, Logroño R (2007) Role of FNA cytology and immunochemistry in the diagnosis and management of medullary thyroid carcinoma: report of six cases and review of the literature. Diagn Cytopathol 35:285–292.
97. Us-Krasovec M, Golouh R, Auersperg M et al (1996) Anaplastic thyroid carcinoma in fine needle aspirates. Acta Cytol 40:953–8.
98. Lowhagen T, Sprenger E (1974) Cytological presentation of thyroid tumors in aspiration biopsy smears: a review of 60 cases. Acta Cytol 18:192–197.
99. Friedman M, Shimaoka K, Lopez CA, Shedd DP (1983) Parathyroid adenoma diagnosed as papillary carcinoma of thyroid on needle aspiration smears. Acta Cytol 27:337–340.
100. Tseng FY, Hsiao YL, Chang TC (2002) Ultrasound-guided fine needle aspiration cytology of parathyroid lesions. A review of 72 cases. Acta Cytol 46:1029–1036.
101. Liu F, Gnepp DR, Pisharodi LR (2004) Fine needle aspiration of parathyroid lesions. Acta Cytol 48:133–136.
102. Gherardi G, Scherini P, Ambrosi S (1985) Occult thyroid metastasis from untreated uveal melanoma. Arch Ophthalmol 103:689–691.

Lymph Nodes: Diagnosis of Malignant Lymphoma

4

4.1 Introduction

Fine-needle biopsy (FNB) is a convenient and reliable first-line diagnostic procedure for the investigation of superficial and deep seated lymphadenopathies. Its application can vary according to the clinical context, the age of the patient, and the anatomic site of the lesion [1–3]. Morphological assessment of the cellular sample serves as the basis for identifying several inflammatory conditions of the lymph nodes, as well as most high-grade lymphoid malignancies and non-lymphoid metastatic tumors, but it has significant limitations in the study of low-grade lymphomas as it does not allow their differentiation from several reactive conditions [4–7]. However, this limitation can be overcome by the use of ancillary laboratory techniques in FNB samples, as these often reveal important immunophenotypic and biomolecular information that assists in obtaining a definitive diagnosis. Finally, a tissue incisional biopsy, using cutting needles, can be performed in parallel with FNB sampling of the lymph node. This approach may add relevant morphological data to the cytological evaluation as well as provide a significant amount of cellular sample for ancillary techniques.

FNB sampling is easily accomplished in experienced hands. The procedure is very well-tolerated by the patient; it is virtually risk-free, inexpensive, simple, and immediately repeatable if required. The main practical limitation is that the diagnostic yield is strongly operator-dependent, which influences the use of FNB in clinical practice. In addition, interpretation of the cellular sample requires considerable expertise and an extensive knowledge of the histopathology of lymphoid lesions. Both these factors represent significant potential disadvantages that, in practice, narrow the wider use of FNB [4,5,8].

4.2 Histological vs. Cytological Approach to Lymphoid Lesions

The conventional histopathological approach to the morphological analysis of lymph node lesions consists of: (1) evaluation of possible effacement of lymph node structure, (2) morphological recognition of the lymph node's cellular components, with their relative quantification, and (3) identification of the cellular distribution within the different lymph node compartments. These steps serve as the basis for the conventional tissue diagnosis of lymphoid malignancies and for planning additional studies, if required, for further evaluation and diagnostic confirmation. It is important to point out that the cytological evaluation of a lymph node cellular sample collected by FNB and smeared onto a slide cannot provide the same data as the conventional approach, because it is not possible to determine the actual structure of the lymph node. Also, the cellular population is not representative of all the cellular components present within the sampled lymph node, nor is it possible to define the location of each cellular component within the different lymph node compartments because they are haphazardly mixed on the smear. Since the cellular population of most lymphomas of low-grade malignancy is qualitatively the same as that seen in reactive conditions, a definitive diagnosis of lymphomas of this type is practically not feasible by FNB alone. Instead, the diagnosis of malignant lymphoma should rely on non-morphological criteria, such as the monoclonality of the cell population and/or peculiar chromosomal translocations, both of which can be determined by ancillary techniques [9–22].

Nonetheless, FNB allows examination of the fine

morphology of all the cells in cytological smears prepared from representative samples of lymphoid proliferations, with prompt and precise identification of each cellular component within the harvest. This offers an advantage in that a definitive diagnosis of high-grade non-Hodgkin's lymphomas and several variants of Hodgkin's lymphoma can be made by FNB sampling [12–14]. These latter malignancies are characterized by an abnormal prevalence of large cells or the presence of peculiar cell types, such as Reed-Sternberg cells, which are not seen in reactive lymphoid proliferations. Concurrent microhistological sampling of the lesional lymph node can amplify the diagnostic yield of the procedure and provides an invaluable opportunity to perform ancillary studies [23]. Table 4.1 summarizes the main lymphoma variants according to the 2008 World Health Organization (WHO) classification [24].

Table 4.1 2008 WHO classification of lymphomas [24]

Precursor lymphoid neoplasms

B lymphoblastic leukemia/lymphoma NOS
B lymphoblastic leukemia/lymphoma with recurrent genetic abnormalities
B lymphoblastic leukemia/lymphoma with t(9;22); bcr-abl1
B lymphoblastic leukemia/lymphoma with t(v;11q23); MLL rearranged
B lymphoblastic leukemia/lymphoma with t(12:21); TEL-AML1 & ETV6-RUNX1
B lymphoblastic leukemia/lymphoma with hyperploidy
B lymphoblastic leukemia/lymphoma with hypodiploidy
B lymphoblastic leukemia/lymphoma with t(5;14); IL3-IGH
B lymphoblastic leukemia/lymphoma with t(1;19); E2A-PBX1 & TCF3-PBX1
T lymphoblastic leukemia/lymphoma

Mature B-cell neoplasms

Chronic lymphocytic leukemia/small lymphocytic lymphoma
B-cell prolymphocytic leukemia
Splenic marginal zone lymphoma
Hairy cell leukemia
Lymphoplasmacytic lymphoma/Waldenstrom macroglobulinemia
Heavy-chain disease
Plasma cell myeloma
Solitary plasmacytoma of bone
Extraosseous plasmacytoma
Extranodal marginal zone B-cell lymphoma of mucosa-associated lymphoid tissue (MALT) type
Nodal marginal zone lymphoma
Follicular lymphoma
Primary cutaneous follicular lymphoma
Mantle cell lymphoma
Diffuse large B-cell lymphoma, NOS (T-cell/histiocyte-rich type; primary CNS type ; primary leg-skin type & Epstein-Barr virus+ elderly type)
Diffuse large B-cell lymphoma with chronic inflammation
Lymphomatoid granulomatosis
Primary mediastinal large B-cell lymphoma
Intravascular large B-cell lymphoma
ALK+ large B-cell lymphoma
Plasmablastic lymphoma
Large B-cell lymphoma associated with HHV8 + Castleman disease
Primary effusion lymphoma
Burkitt's lymphoma
B-cell lymphoma, unclassifiable, Burkitt-like
B-cell lymphoma, unclassifiable, Hodgkin's lymphoma-like

Mature T-cell and natural killer (NK)-cell neoplasms

T-cell prolymphocytic leukemia
T-cell large granular lymphocytic leukemia
Chronic lymphoproliferative disorder of NK cells
Aggressive NK-cell leukemia
Systemic Epstein-Barr virus + T-cell lymphoproliferative disorder of childhood
Hydroa-vacciniforme-like lymphoma
Adult T-cell lymphoma/leukemia
Extranodal T-cell/NK-cell lymphoma, nasal type
Enteropathy-associated T-cell lymphoma
Hepatosplenic T-cell lymphoma
Subcutaneous panniculitis-like T-cell lymphoma
Mycosis fungoides
Sézary syndrome
Primary cutaneous CD30+ T-cell lymphoproliferative disorder
Primary cutaneous $\gamma\delta$-T-cell lymphoma
Peripheral T-cell lymphoma, NOS
Angioimmunoblastic T-cell lymphoma
Anaplastic large-cell lymphoma, ALK+-type
Anaplastic large-cell lymphoma, ALK-type

Hodgkin's lymphoma (Hodgkin's disease)

Nodular lymphocyte-predominant Hodgkin's lymphomas
Classic Hodgkin's lymphomas
Nodular sclerosis Hodgkin's lymphoma
Lymphocyte-rich classic Hodgkin's lymphoma
Mixed cellularity Hodgkin's lymphoma
Lymphocyte depletion Hodgkin's lymphoma

Post-transplant lymphoproliferative disorders (PTLD)

Plasmacytic hyperplasia
Infectious-mononucleosis-like PTLD
Polymorphic PTLD
Monomorphic PTLD (B- and T-/NK-cell types)
Classic Hodgkin's Disease-type PTLD

Histiocytic and dendritic cell neoplasms

Histiocytic sarcoma
Langerhans cell histiocytosis
Langerhans cell sarcoma
Interdigitating dendritic cell sarcoma
Follicular dendritic cell sarcoma
Fibroblastic reticular cell tumor
Indeterminate dendritic cell sarcoma
Disseminated juvenile xanthogranuloma

4.3 Indications for Fine-Needle Biopsy of Lymph Nodes

The use of FNB in the diagnostic work up of a lymphadenopathy is variable according to the clinical scenario and the diagnostic expectations. It can serve as a first-line screening test aimed simply at assessing whether lymph node enlargement is due to a lymphoid proliferation or a metastatic malignancy. While FNB is not expected to provide a conclusive diagnosis, it is used to support further clinical and pathological assessment. At the opposite end of the spectrum, and keeping a higher profile, FNB may be used to provide a conclusive diagnosis in the context of therapeutic decision-making; for example, in the evaluation of a deep-seated lymph node enlargement in a patient who presents in poor condition such that the use of any alternative diagnostically invasive procedure is contraindicated. In such cases, FNB is often complemented by microhistological core-needle biopsy (CNB) sampling of the lymph node.

Based on these considerations, the indications for lymph-node FNB are the following:

- Diagnosis of inflammatory granulomatous conditions or acute inflammation.
- Staging of malignant lymphoma (when the disease has been already diagnosed by means of a conventional excisional biopsy).
- Diagnosis of lymphoma relapse.
- Primary diagnosis of malignant lymphoma in patients with rapidly progressive disease (high-grade lymphoma) or deep-seated and poorly accessible lymph node involvement, especially in patients in poor clinical condition [25].
- Diagnosis of lymph node involvement by non-lymphoid metastatic malignancies (see Chapter 5).

4.4 Evaluation of the Cellular Sample

4.4.1 Cellularity

The cellularity should be first evaluated microscopically at a low power view. FNB sampling of an enlarged lymph node that is the site of a lymphoid proliferation, whether benign or malignant, generally yields a highly cellular harvest. Sparse cellularity can be due to intranodal sclerosis, necrosis, or blood contamination and contraindicates any further assessment; instead, a repeat biopsy should be performed to obtain a more representative sample. Intranodal sclerosis can occur in some variants of malignant lymphoma as well as in metastatic carcinoma. Coagulative necrosis can develop in granulomatous inflammation or as a consequence of lymph node infarction, the latter being a common complication of some high-grade lymphomas. Blood contamination is often seen in inguinal lymph nodes and is due to vascular transformation of the sinuses.

4.4.2 Lymphoglandular Bodies

The detection of lymphoglandular bodies in the smear is required to establish that the sample has been obtained from a lymphoid organ. Lymphoglandular bodies consist of fragments of the cytoplasmic content of lymphoid cells and are totally delimited by a plasma membrane (Fig. 4.1). They are characterized by a globular mophology and their size is less than the diameter of a red blood cell. It should be noted that similar structures can be observed in samples from small-cell carcinoma of the lung and from metastatic seminoma [26].

4.4.3 Identification of Cell Type

Examining the smear at an intermediate magnification allows lymphoid cells and non-lymphoid ancillary

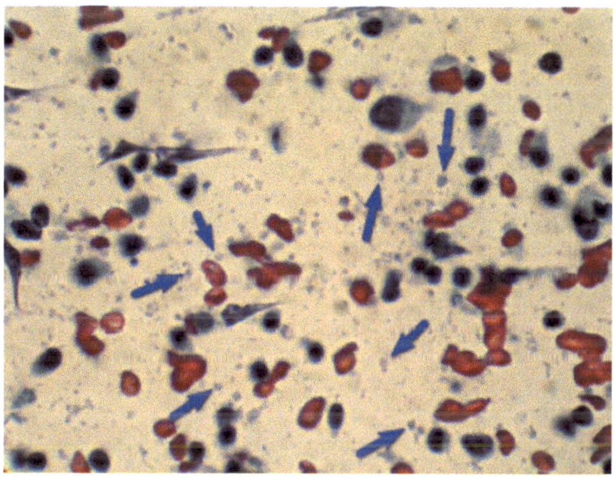

Fig. 4.1 High-magnification view of lymphoglandular bodies (*blue arrows*), which appear as globoid structures interspersed in the background among red blood cells and lymphocytes. Papanicolaou (P) stain, ×1000

elements to be identified. The latter represent an integral part of the lymph node parenchyma. All of the cell types that may be recognizable in a cytological smear are listed in Table 4.2. Lymphoid cells are very well visualized in ethanol-fixed smear preparations stained according to the Papanicolaou method, and cytomorphology correlates well with the appearance of cells in paraffin tissue sections. Conversely, the morphology of cells in air-dried smears stained according to the May Grünwald Giemsa method correlates poorly with the appearance of the same cells in routine histopathological preparations. Based on these considerations, Papanicolaou staining of ethanol-fixed smears is considered to provide better insight into the cytopathology of lymphomas and is preferred over the May Grünwald Giemsa method. *Lymphoid cells* commonly appear as dispersed and non-cohesive, although there may be a sort of pseudoaggregation (see below). *Non-lymphoid cells* consist of the supportive stromal components of each lymph node compartment and several elements appearing in inflammatory or regressive conditions. The third cellular component that may be detected in a FNB lymph node sample is the so-called *alien cellular population* and is due to lymph node colonization by a metastatic malignancy. The approach to metastatic malignancies appearing in lymph nodes and in other anatomic sites, such as viscera and soft tissues, is beyond the scope of this chapter but is described elsewhere in this book.

4.4.3.1 Lymphoid Cells

A smear of the lymph node sample obtained by FNB allows for the identification of a large variety of cell types of lymphoid lineage, most of which are seen both in reactive conditions and in various malignant non-Hodgkin's lymphomas of the "low grade" category (Table 4.2). Since only a minority of cell types appears exclusively in malignant lymphomas, such cells represent the key diagnostic feature of these malignancies. Table 4.3 schematically outlines the main features distinguishing the large majority of the elements of lymphoid lineage in Papanicolaou-stained smears. The approach to classification is based on the evaluation of the size of the cells and on the

Table 4.2 Cell types of the lymph node

Cell types seen in reactive and neoplastic conditions	Cell types seen only in neoplastic conditions
Cortical compartment	Burkitt-type blastic B-cells
Small B lymphocytes, lymphoplasmacytoid B-lymphocytes, plasma cells	Reed-Sternberg and Hodgkin's cells
Follicular center cells: centrocytes, centroblasts, immunoblasts	Pleomorphic and anaplastic T-cells
Tingible-body histiocytes	B- and T-lymphoblasts
Follicular dendritic cells	
Intrafollicular small T-lymphocytes	
Mantle zone lymphocytes	
Marginal zone lymphocytes (spleen)	
Paracortical compartment	
Small T-lymphocytes	
Histiocytes (including epithelioid and multi-nucleated histiocytes)	
Small B lymphocytes, lymphoplasmacytoid B-lymphocytes, plasma cells	
Langerhans' cells	
Endothelial cells	
Plasmacytoid monocytes	
Medullary compartment	
Small T-lymphocytes	
Histiocytes (including epithelioid and multi-nucleated histiocytes)	
Endothelial cells	
Mast cells	

Table 4.3 Main morphologic features distinguishing the large majority of the elements of lymphoid lineage in Papanicolaou-stained smears

Cell type	Size (fold difference with the diameter of a RBC)	Morphological features	Corresponding cell type
Small lymphocyte	1.2–1.5	Small nucleus, round nuclear outline, dense chromatin, no nucleoli, sparse or minimal cytoplasm	Small B-lymphocyte Small T-lymphocyte
Small centrocyte and centrocyte-like cells	1.5–2.0	Small nucleus, irregular nuclear profile (cleaved), dense chromatin, no nucleoli, sparse cytoplasm	Follicular center small centrocyte, mantle zone lymphocyte, marginal zone lymphocyte
Large centrocyte	2.1–3.0	Medium-sized nucleus, irregular nuclear outline (cleaved), dense or finely granular chromatin, no or small nucleoli, sparse cytoplasm	Follicular center large centrocyte Normal activated mantle cell lymphocyte Mantle cell lymphoma elements
Plasma cell	2.1–3.2	Medium-sized nucleus (may be eccentrically placed), round nuclear profile with a central nucleolus of variable size, finely granular to clumped chromatin, moderate to abundant cytoplasm with Golgi zone	Resting and activated plasma cells Lymphoplasma-cytic/cytoid cells in some B-cell lymphomas
Centroblast	2.6–3.2	Medium-sized nucleus, round or multilobated nuclear outline, vesicular or finely granular chromatin, 2–4 nucleoli (at least one attached to the nuclear membrane), sparse cytoplasm	Follicular center centroblast Centroblast cells in follicular lymphoma Large-cell, B-cell-type lymphoma elements
Immunoblast	3.0–3.9	Large nucleus, round nuclear outline, single centrally located and prominent nucleolus, basophilic and abundant cytoplasm	B- and T-immunoblasts Large cell, B-cell type lymphoma elements Large cells in PTCL, unspecified
Lymphoblast (non-convoluted or convoluted)	2.0–4.5	Intermediate to large nucleus, round to irregular to convoluted nuclear profile (pleomorphic), dense to grossly granular chromatin, no nucleoli, sparse and vacuolated cytoplasm (MGG stain)	B-, null-, or T-phenotype lymphoblast in precursor cell lymphomas
Burkitt-type blast cell	2.2–3.5	Intermediate to large nucleus, round nuclear profile, coarsely granular chromatin, multiple nucleoli, sparse cytoplasm	Burkitt-type lymphoma cell Large-cell, B-cell lymphoma elements
Anaplastic	> 4.0	Giant, possibly polylobated, nucleus or polynucleation, vesicular chromatin, multiple sometimes prominent and bizarre nucleoli, variable amount of cytoplasm, indistinct plasma membrane	PTCL, anaplastic large-cell lymphoma elements Lacunar type Reed-Sternberg cell Large-cell B-cell lymphoma elements Mantle cell lymphoma, blastoid variant elements Large cells in PTCL, unspecified
Polynucleated Reed-Sternberg cell	> 4.0	Large, possibly polylobated nucleus prominent, eosinophilic and multiple nucleoli, vesicular to finely granular chromatin, microvacuolated or partially disintegrated cytoplasm, barely evident external membrane	Reed-Sternberg cell, diagnostic type Reed-Sternberg-like cells in various non-Hodgkin's lymphoma types
Mononuclear Reed-Sternberg cell	> 4.0	Intermediate to large, non-lobated, nucleus, prominent eosinophilic nucleolus with a clear halo, vesicular chromatin, microvacuolated or partially disintegrated cytoplasm, barely evident external membrane	Reed-Sternberg cell, lymphohistiocytic type Reed-Sternberg-like cells in various non-Hodgkin's lymphoma types

PTCC = peripheral T-cell lymphoma

morphological features of their nuclei and the cytoplasm. Figures 4.2–4.12 provide examples of the cytomorphological features of the listed cell types.

Cell size is approximately determined by comparing the median cellular diameter to the diameter of red blood cells (RBCs) detected in the smear. This approach provides a distinction in three broad categories: *small cells*, with diameters ≤2×RBC; *large cells*, with diameters between >2×RBC and ≤4×RBC; and *atypical blastic elements*, which mostly appear larger than 4×RBC. The first category basically includes the following cells, which appear both in normal and neoplastic conditions: reactive small lymphocytes of B and T lineage; centrocytes present in reactive follicles; the lymphoid elements of the follicular mantle in normal conditions; the population of cells seen in small lymphocytic non-Hodgkin's lymphoma/B-cell chronic lymphocytic leukemia, in B-cell mantle cell non-Hodgkin's lymphoma (classical variant), and in nodal and extranodal marginal zone B-cell non-Hodgkin's lymphoma; and the neoplastic follicular center cells with centrocytic features

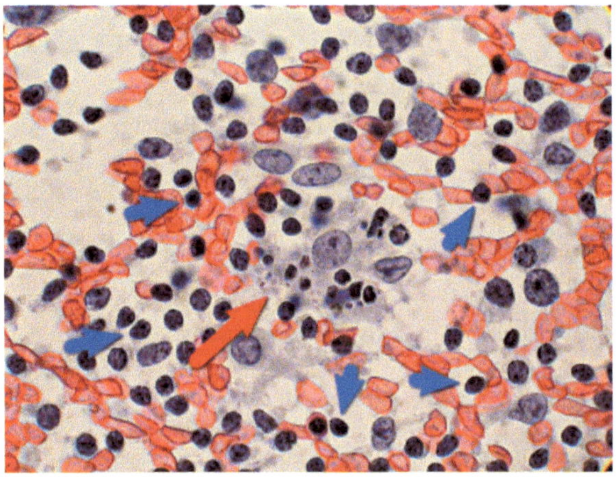

Fig. 4.2 A tingible-body hystiocyte is indicated by the *red arrow*. The cell is characterized by an abundant cytoplasm containing numerous phagocytosed basophilic fragments representing nuclear debris. *Blue arrows* point to characteristic small lymphocytes. P stain, ×1000

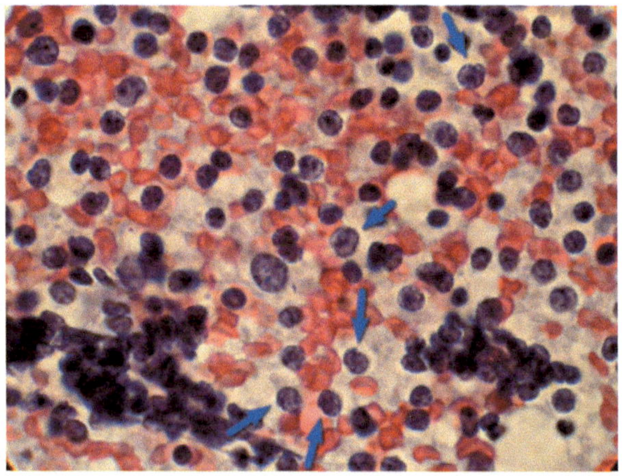

Fig. 4.3 Small centrocytes (*blue arrows*) contain a small nucleus characterized by variably deep infoldings. These cells are interspersed with small lymphocytes and apparently clustering cells forming pseudoaggregates. P stain, ×1000

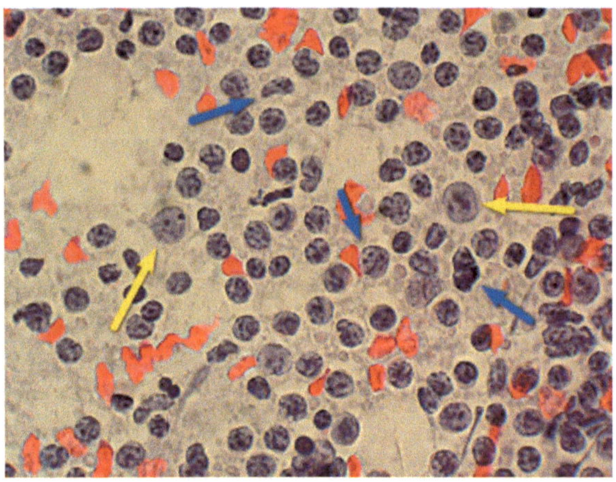

Fig. 4.4 Centroblasts (*yellow arrows*) and large centrocytes (*blue arrows*). The background contains numerous lymphoglandular bodies. P stain, ×1000

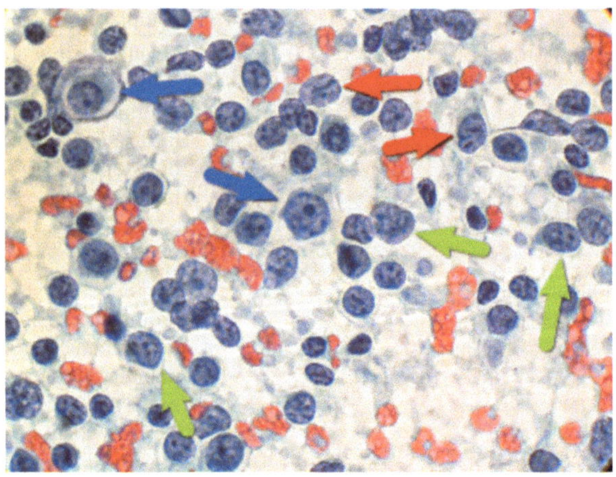

Fig. 4.5 Cytological appearance of immunoblasts (*blue arrows*), centroblasts (*green arrows*), and large centrocytes (*red arrows*). P stain, ×1000

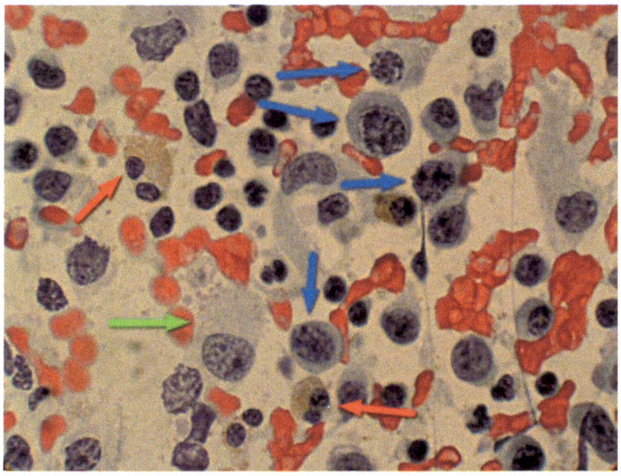

Fig. 4.6 Cytological appearance of plasma cells (*blue arrows*), seen interspersed with eosinophilic granulocytes (*red arrows*) and histiocytes (*green arrow*). P stain, ×1000

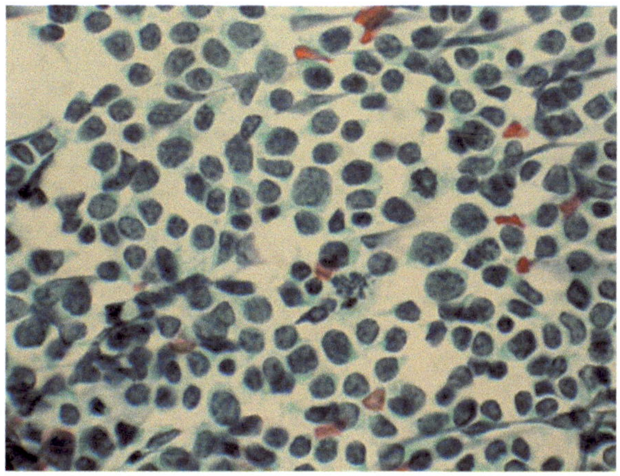

Fig. 4.7 Cytological appearance of lymphoblasts in a sample obtained from a patient with precursor cell lymphoma, T-cell type. Note that the chromatin texture is markedly monotonous in these cells but the size and shape of the nucleus are markedly variable, depicting cellular pleomorphism. P stain, ×1000

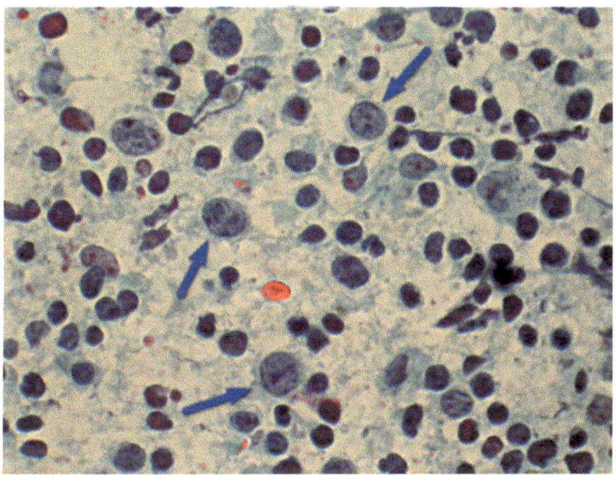

Fig. 4.8 Several Burkitt-type blasts. These cells (indicated by *blue arrows*) are characterized by a large nucleus containing multiple basophilic nucleoli that only rarely are close to the nuclear membrane. P stain, ×1000

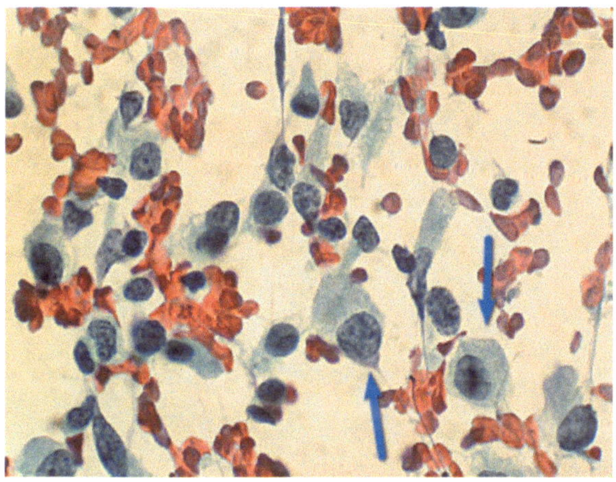

Fig. 4.9 Cytological appearance of the cellular harvest in a sample obtained from a patient with peripheral T-cell lymphoma, anaplastic type. The cells (indicated by *blue* arrows) are pleomorphic and contain a moderate amount of cytoplasm. P stain, ×1000

appearing in follicular type B-cell non-Hodgkin's lymphoma [12–14]. In fact, all these elements have in common a small nucleus with a round or cleaved profile, a finely granular or dense chromatin with no prominent nucleoli, and sparse cytoplasm. The second category comprises large centrocytes, centroblasts, and the immunoblasts appearing in reactive follicular centers as well as in several types of B-cell non-Hodgkin's lymphoma; activated plasma cells; the large cells proliferating in different types of peripheral T-cell lymphomas; and in B-cell and T-cell lymphoblastic lymphomas. These elements have in common a large nucleus and a variable amount of cytoplasm. The nuclear profile can be round, cleaved, or convoluted. Nucleoli can be single or multiple and their position within the nucleus is relevant to the identification of the cell type. The chromatin is finely to coarsely granular. The cytoplasm in Papanicolaou-

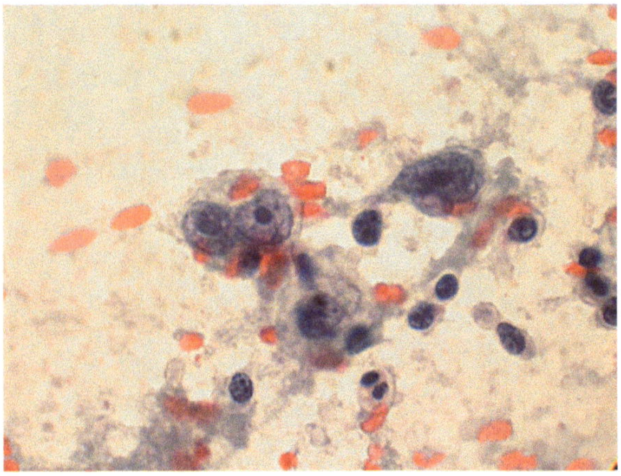

Fig. 4.10 Cytological appearance of a Reed-Sternberg cell, diagnostic type; the cell is large and apparently contains two nuclei, each containing a prominent centrally placed nucleolus. An additional cell on the right side of the figure contains a single nucleus with multiple infoldings of the external membrane. P stain, ×1000

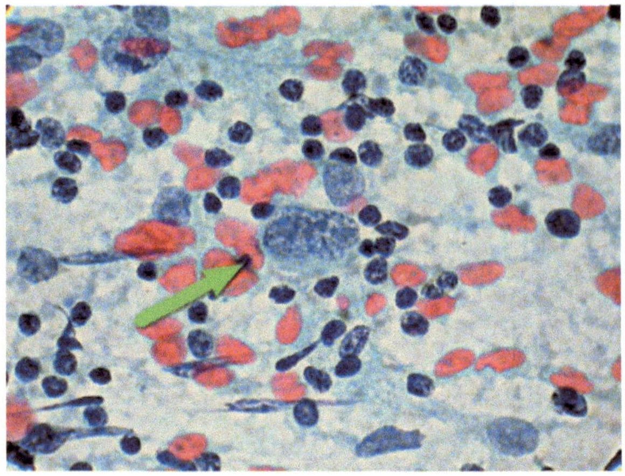

Fig. 4.11 Cytological appearance of a mononuclear Reed-Sternberg cell. The cell contains a large nucleus with a bizarre nucleolus (*green arrow*). Small lymphocytes are seen in the background. P stain, x100

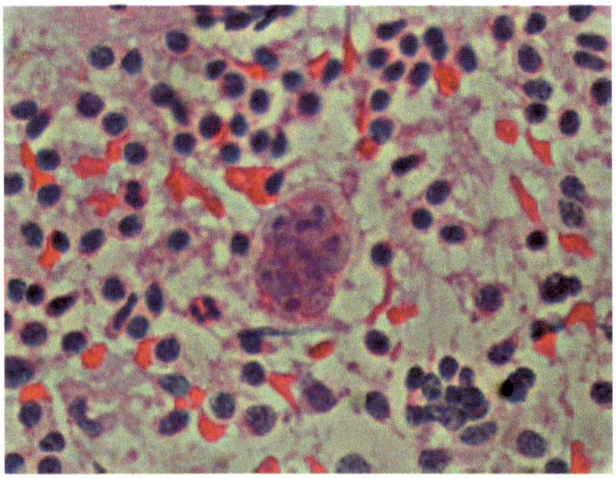

Fig. 4.12 Cytological appearance of a mononuclear Reed-Sternberg cell with a voluminous single nucleus that is characterized by multilobation. Each lobe contains a basophilic nucleolus. Hematoxylin & eosin (H&E) stain, ×1000

stained smear preparations is amphiphilic or clear or finely vacuolated. The third category of atypical blastic elements includes Reed-Sternberg cells and their variants, anaplastic cells of some peripheral T-cell lymphomas and large B-cell lymphomas, and the large bizarre cells seen in the blastoid variant of mantle cell lymphoma [12–14]. The nuclei of these cells are very large and their shape is variable. The nuclear outline can be round and irregular, multilobed simulating multinucleation, or absolutely bizarre. The chromatin generally appears finely granular. Nucleoli are generally prominent and can be single or multiple. Atypical blastic cells occur almost exclusively in lymphoid malignancies and their recognition, irrespective of their quantity, is a key factor in the diagnosis of these tumors.

4.4.3.2 Ancillary Cellular Components

The ancillary cells can vary in amount and type in FNB samples of lymph nodes, reflecting their different activation states in reactive and neoplastic conditions. Histiocytes are intermediate to large in size and contain a large nucleus with a finely granular chromatin and a small nucleolus. The cytoplasm is abundant and multiple phagocytic vacuoles are seen that contain irregularly shaped highly basophilic bodies measuring <1×RBC (Fig. 4.2). These "tingible bodies" consist of nuclear fragments that are basophilic due to their content of densely stained chromatin substance. *Tingible-body histiocytes* are an integral cellular component of the follicular center of the lymph node and in FNB samples they can be considered as a reliable indicator of the presence of hyperplastic lymphoid follicles within the lymph node. True tingible bodies are, as noted above and by definition, only fragments of nuclei; they should not be confused with entire nuclei, the presence of which, conversely, indicates active apoptosis within the cellular proliferation. Active apoptosis is infrequent in benign conditions and is much more commonly observed in some variants of malignant lymphoma, such as Burtkitt's and Burkitt-like B-cell non-Hodgkin's lymphoma (see below). For this reason, histiocytes containing entire nuclei or entire apoptotic cells are not to be defined as tingible-body histiocytes, and the implications of their detection are completely different. True tingible-body histiocytes should also be distinguished from the mononucleated or multinucleated histiocytes that appear to engulf entire non-apoptotic lymphocytes or plasma cells and which are seen in Rosai-Dorfman disease (see below). Other types of histiocytes have a nuclear morphology resembling that of tingible-body histiocytes but they contain lipid vacuoles, phagocytosed hemosiderin, or melanin pigment within their cytoplasm. *Epithelioid histiocytes* are cells of intermediate size, with a round to oval nucleus containing vesicular chromatin and sometimes a small nucleolus. The cytoplasm is amphiphilic or slightly eosinophilic, may contain small vacuoles, and appears somewhat fragile (Fig. 4.13). These cells occur in granulomatous inflammatory conditions and in various types of malignant lymphomas [27]. In addition, they are activated in lymph nodes draining carcinoma or seminoma. *Reticular dendritic cells* are difficult to discern from endothelial cells. In smears from reactive lymphoid hyperplasia or follicular B-cell lymphomas, they generally are seen to entrap follicular center cells (centrocytes and centroblasts). *Endothelial cells* have a vesicular nucleus and, albeit rarely, show a prominent nucleolus; they are easily recognized delimiting capillary walls. *Fibrocytes* may be present in stromal fragments but are rarely prominent in lymph node samples. They may be admixed with epithelioid histiocytes (Fig. 4.13).

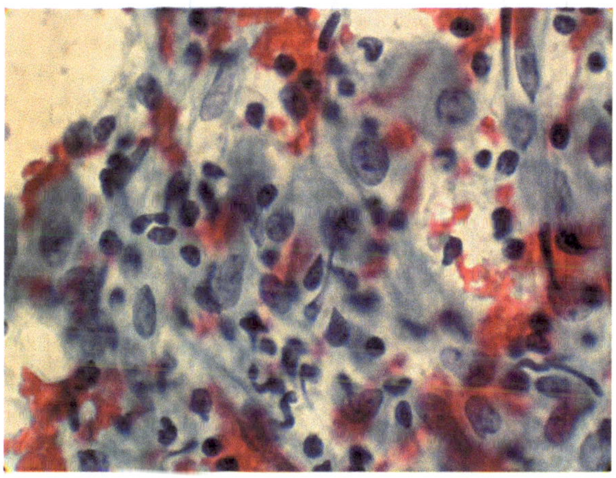

Fig. 4.13 Cytological appearance of typical epithelioid cells. These medium to large cells contain a round nucleus with finely granular chromatin. A small nucleolus is occasionally seen. P stain, ×1000

4.5 Pattern Profiling of FNB Samples

The interpretation and pattern profiling of representative FNB samples of lymphoid lesions is based on two key features: (1) cytomorphological characterization of all the lymphoid cellular components in the smear, and (2) recognition of the possible prevalence of one or more cellular component(s) over the others in the harvest, quantifying it in relative terms. The first and basic result of this analytical process leads to the identification of the potential monomorphism, polymorphism, or pleomorphism of the cellular harvest. The term *monomorphism* implies that the large majority of cells (approximately >80–90%) are similar in appearance; that is, the cellular changes mostly coincide and a single cell type is absolutely prevalent. The term *pleomorphism* is meant to indicate that within the homogeneous cellular population, which is equally prevalent in the sample (approximately >80–90%), a significant morphological variability is detected. Thus, in both monorphism and pleomorphism a single cell type strongly prevails, but in monomorphism the cells retain a strikingly similar morphological appearance, while in pleomorphism the cellular changes do not completely coincide due to, for example, variability in the chromatin pattern, nuclear outline, nucleolar features, etc. Nonetheless, this variability does not prevent the characteristic morphology of that cell type to be fully recognized. The term *polymorphism* is used when in a given cellular population multiple cell types are easily recognized and no absolute prevalence of a single component is detected. A polymorphic cellular population can, however, contain a dominant cell type but it is lesser than 80% of the harvest. Thus, according to the above definitions, the terms polymorphism and pleomorphism denote completely different situations.

Pattern profiling of FNB samples is based on recognition of the monomorphism, pleomorphism, or polymorphism of the cellular population and upon

Table 4.4 Pattern profiling of lymph node samples

Polymorphous small- and large-cell pattern, tingible-body histiocytes present
Polymorphous small- and large-cell pattern, tingible-body histiocytes absent
Polymorphous cell pattern, large-cells prevalent
Polymorphous cell pattern, small lymphocytes prevalent, with atypical/blastic cells
Monomorphous small lymphocytic pattern
Pleomorphic small- and/or large-cell pattern

recording the presence or absence of tingible-body histiocytes and atypical blastic cells. This approach produces a tiered system for classifying lymph node FNB samples that comprises six diagnostic categories, as seen in Table 4.4. The scheme reflects the different risks of possible malignancies and delineates different disease groups with intrinsically homogeneous cytomorphological features.

4.5.1 Polymorphous Small- and Large-Cell Pattern, Tingible-Body Histiocytes Present

Observations at low-power magnification commonly show an intermediate to abundant cellularity in the harvest, which is an essential prerequisite for the definition of this pattern. The detection of sparse cellularity may be due to improper sampling or reflect intranodal fat substitution, sclerosis, or even a metastatic malignancy; it therefore represents a contraindication to making a definitive diagnosis. The cellular population in representative samples consists of a large variety of cell types, including follicular center cells (centrocytes and centroblasts), small lymphocytes, plasmacytoid lymphocytes, plasma cells, immunoblasts, and inflammatory cells (neutrophilic and eosinophilic granulocytes, histiocytes) (Fig. 4.14). By definition, the large-cell component (centroblasts and immunoblasts) in the harvest ranges between 10% and 40%, and the small-cell component (small lymphocytes, plasmacytoid cells, plasma cells, centrocytes) between 60 and 90%. Tingible-body histiocytes are always seen, although their amount varies considerably. Atypical blastic cells are absent, by definition. The background contains other cell types, such as endothelial cells, reticular dendritic cells, fibrocytes, and mononuclear and multinucleated histiocytes, and, possibly, necrotic debris. Epithelioid cells may also be present and tend to aggregate in loose sheets or even in well-defined granulomata. Amorphous accumulations of a highly basophilic substance are probably to be interpreted as necrotic sheets of follicular center cells. When the described polymorphous small- and large-cell pattern is complemented by the presence of the characteristic tingible-body histiocyte component, the cytological picture can be confidently considered as diagnostic of *follicular lymphoid hyperplasia* of the lymph node [28]. Clinical findings and ultrasound examination of the enlarged lymph node generally support this diagnosis. Different etiologies should be taken into account in the clinical work-up of the patient (toxoplasmosis, infectious mononucleosis, etc.). Lymph node excision for histological examination should be considered for a more definite diagnosis if after 4–6 weeks following the cytological diagnosis no possible etiological factor has been found and, more importantly, lymph node enlargement persists and is not modified despite treatment. Surgical biopsy can confirm the diagnosis of reactive follicular hyperplasia in most cases, although sometimes, especially in young patients, a diagnosis of lymphocyte-predominant Hodgkin's disease is established.

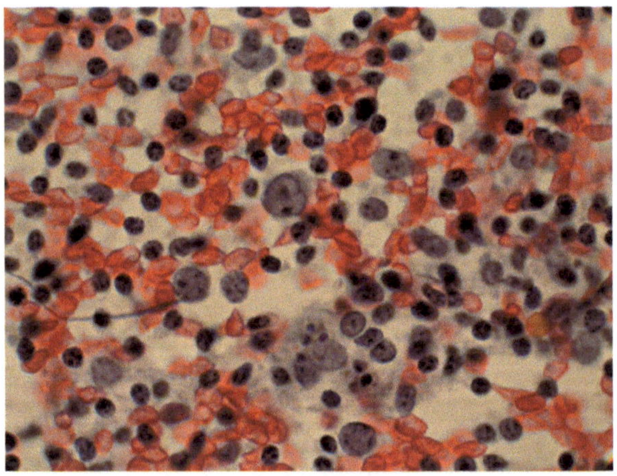

Fig. 4.14 Typical microscopic view of a lymphoid sample with a polymorphous cell pattern, including the presence of tingible-body histiocytes. The cells consist of small lymphocytes, centroblasts, and centrocytes. A tingible-body histiocyte is seen in the lower half of the image. P stain, ×1000

4.5.2 Polymorphous Small- and Large-Cell Pattern, Tingible-Body Histiocytes Absent

The cytological picture seen in the smear is similar to that previously described, as far the cellularity and the composition of the cellular population are concerned, but no tingible-body histiocytes are detected (Fig. 4.15). A significant histiocytic component can be observed but these cells contain lipoid material, hemosiderin pigment, or other phagocytosed products. The absence of tingible-body histiocytes within the sample deprives the observer of a reliable indication that the lesion is benign. In fact, in this author's experience, about 40% of the patients presenting with this pattern have a lymphoma, generally of low-grade malignancy. This pattern represents the real "gray zone" of FNB of the lymph nodes because its negative predictive value is very low; thus, the overall picture should be considered as indeterminate for possible malignancy. Proper clinical correlation is of paramount importance to decide whether or not investigation of the enlarged lymph node should be immediately pursued by surgical biopsy. Since malignant lymphomas with this cytological pattern are rare in patients under the age of 20 years, a reasonable approach is to postpone surgical biopsy for 4–6 weeks only in this age group. Surgical excision of the lymph node for histological examination should be performed after the elapsed time, provided that an extensive clinical and laboratory investigation of possible causal factors has yielded negative results and, most importantly, the lymph node tumefaction has not subsided. Cytohistological correlation shows that several pathological conditions can be responsible for this pattern. These are described below.

4.5.2.1 Non-Specific Reactive Lymph Node Hyperplasia

The lack of tingible-body histiocytes in the FNB sample of an enlarged lymph node with reactive lymphoid hyperplasia is generally due to poor or no activation of the follicular B-cell compartment and, conversely, to an expansion of the paracortical T-dependent areas and a consequent "diffuse" pattern on histological examination. This histological picture is typical of several conditions and the exact causal factor often remains undiscovered despite an extensive clinical work-up. The presence of a significant histiocytic component in which these cells contain lipid or hemosiderin in their cytoplasm is not unusual in FNB samples but often of no diagnostic significance. The detection of melanin pigment can suggest the diagnosis of dermatopathic lymphadenopathy, in the proper clinical context (Fig. 4.16) [29]. In addition, Rosai-Dorfman disease can present with this cytological pattern, in which case the diagnosis is based on detection of the characteristic histiocytes showing prominent lymphophagocytosis [30].

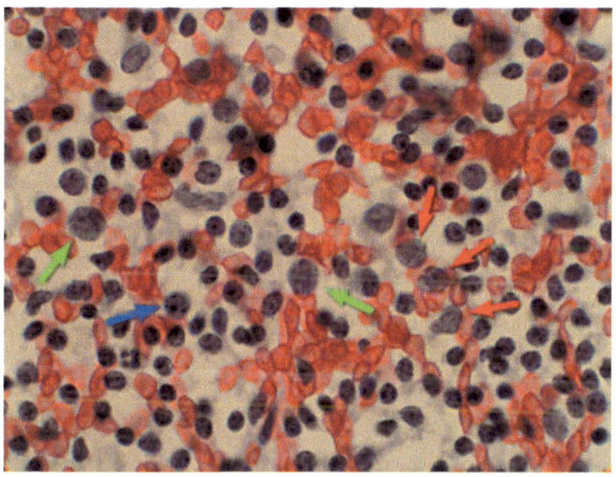

Fig. 4.15 A polymorphous cellular population consisting of small lymphocytes (*blue arrows*), large centrocytes (*red arrows*), and centroblasts (*green arrows*). Tingible-body histiocytes are absent. P stain, ×1000

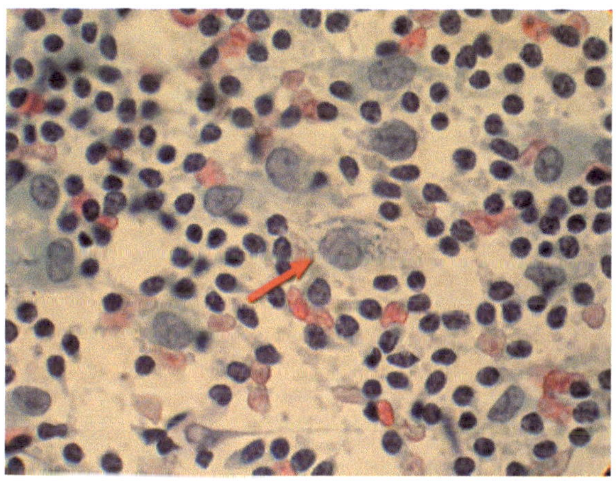

Fig. 4.16 Histiocyte-like cells admixed to small lymphocytes are seen in FNB smears from dermatopathic lymphadenopathy. The *arrow* points to a cell containing melanin granular pigment in the cytoplasm. P stain, x1000

4.5.2.2 Reactive Lymph Node Hyperplasia with Florid Immunoblastic Proliferation

FNB sampling of enlarged lymph nodes in patients with infectious mononucleosis [31,32] or HIV infection [33,34] can show this cytological pattern, in which there may also be a significant proliferation of immunoblasts–otherwise unusual in a conventional reactive lymph node. The proportion of immunoblasts in the cellular harvest should not exceed, by definition, 40%. Proper correlation with serological and clinical findings is generally required to make a correct diagnosis, obviating the need for tissue biopsy and allowing the prompt initiation of treatment.

4.5.2.3 Necrotizing Histiocytic Lymphadenitis, Kikuchi Type

Kikuchi-Fujimoto lymphadenitis is typically seen in laterocervical and supraclavicular locations in young patients and is generally a localized disease [35]. It is self-limited and may be associated with systemic symptoms. Histologically, the affected lymph node shows a necrotizing process characterized by patchy or confluent coagulative necrosis, with karyorrhexis and an absence or paucity of granulocytes. There is also a proliferation of large cells consisting of a mixture of T-lymphocytes and histiocytes. On FNB, the cytological picture is that of a polymorphous lymphoid population with abundant karyorrhectic debris and histiocytes, many of which show a small and eccentrically placed crescent-shaped nucleus (Fig. 4.17) [36–38]. In many cases, however, these diagnostic features are lacking such that these samples are indistinguishable from those of other nonspecific reactive lymphadenopathies. Because of the morphological similarities between lupus lymphadenitis and Kikuchi's lymphadenitis, however, serology studies are warranted to exclude systemic lupus erythematosus [35].

4.5.2.4 Non-Hodgkin's Lymphomas, B-Cell Type

In FNB samples, some variants of mature B-cell neoplasms, namely, low-grade variants of follicular lymphoma and diffuse large B-cell lymphoma, can show a polymorphous small- and large-cell pattern in which tingible-body histiocytes are absent. The harvest from lymph nodes harboring follicular lymphomas grade 1 or 2 consists of small lymphocytes, small centrocytes, centroblasts, and, rarely, immunoblasts [28]. The relative amount of centroblasts and immunoblasts, which account for the large-cell component, is definitely <40% (Fig. 4.18). The only suggestion of possible lymphoma in the smear is the frequent detection of pseudoaggregations of lymphoid cells. Cells with larger vesicular nuclei are intimately admixed with lymphoid cells within these

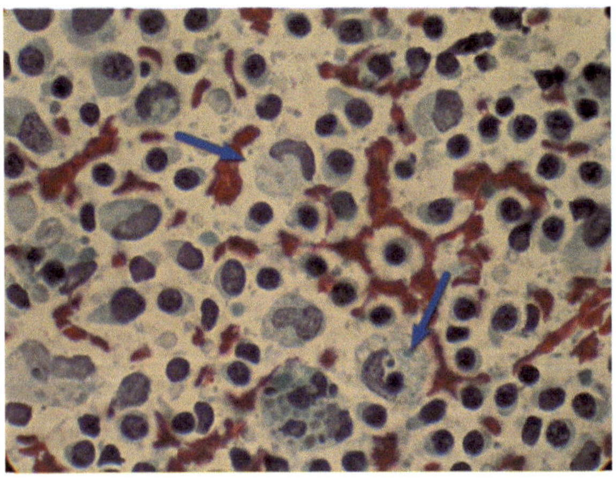

Fig. 4.17 Numerous histiocytic cells, each with a large and sometimes crescenteric nucleus (*blue arrows*). The cells contain phagocytosed globoid structures in their cytoplasm, a characteristic finding in necrotizing Kikuchi-type lymphadenitis. P stain, ×1000

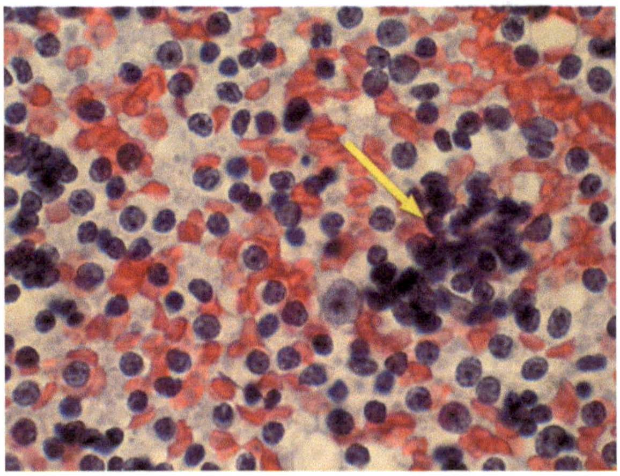

Fig. 4.18 Cytological appearance of follicular lymphoma. The harvest contains centroblasts and centrocytes that sometimes appear in pseudoaggregates (*yellow arrow*). P stain, ×1000

aggregations and correspond to reticular dendritic cells. Likewise, FNB sampling of diffuse large B-cell lymphomas often fails to disclose a significant component of large cells, and the cytological picture falls in the category of the polymorphous small- and large-cell pattern.

4.5.2.5 Nodular, Lymphocyte-Predominant Hodgkin's Lymphoma

This variant of Hodgkin's lymphoma mostly occurs in young and middle-aged patients. The clinical onset is marked by localised lymph node involvement (mainly in the neck, inguinal area, and axilla), and the patient reports a history of a slowly growing and asymptomatic mass [39]. Histologically, the tumor consists of a nodular proliferation of small lymphocytes admixed with intermediate-size histiocyte-like cells with a vesicular nucleus that looks multilobed due to multiple deep membrane foldings and contains small nucleoli [37,39]. These cells represent lymphohistiocytic (LH) Hodgkin's cells. Classical Reed-Sternberg cells are not present. In FNB samples, LH cells can be completely lacking [40]. When present, they are easily misinterpreted as conventional histiocytes or hypertrophic endothelial cells and generally are overlooked (Fig. 4.19). Tingible-body histiocytes are never seen. The cellular harvest may include small lymphocytes, plasma cells, centroblast-like cells, and the overall morphological picture is classified within a polymorphous small- and large-cell pattern. The diagnosis of Hodgkin's lymphoma is generally obtained upon histological investigation of the excised lymph node.

4.5.3 Polymorphous Cell Pattern, Large Cells Prevalent

The cytological picture is characterized by a mixture of small lymphocytes and large lymphoid elements, with the latter component representing >40% of the harvest population. When examining the smear at high-power magnification, one should pay close attention to the size of each cell type present and evaluate the prevalence of cells measuring >2×RBC in their largest diameter in at least ten high-power fields. Large lymphoid elements may consist of large centrocytes, centroblasts and/or immunoblasts, plasmablasts or immature plasma cells, Burkitt-type blasts, or large unclassified blastic cells. By definition, the size of these cells almost never exceeds 4×RBC. They are intimately admixed with small lymphocytes and small centrocytes (Fig. 4.20). A marked morphological similarity among the large cells may occur, which confers an overall monomorphous appearance to the cellular harvest. Ancillary cells may even include occasional tingible-body histiocytes or histiocytes containing lipoid material, hemosiderin pigment, or other phagocytosed products, as well as endothelial cells. In some actively growing tumor

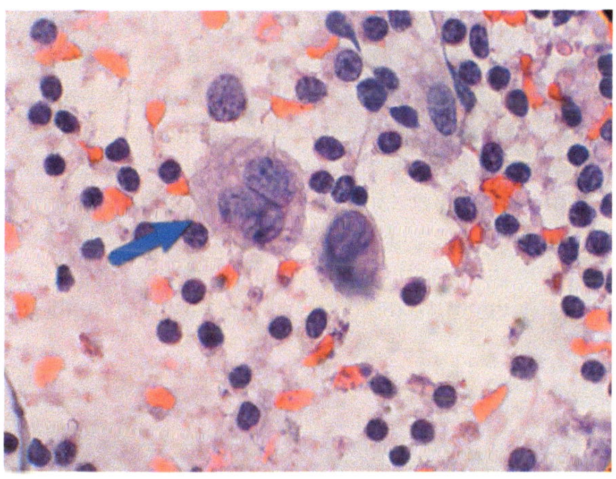

Fig. 4.19 Cytological appearance of a lymphohistiocytic (LH) Hodgkin's cell (*blue arrow*). The cell is large and contains a voluminous nucleus, with multiple infoldings of the nuclear membrane and small nucleoli. P stain, ×1000

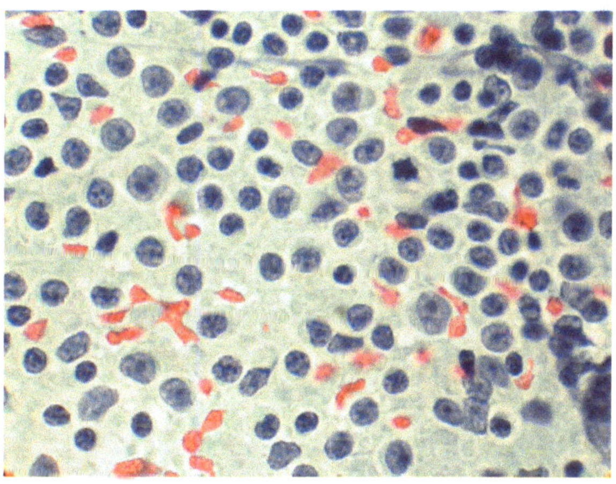

Fig. 4.20 A polymorphous cell population with a prevalence of large cells representing >40% of the harvest. Scattered small lymphocytes are seen in the background. P stain, ×1000

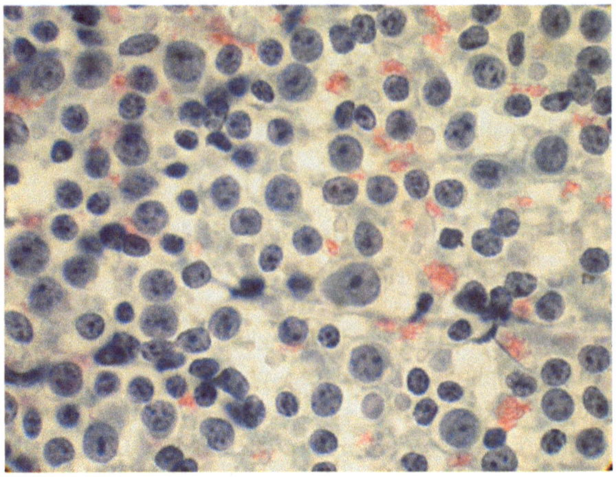

Fig. 4.21 The large majority of cells shown here are immunoblasts and centroblasts. P stain, ×1000

variants, a large number of histiocytes containing entirely apoptotic lymphocytes can be observed; these are not to be confused with tingible-body histiocytes. The background often contains apoptotic bodies, necrotic debris, and aggregates of amorphous highly basophilic material (Fig. 4.21).

Cytohistological correlation discloses that the polymorphous cell pattern with prevalent large lymphoid cells is typical of malignant lymphoma. In fact, reactive lymphoid hyperplasia hardly ever contains a large-cell component exceeding 40% of the harvest. By far, the most commonly detected lymphomas presenting with this pattern belong to the group of mature B-cell neoplasms and are represented by the diffuse large B-cell non-Hodgkin's lymphoma and its variants, large B-cell lymphoma of the mediastinum, and Burkitt's lymphoma.

4.5.3.1 Diffuse Large B-Cell Non-Hodgkin's Lymphoma

Diffuse large B-cell non-Hodgkin's lymphoma is the most frequently detected lymphoid malignancy worldwide, accounting for just over 30% of all cases [41]. The peak incidence is in the seventh decade of life, with a slight prevalence of males over females; the disease almost never occurs in pediatric patients. Patients can present with nodal or extranodal involvement. The clinical onset is generally marked by a rapidly progressive disease associated with "B symptoms" (slight fever, night sweating, asthenia, etc.). Histologically, the tumor is characterized by a diffuse proliferation of medium to large lymphoid cells with a large nucleus displaying a round, cleaved, multilobed, or "floret-like" profile, and containing two to three nucleoli or a single and prominent and centrally located nucleolus. The counterparts of these cells in cytological preparations are large centrocytes, centroblasts, and immunoblasts. In some variants, the cells can contain up to five nucleoli and appear definitely bizarre (Burkitt-like and anaplastic variants). Immunohistochemically, the tumor cells display a B-cell phenotype (CD20+/CD79a+/CD3-) and are consistently positive for CD10, inconsistently positive for bcl-2, and infrequently positive for CD5 [42]. Co-expression of these latter two markers seems to confer a worse prognosis [43]. CD30 can be expressed in the anaplastic variant [42]. Genetic studies are not required for the diagnosis. Since the differential diagnosis includes several entities, immunohistochemistry is of help in problem solving (Table 4.5).

The *mediastinal large B-cell lymphoma* is a subtype of diffuse large B-cell lymphoma of putative thymic B-cell origin [41,44]. It is seen in young adults, with a slight female prevalence. Patients generally present with signs and symptoms relating to a large anterior mediastinal mass, often causing superior vena cava syndrome. The tumor is frequently diffusely necrotic and/or undergoes massive sclerosis, thus precluding a definitive diagnosis by percutaneous FNB [45]. The tumor cells are large and pleomorphic with an amphiphilic cytoplasm (Fig. 4.22) that looks clear only in tissue sections prepared from a core biopsy.

Early intensive treatment of this form of lymphoma

Table 4.5 Differential diagnosis of large B-cell lymphoma

Carcinoma	CD45-/CK+ or CK-/EMA+
Melanoma	CD45-/CK-/S100P+/HMB45+ and/or Melan-A+
Anaplastic large-cell lymphoma T-cell type	CD45+/CD3+/CD30+/CD20-/EMA+ or -/CK-
Plasma cell myeloma	CD45±/CD20-/CD3-/CD138+/CD31+
Myeloid sarcoma	CD45-/CD20-/CD3-/CK-/S100P-/MPO+/CD68+

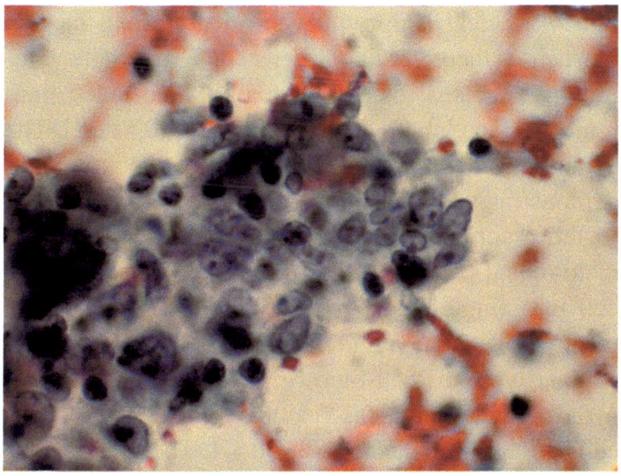

Fig. 4.22 In large cell B-cell lymphoma of the mediastinum, the neoplastic elements tend to form syncytial-like aggregates and are characterized by a vesicular chromatin with prominent nucleoli. P stain, ×1000

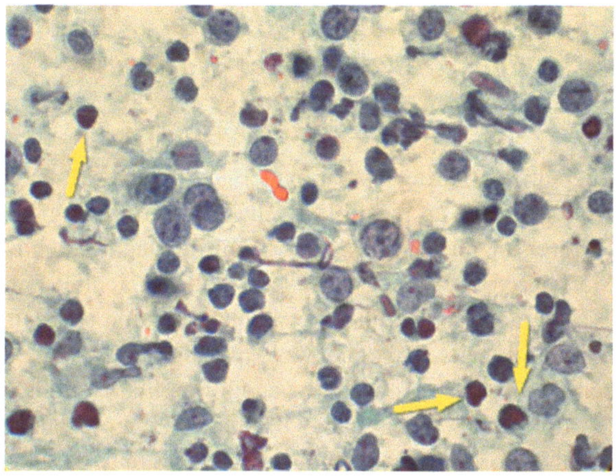

Fig. 4.23 In samples from Burkitt lymphoma, numerous blast cells are admixed with apoptotic nuclei (*yellow arrows*) and small lymphocytes. P stain, ×1000

is generally followed by a good response and complete remission [44], making prompt diagnosis by FNB of paramount importance.

In FNB samples, *follicular lymphoma grade 3* is practically indistinguishable from diffuse large B-cell lymphoma because of the enormous component of proliferating centroblasts. The smear may also contain an additional polymorphous cellular population, including small lymphocytes and small and large centrocytes, perhaps with pseudoaggregation. This picture is also seen in cases of diffuse large B-cell lymphoma arising secondarily in patients with follicular lymphoma.

4.5.3.2 Burkitt's Lymphoma

This highly aggressive malignancy occurs endemically in equatorial Africa and sporadically throughout the world in children and young adults [46]. An AIDS related variant has also been described [47]. The tumor consists of a diffuse proliferation of intermediate to large blast cells somewhat monotonous in appearance. In FNB samples, the nuclei of these cells are round, the chromatin is coarsely granular, and two to five basophilic nucleoli are detected (Figs. 4.8, 4.23) [48]. The cytoplasmic rim is minimal and looks basophilic or slightly vacuolated. Cytoplasmic vacuoles are much better seen on air-dried smears stained with May Grünwald Giemsa stain. There is evidence of apoptosis and mitotic figures are frequent as well (Fig. 4.23). Other lymphoid elements include small lymphocytes and rare plasma cells. Eosinophils are not infrequently detected. Ancillary cells consist of abundant histiocytes that have ingested apoptotic cells; as noted above, these cells are not to be confused with tingible-body histiocytes.

4.5.3.3 Lymph Node Involvement by Plasma Cell Myeloma

Multiple myeloma in patients with disease of advanced stage can localize within lymph nodes. Although a rare occurrence, it is well-documented in the literature and several cases have been diagnosed by FNB. The medium to large tumor cells are characterized by large nuclei with a prominent centrally located nucleolus and a sparse cytoplasm. Necrosis may be prominent. The overall morphology of the cellular infiltrate is much more similar to that of diffuse large B-cell neoplasms. Lymph node involvement by plasma cell myeloma should be differentiated from primary extramedullary plasmacytoma arising in the lymph nodes [49]. The latter tumors are differentially distinguished by the characteristic proliferation of mature plasma cells [50].

4.5.4 Polymorphous Cell Pattern, Small Cells Prevalent, with Scattered Large Atypical Blasts

The salient finding in this pattern is the presence of scattered large atypical blast cells with morphological features of mononucleated or multinucleated Reed-Sternberg cells as well as large and atypical B- or T-immunoblasts within a prevalent population of small lymphoid cells (lymphocytes, plasma cells, small centrocytes, rare centroblasts, and inflammatory cells). By definition, the atypical blastic cells represent a small minority of the cellular harvest and may be very sparse, detected after an extensive search. In fact, atypical blast cells are the only malignant cell component within the harvest whereas the polymorphous small-cell population is reactive in nature. FNB sampling reveals three main disease entities with this cytological pattern. Their overlapping morphological features often preclude their distinction unless proper immunohistochemical studies are performed.

4.5.4.1 Classical Hodgkin's Lymphoma

The four subtypes of classical Hodgkin's lymphoma differ with respect to the site of disease involvement, clinical presentation, growth pattern, composition of the cellular background, number of atypical neoplastic cells, and/or their degree of atypia [39]. In all four subtypes, the neoplastic cell component, i.e., mononuclear Hodgkin's cells and multinucleated Reed-Sternberg cells, resides in a reactive infiltrate containing a polymorphous population of small lymphocytes, plasma cells, and inflammatory cells. The subtypes vary widely in the morphology of their component neoplastic cells and the composition of the reactive infiltrate. The morphology of Reed-Sternberg cells differs in cytological preparations depending on whether the tissue section has been formalin-fixed or paraffin embedded. In particular, in histological preparations, at least four variants of these cells have been recognized (diagnostic, mononuclear, lacunar, and pleomorphic) according to their nuclear profile, nucleolar appearance and size, nuclear membrane thickness, and cytoplasmic features [37,39]. In smears, the likelihood of examining the cells in their entirety allows for a better and more accurate evaluation of nuclear and cytoplasmic features. In fact, in most cases these very large cells contain a single voluminous nucleus that is actually subdivided into multiple deep lobes (Figs. 4.10–4.12) [40,51,52]. The examination of such cells on multiple focus planes demonstrates that each lobe is nonetheless connected to the others such that the multinucleation seen in histological preparations is an artifact of viewing the cell in a single tissue section. Moreover, in smears, the cytoplasm never looks clear or empty; thus, a lacunar type of Reed-Sternberg cell cannot be recognized. The cytological features of Reed-Sternberg cells are listed in detail in Table 4.4. These large cells with their voluminous nuclei appear as isolated elements in the smear and stand out, due to their size and peculiar morphology, against a background of reactive small cells (Figs. 4.10–4.12). Each nuclear lobe or each nucleus contains a prominent nucleolus surrounded by clear chromatin. The size and number of the nucleoli can vary greatly. Pleomorphic and bizarre cells are also recognized (Fig. 4.24). The background may contain numerous plasma cells, eosinophilic granulocytes, endothelial cells, and fibroblasts but characteristically lacks a significant component of follicular center cells (especially centroblasts) or tingible-body histiocytes. There may be numerous epithelioid cells, imparting a typical lymphoepithelioid appearance to the harvest. Stromal fragments composed of fibrocytes and collagen are commonly present. The cellular harvest is often poor due to intralesional sclerosis and/or necrosis, such that a diagnosis cannot be rendered. The above considerations

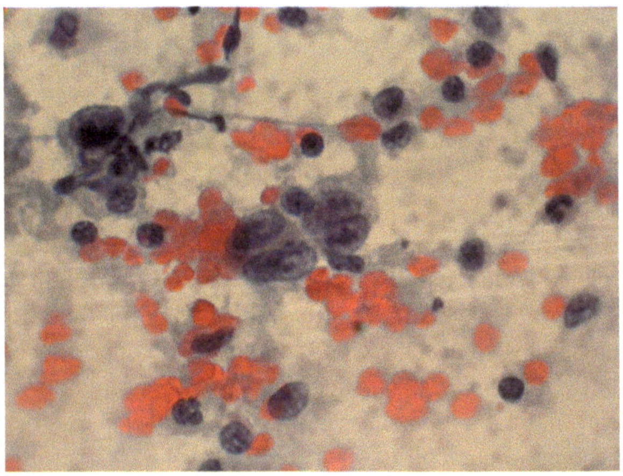

Fig. 4.24 A pleomorphic Reed-Sternberg cell containing multiple nucleoli and a fragile cytoplasm. P stain, ×1000

explain why FNB sampling does not distinguish among the four subtypes of classical Hodgkin's lymphoma: lymphocyte-rich, nodular sclerosis, mixed cellularity, and lymphocyte depleted. In general, in FNB samples these subtypes differ regarding the number of atypical blast cells, the composition of the reactive infiltrate, and the amount of cellularity, although these differences do not play a relevant diagnostic role. A cytohistological correlation demonstrates only that the nodular sclerosis and mixed cellularity subtypes are characterized by a more polymorphous reactive component and a sufficient number of diagnostically atypical cells, while the lymphocyte-depleted subtype is characterized by the poor cellularity of the harvest, which includes pleomorphic and bizarre cells against a necrotic background. Finally, the lymphocyte-rich subtype can be marked by sparse or no Reed-Sternberg cells, entering the differential diagnosis with other lymphomas. Since a conclusive diagnosis of Hodgkin's lymphoma relies on a demonstration of the peculiar immunohistochemical reactivity of Reed-Sternberg cells, a concomitant CNB of the lymph node and a representative cellular sample are needed. Reed-Sternberg cells display the unusual CD45-/CD30+ profile and coexpress CD15 and CD20 in, respectively, about 75 and 50% of cases [39,53]. CD30 immunohistochemical positivity is typically accentuated along the external membrane and appears as a dot-like cytoplasmic accumulation. PAX-5 positivity in these cells is an additional finding with a promising diagnostic role [54].

4.5.4.2 T-Cell/Histiocyte-Rich Large B-Cell Lymphoma

In this variant of large B-cell lymphoma, the majority of the cells are small lymphocytes of T-cell lineage, with or without a significant number of histiocytes; neoplastic B-cells comprise <10% of the entire population [41]. The large cells may resemble large centroblasts, immunoblasts (Fig. 4.25), or Reed-Sternberg-like cells, and the reactive ancillary component consists of small lymphocytes and rare plasma cells. This variant can be accurately diagnosed by FNB complemented by ancillary techniques aimed at identifying the clonality of the large cells of B-cell lineage [15,17,23]. The differential diagnosis includes nodular lymphocyte-predominant Hodgkin's lymphoma and the lymphocyte-rich subtype of classical Hodgkin's lymphoma.

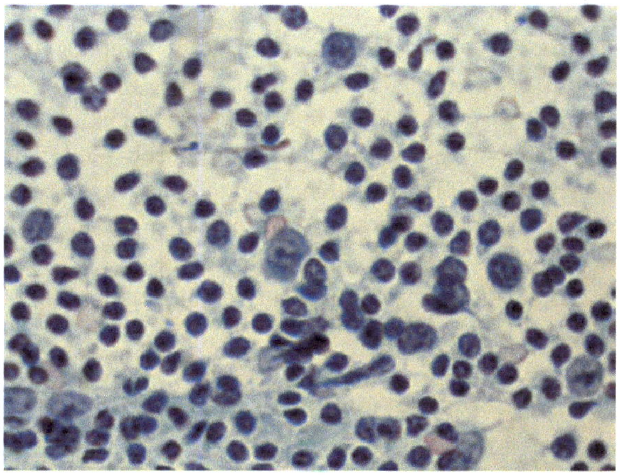

Fig. 4.25 In samples from T-cell-rich B-cell lymphomas, the harvest is characterized by scattered large cells of immunoblastic type and a prevalent population of small lymphocytes. P stain, ×1000

4.5.4.3 Peripheral T-Cell Lymphoma, Anaplastic Large-Cell Type

CD30+ anaplastic large-cell lymphoma can overlap morphologically with Hodgkin's lymphoma, especially when the neoplastic elements simulate pleomorphic Reed-Sternberg cells and appear in the smear scattered within a polymorphous lymphoid infiltrate mainly composed of small lymphocytes and plasma cells [52]. A correct diagnosis is based on the immunohistochemical typing of tumor cells, which show a CD45+/CD15-/CD30+/CD3+/CD20- profile [39].

4.5.5 Monomorphic, Small Lymphoid Cell Pattern

The main feature of this pattern is the marked prevalence (>80–90%) within the sample of a cellular component consisting of small lymphoid cells showing moderate to marked monomorphism. There is abundant cellularity against a background that is clean or moderately contaminated by blood. A survey of the smear at intermediate to high power demonstrates that the harvest is dominated by a single cellular component composed of small cells (<2×RBC) with the cytological features of small lymphocytes, small centrocytes, or lymphoplasmocytoid lymphocytes. These cells are admixed with a small minority of plasma cells, granulocytes, or epithelioid histiocytes. The monomorphous, small lymphoid cell pattern is seen in about 90% of malignant lymphomas of different types but in no more than 10% of benign conditions, specifically, reactive lymphoid hyperplasia. The positive predictive value of this pattern thus is about 90%.

4.5.5.1 Chronic Lymphocytic Leukemia/Small Lymphocytic Lymphoma

This type of mature B-cell neoplasm is typically seen in patients older than 50 years of age and has a definite male prevalence. The clinical onset is marked by a generalized lymphadenopathy, with splenomegaly and involvement of the bone marrow and peripheral blood. The lymphocyte count is generally $>10\times10^9$/L [55]. Histologically, the architecture of the involved lymph node is totally obliterated by the presence of a diffuse or focally pseudofollicular proliferation of small lymphocytes of monotonous morphology. Both in tissue sections and FNB samples, the neoplastic cell population consists of small lymphocytes with round nuclei, dense chromatin, and a barely evident cytoplasmic rim (Fig. 4.26). Pseudofollicles in tissue sections represent foci of cellular proliferations in which the cells are slightly pleomorphic and larger than the surrounding small and monomorphic neoplastic cells. In smears, these latter elements, referred to as "paraimmunoblasts," are easily discerned and appear to be randomly dispersed within the cellular harvest. The diameter of these cells can exceed 2×RBC; the chromatin is dispersed within the nuclei, which contain small nucleoli, and the cytoplasm is sparse but easily recognizable (Fig. 4.27). Immunohistochemical examination of CNB or needle-rinse samples shows small lymphoid cells positive for the B-cell markers CD20 and CD79a and with the additional profile CD5+/CD10-/CD23+/CD43+. Follicular dendritic cells expressing CD21 are sparse or absent [55]. Molecular studies, which can be performed in cytological preparations or core biopsies, show a monoclonal IgH rearrangement [18,19,23].

4.5.5.2 Lymphoplasmacytic Lymphoma/ Waldenstrom 's Macroglobulinemia

This neoplasm of mature B-cells consists of a proliferation of small lymphocytes, plasmacytoid lymphocytes, and plasma cells. The lymph nodes, bone marrow, and spleen are usually involved and there is a characteristic production of a monoclonal IgM serum paraprotein [55,56]. In FNB samples collected from affected lymph nodes, the cellular harvest is

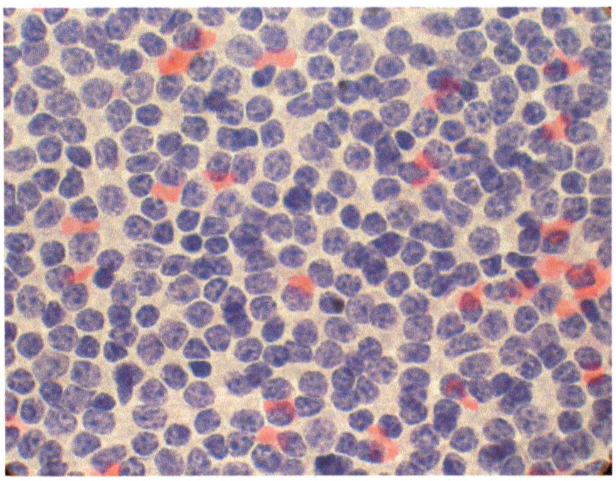

Fig. 4.26 In samples from B-cell-type small lymphocytic lymphoma/chronic lymphocytic leukemia. the harvest is composed of a monotonous population of small lymphocytes with a round nucleus, a finely granular or stippled chromatin, and sparse cytoplasm. P stain, ×1000

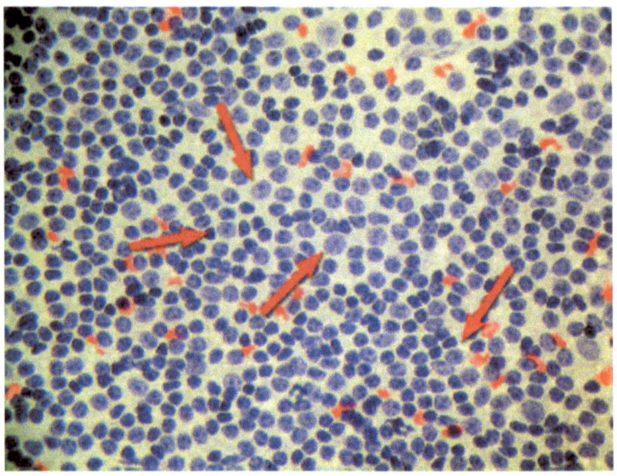

Fig. 4.27 In samples from B-cell-type small lymphocytic lymphoma/chronic lymphocytic leukemia, it may be possible to observe scattered larger cells displaying a small nucleolus and a larger amount of cytoplasm (*red arrows*). P stain, ×600

dominated by a monotonous population of small lymphocytes as well as plasmacytoid lymphocytes and a significant component of mature plasma cells (Fig. 4.28). Cells express the B-cell associated antigens CD20 and CD79a and are CD5-/CD10-/CD23-. Positivity for CD138 is an additional immunohistochemical finding [57].

4.5.5.3 Mantle Cell Lymphoma, Classical Variant

Mantle cell lymphoma is a mature B-cell neoplasm generally occurring in middle-aged and older adults, with a male predominance. A marked and disseminated lymph node involvement dominates the clinical picture at disease onset and is generally associated with splenomegaly, bone marrow involvement, and possible extranodal disease [58]. In FNB samples (Fig. 4.28), the neoplastic population mainly consists of monomorphic lymphoid cells with markedly irregular nuclear profiles due to multiple and deep clefts. The chromatin is rather dense or coarsely granular, no prominent nucleoli are detected in the nucleus, and the cytoplasm is sparse or barely evident. The size of these cells generally does not exceed 2×RBC. Additional cell components are small lymphocytes, plasma cells, endothelial cells, and histiocytes. The general appearance of the smear is that of a marked cellular monomorphism (Fig. 4.28). Immunohistochemical evaluation in CNB or needle-rinse samples discloses, other than expression of the B-cell associated markers CD20 and CD79a, the profile CD5+/CD10-/CD23- [59]. The additional expression of cyclin D1 or, better, demonstration of the t(11;14)(q13;q32)(bcl-1) translocation by molecular genetic analyses provides confirmatory evidence for the diagnosis [16,17]. As mantle cell lymphoma is a rather aggressive malignancy, its distinction from other lymphomas composed of small lymphocytes is of utmost importance.

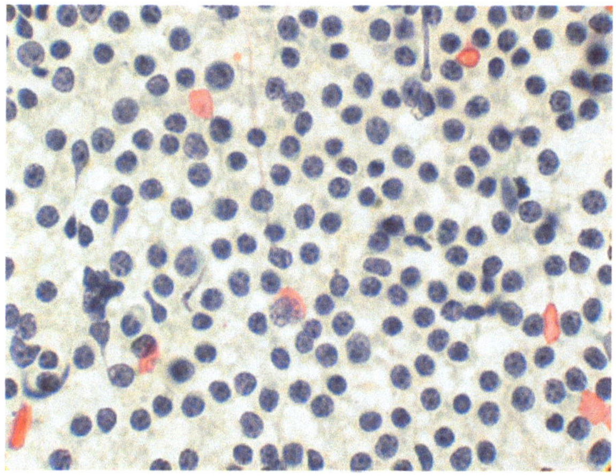

Fig. 4.28 In B-cell non-Hodgkin's lymphoma, mantle cell type, the harvest consists of a monotonous population of small cells with an irregularly shaped and cleaved nucleus. P stain, ×1000

4.5.5.4 Follicular Lymphoma, Grades 1 and 2

Follicular lymphoma mainly affects middle-aged adults and without a sex predominance. The clinical onset is characterized by lymph node enlargement in multiple sites (mainly the neck and retroperitoneum) and frequently by concomitant splenomegaly and bone marrow involvement [60]. Histologically, the lymph node architecture is effaced by a nodular, or nodular and diffuse proliferation of centrocytes and centroblasts. In FNB samples, the cellular population is similarly composed of small lymphocytes, plasmacytoid lymphocytes, small and large centrocytes, centroblasts, and occasional immunoblasts [7,8,12,14,59]. The prevalence of cell types is variable according to the histological grade of the tumor [60]. The three-grade system is based on the absolute number of centroblasts in ten neoplastic follicles counted per 40× high-power microscopic field (hpf). Grade 1 and 2 lesions have, respectively, 0–5 and 6–15 centroblasts/hpf. In fact, the cytological harvest obtained from tumors of histological grade 1 or 2 can show an overwhelming component of small cells (centrocytes and small lymphocytes) with sparse or absent centroblasts; thus, it is best classified within the monomorphic, small-cell-predominant cytological pattern (Fig. 4.29). The tendency of centrocytes to pseudoaggregation may be the only hint as to the diagnosis of follicular lymphoma (Fig. 4.30). A definitive diagnosis relies on the demonstration of the t(14;18)(q32;q21)bcl-2 translocation by means of molecular genetic studies in cytological or microhistological specimens [17,61]. Immunohistochemically, small cells express the B-cell markers CD20 and CD79a as well as the profile CD5-/CD10+/CD23±. Immunohistochemical and DNA-ploidy studies can contribute to determining the grade of this lymphoma also on cytological samples [62].

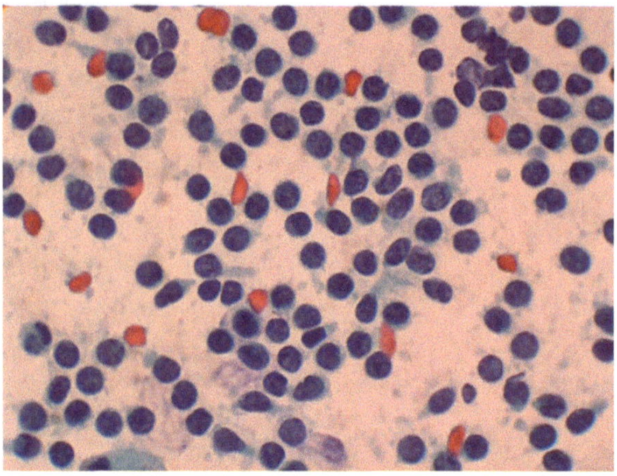

Fig. 4.29 In follicular B-cell lymphoma, grade 1, the harvest mainly consists of a population of small centrocytes and lymphocytes. P stain, ×1000

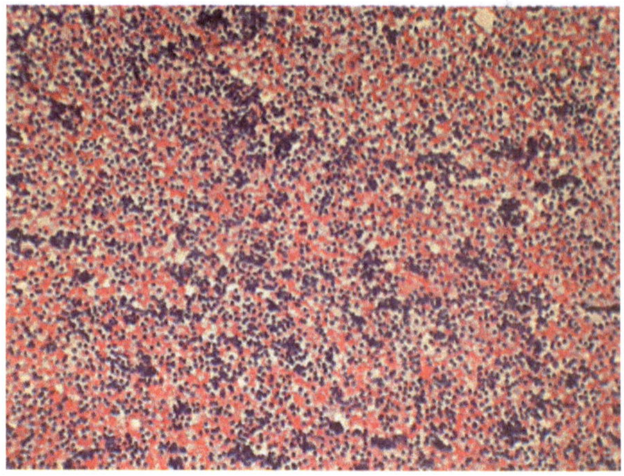

Fig. 4.30 In follicular B-cell lymphoma, grade 1, the only hint to the correct diagnosis is obtained by observing, at medium microscopic power, the tendency of cells to form pseudoaggregates. P stain, ×400

4.5.5.5 Marginal Zone Lymphoma

Marginal zone lymphoma is mainly an extranodal malignancy; a concomitant lymph node involvement occurs in only a small minority of cases. Primary sites of involvement include the mucosa-associated lymphoid tissue in the gastrointestinal tract, the lung, ocular adnexae, thyroid, salivary glands, and breast [39,40,63]. A primary splenic involvement is also recognized [41]. Significant lymph node enlargement occurs late in the course of the disease [64]. Retroperitoneal lymph nodes may be sampled by FNB even if a primary lesion in the stomach or small intestine has not been recognized yet [32]. Likewise, a concomitant cervical lymph node enlargement may be detected in patients with marginal zone lymphoma in the thyroid or salivary glands and the sampling of these lymph nodes contributes to a definitive diagnosis. The appearance of the cellular harvest is best classified within the monomorphic, small-cell-predominant pattern (Fig. 4.31). In fact, the cellular harvest consists of small lymphocytes with irregular nuclei resembling those of centrocytes, finely granular chromatin, inconspicuous nucleoli, and sparse cytoplasm. Additional cells include small monocytoid cells, small lymphocytes, but few if any plasma cells. Immunohistochemically, the cells express the B-cell markers CD20 and CD79a and are non-reactive for CD5, CD10, and CD23 [65]. A conclusive diagnosis is based upon demonstration of a monoclonal IgH gene rearrangement by molecular studies.

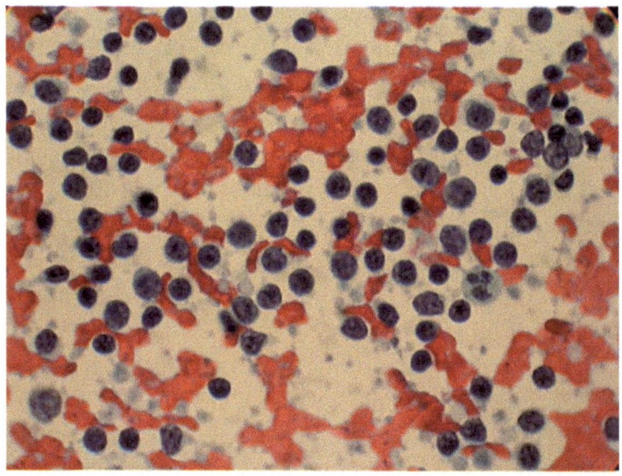

Fig. 4.31 In B-cell lymphoma, marginal zone type, the harvest contains a monotonous population of small to medium-sized cells with an irregularly shaped (centrocyte-like) nucleus and very sparse cytoplasm. P stain, ×1000

4.5.5.6 Nodular Lymphocyte-Predominant Hodgkin's Lymphoma

The clinical and pathological features of this variant of Hodgkin's lymphoma were discussed in an earlier section of this chapter. Nonetheless, it is worth

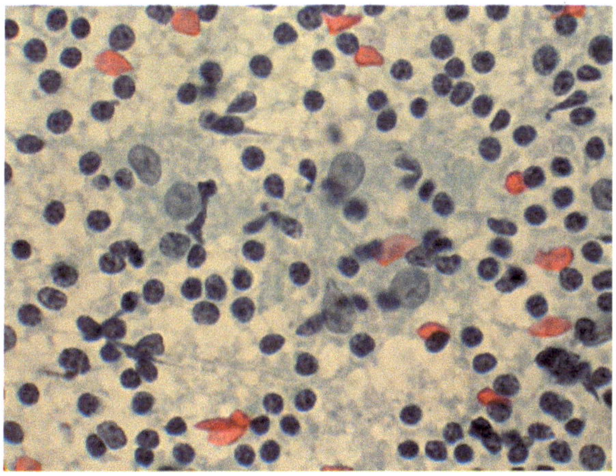

Fig. 4.32 In this FNB sample obtained from a patient with lymphocyte-predominant Hodgkin's lymphoma, the cellular harvest consists of abundant epithelioid histiocytes and small lymphocytes with a "lymphoepithelioid" appearance. P stain, ×1000

emphasizing that the cellular infiltrate collected by FNB typically consists of an entirely monomorphic population of small lymphocytes [39], with only the occasional presence of larger cells expressing the features of LH cells, which, however, are often not recognized or are confused with conventional histiocytes or endothelial cells (Fig. 4.19). The morphological picture is thus of a monomorphic, small lymphoid cell pattern. There may also be a significant component of epithelioid histiocytes, thus imparting a lymphoepithelioid appearance to the cellular harvest (Fig. 4.32).

4.5.5.7 Diffuse Reactive Lymphoid Hyperplasia

A minority of samples with a monomorphic, small lymphoid cell pattern on FNB turn out to be reactive lymphoid hyperplasia upon histological evaluation of the excised lymph node. In these cases, there is prominent activation of the T-cell-dependent paracortical compartment of the lymph node. Histological criteria allow the benign nature of the lesion to be easily identified mainly because the lymph node architecture is not effaced. By contrast, cytological evaluation discloses a monomorphic population of small lymphocytes with a minor component of plasma cells. The ancillary cellular component may be made up of endothelial cells and histiocytes, with the latter sometimes containing melanin pigment granules in their cytoplasm (dermatopathic lymphadenopathy) [29].

4.5.6 *Pleomorphic, Small- and/or Large-Cell Pattern*

A pleomorphic sample contains a continuum of cells that differ in size, shape, or nuclear morphology but which are still recognizable as a single neoplastic cell type. Pleomorphism refers, for example, to cellular and nuclear size and thus to a continuum of small to medium-sized to large cells that share the same chromatin texture, nuclear profile, and nucleolar features. As an alternative, the cells may be approximately the same size and retain the same chromatin texture but their nuclei vary significantly in shape due to different extents of cleavage and convolution of the external membrane. FNB samples showing the above-described pleomorphic cell pattern represent malignant lymphomas of different types. Pleomorphism is associated with increased cell proliferation, apoptosis, and mitotic activity. The background often includes necrotic debris and the cells show frequent basophilic changes, with massive nuclear disintegration and fusion due to smearing artifacts.

4.5.6.1 Peripheral T-Cell Lymphoma, Unspecified

This is a heterogeneous group of malignant non-Hodgkin's lymphomas most often occurring in the elderly and in association with immune disorders [66]. The clinical onset is marked by the involvement of lymph nodes at multiple sites and concomitant general symptoms, including fever, weight loss, asthenia, and malaise. In FNB samples, the cellular harvest consists of atypical lymphoid cells showing slight to moderate variability in size, with variably convoluted nuclei containing coarsely granular chromatin and small nucleoli (Fig. 4.33) [67,68]. The amount of cytoplasm is also variable but tends to be sparse. Necrotic changes are seen, as are apoptotic bodies. Occasional large cells simulate Reed-Sternberg cells. The ancillary cell component comprises plasma cells, eosinophils, and endothelial cells. In some cases, there is a significant component of epithelioid histiocytes that may outnumber the lymphoid cells, thus

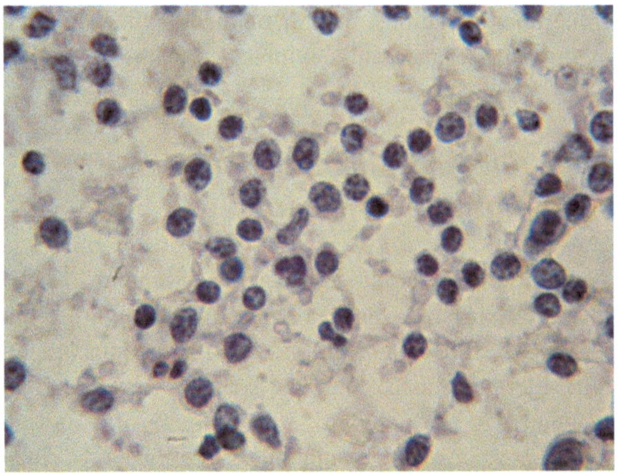

Fig. 4.33 In peripheral T-cell lymphoma, unspecified type, the harvest consists of a pleomorphic population of medium-sized cells showing a variably shaped nucleus with a coarsely granular chromatin. P stain, ×1000

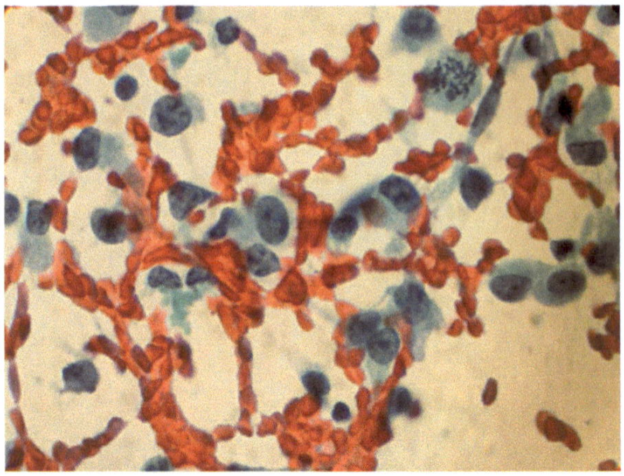

Fig. 4.34 In peripheral T-cell lymphoma, anaplastic cell type, the harvest consists of a pleomorphic population of large cells with large nuclei and well-evident cytoplasm. A mitotic figure is seen in the upper right side of the image. P stain, ×1000

producing a lymphoepithelioid smear. Immunohistochemically, the lymphoid cells variably express the T-cell markers CD3, CD4, and CD8 while larger cells may express CD30. A conclusive diagnosis relies on the detection of a T-γ gene rearrangement in microhistological specimens.

4.5.6.2 Peripheral T-Cell Lymphoma, Anaplastic Large-Cell Type

This lymphoma variant shows a peak of age incidence in the second and third decades of life. At clinical onset, there is a disseminated lymph node involvement as well as concomitant extranodal disease (in the skin, bone, soft tissues, and gastrointestinal tract). The bone marrow is also frequently involved [69]. In FNB samples, the lymphoid cells are medium to large in size with a moderate amount of cytoplasm. Their nuclei are large and kidney-shaped or more elongated and horseshoe-shaped and appear quite pleomorphic (Fig. 4.34) [70-72]. Multiple nucleoli are present. In a minority of cases, the cells form cohesive aggregates, thus simulating a metastatic epithelial malignancy of undifferentiated type. The background is rich in small lymphocytes, plasma cells, epithelioid histiocytes, eosinophils, and neutrophils. The ancillary component may outnumber the atypical lymphoid cells, giving rise to a cytological picture that may be classified as a polymorphous, small-lymphoid-cell-predominant pattern with scattered large atypical blasts. This picture is seen in the Hodgkin-like variant of anaplastic large-cell lymphoma [52]. A small-cell variant of this tumor is also recognized [73] and the cellular infiltrate in FNB is likely to resemble that of peripheral T-cell lymphoma, unspecified type. Immunohistochemical studies show that the anaplastic large cells have the profile CD45+/CD3+/CD20-/CD15-/CD30+ [69] (Fig. 4.35).

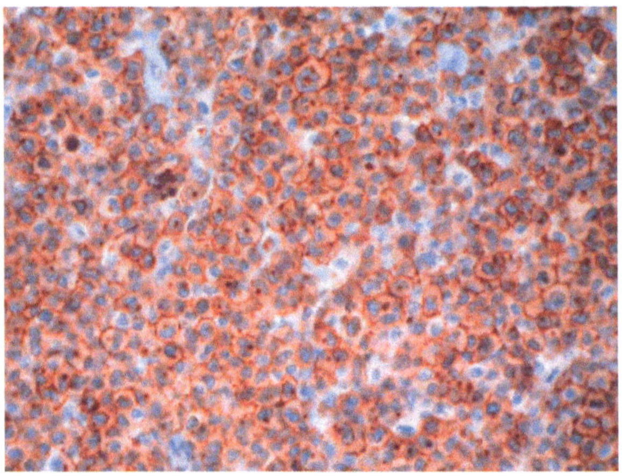

Fig. 4.35 Tissue section from a core biopsy of the same lymph node as shown in Fig. 4.34. Immunostaining for CD30 shows the peculiar membranous and dot-like positivity. Counterstained with hematoxylin, ×1000

In most of the cases occurring in young patients, tumor cells are found to coexpress anaplastic large-cell kinase (ALK) [69]. ALK positivity is more often seen in males and seems to predict a better response to chemotherapy. A T-γ gene rearrangement is detected in 60–70% of patients. The differential diagnosis of this tumor includes metastatic carcinoma, Hodgkin's lymphoma, and, occasionally, reactive lymphoid hyperplasia with florid immunoblastic proliferation.

4.5.6.3 Precursor B- and T-Lymphoblastic Leukemia/Lymphoma

These malignancies are rarely encountered in a non-hematological clinical context [74-76]. The distinction of lymphoma (for cases with predominant lymph node and visceral involvement) vs. leukemia (for cases with bone marrow and peripheral blood involvement) is purely academic since the two modalities always coexist and are variably expressed in the course of the disease. Both the B- and the T-type occur in the pediatric age group but the latter can occur in young adults and even elderly patients [74]. The lymphomatous variant affects the lymph nodes, soft tissues, skin, and viscera in general. An important site of involvement is the retroperitoneum, where a huge mass can be discovered at presentation. Upon FNB sampling, the lymphoid cells appear pleomorphic and of variable size (Fig. 4.36). B-lymphoblasts are generally characterized by round nuclei while T-lymphoblasts manifest varying degrees of convolution, but there are significant exceptions to this rule [12,13]. Apoptotic bodies are frequently detected in the background. Histiocytes containing entire cells or apoptotic bodies are also present. Immunohistochemical studies show that B-immunoblasts variably express the B-cell markers CD20 and CD79a and coexpress TdT and CD10. T-lymphoblasts are instead variably positive for CD3, CD4, and CD8 and may coexpress TdT and CD10. The most frequent sites of FNB sampling of these malignancies are the retroperitoneum, thyroid, and salivary glands [74-76].

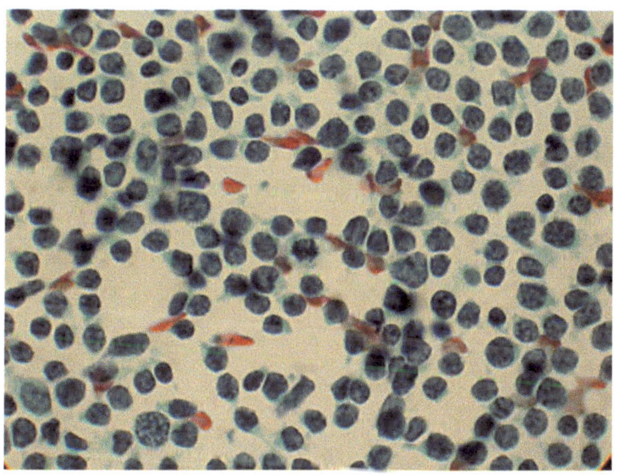

Fig. 4.36 In precursor-type, lymphobastic lymphoma, T-cell type, the cellular harvest is characterized by the prominent cellular pleomorphism. Some elements have a convoluted appearance. P stain, ×1000.

4.5.6.4 Mantle Cell B-Cell Lymphoma, Blastoid Variant

Mantle cell lymphoma can appear at presentation, but more commonly in recurring disease, with a characteristic pleomorphic cell pattern which is defined under the heading of "blastoid" variant. The proliferating cells which are small and resemble centrocytes in the classical variant, are intermediate to large in size in the blastoid variant. Moreover, the nuclei manifest varying degrees of convolution, with deep clefts and pronounced lobation, coarsely granular chromatin, and prominent nucleoli [77]. The occurrence of a concomitant leukemic involvement is intriguing and suggests a precursor B-lymphoblastic lymphoma. Immunohistochemical findings include positivity for CD20 and CD79a and a CD5+/CD10-/CD43+/cyclin D1+ profile. Molecular studies demonstrate a bcl-1 t(11;14) translocation and provide a conclusive diagnosis [16,21].

4.6 Concluding Remarks

The suggested approach to classifying cytological samples of lymph nodes collected by FNB is rooted firmly in morphology as a springboard for selecting the most likely diagnosis. Once the major pattern has been identified, the diagnostic possibilities are dramatically reduced. This is illustrated in Table 4.6, which shows the possible corresponding pattern profile(s) of most lymphoma variants and benign lymphoid proliferations. Pattern profiling of the cytological sample provides a basis to select the diagnostic possibilities

Table 4.6 Lymphoid lesion and possible corresponding cytological pattern profile

	Polymorphous, small- and large-cell, TBH+	Polymorphous, small- and large-cell, TBH-	Polymorphous, large-cell prevalent	Polymorphous, small-cell prevalent with atypical blast	Monomorphic, small-cell	Pleomorphic, small- and large-cell
LH, follicular	•	•				
LH, diffuse					•	
NHL, small lymphocytic/CLL					•	
NHL, lymphoplasmacytoid					•	
NHL, follicular, G2 and G2		•				
NHL, follicular, G3			•			
NHL, marginal zone					•	
NHL, mantle cell, classic v.					•	
NHL, mantle cell, blastoid v.						•
NHL, large B-cell, diffuse		•	•			
NHL, T-cell-rich B-cell type		•		•		
NHL, Burkitt type			•			
NHL, lymphoblastic B- / T-type						•
PTCL, pleom., small- / large-cell						•
PTCL, anaplastic large-cell type				•		•
HL, LP, nodular		•			•	
HL, Classical, MC				•		
HL, Classical, NS				•		
HL, NS, syncitial variant						•
HL, Classical, LR				•	•	
HL, Classical, LD						•

CLL chronic lymphocytic leukemia; *HL* Hodgkin's lymphoma; *LD* lymphocyte depleted; *LH* lymphoid hyperplasia; *LP* lymphocyte predominant; *LR* lymphocyte rich; *MC* mixed cellularity; *NHL* non-Hodgkin's lymphoma; *NS* nodular sclerosis; *PTCL* peripheral T-cell lymphoma; *TBH* tingible-body histiocytes.

and to build up a diagnostic algorithm to reach the most conclusive diagnosis. If required, one can decide to collect additional tissue samples by CNB of the lesion, with the aim of performing ancillary investigations such as immunohistochemistry or molecular biology. The importance of a prudent correlation with all available clinical data, finally, cannot be overemphasized. Figure 4.37 illustrates the most convenient diagnostic algorithm for the three patterns that offer the largest number of diagnostic possibilities.

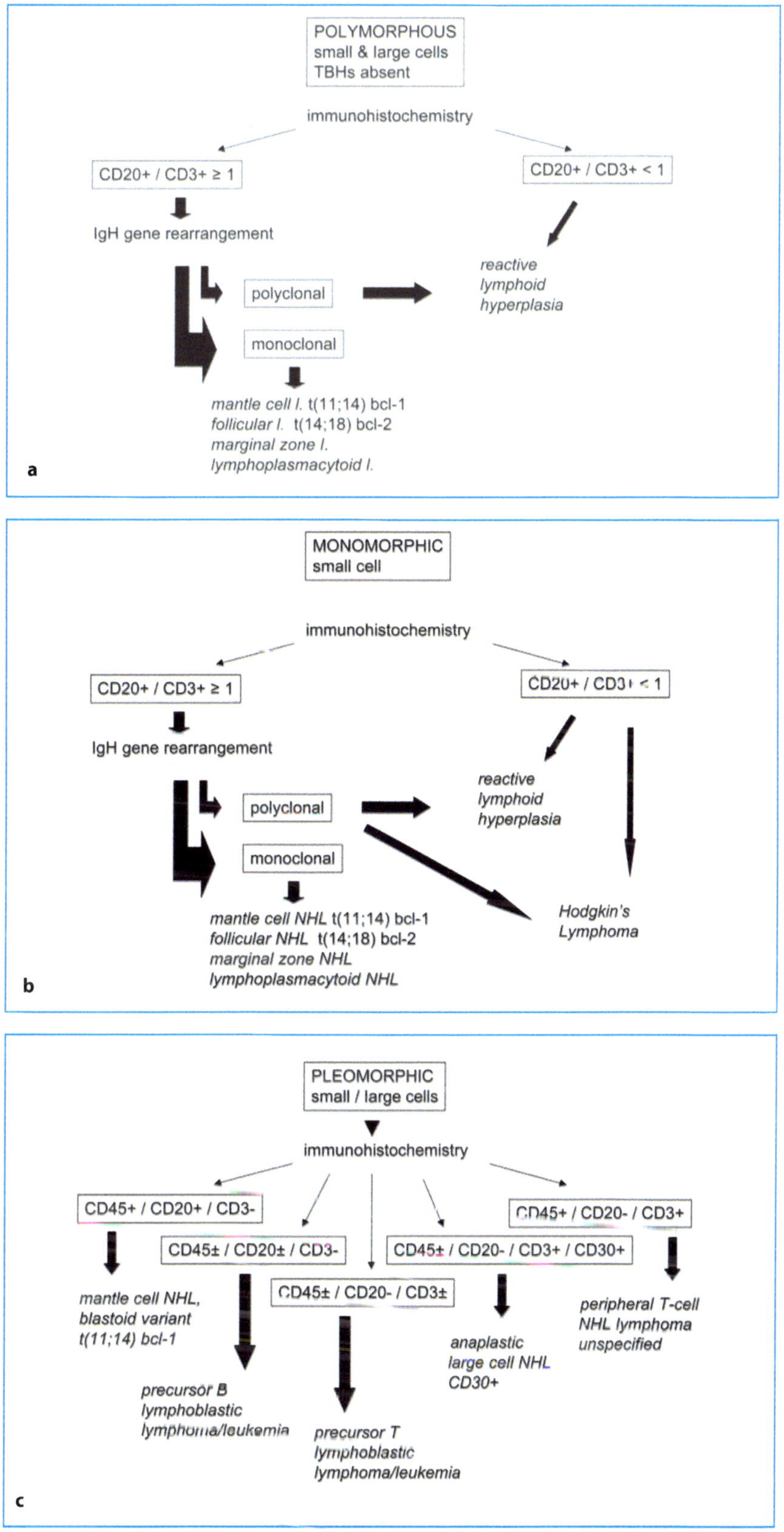

Fig. 4.37 Suggested diagnostic algorithms for evaluation of FNB lymphoid samples with a polymorphous small & large cells, tingible body histiocytes (TBHs) absent pattern (**a**), a monomorphic small cell pattern (**b**), and a pleomorphic small/large cells pattern (**c**)

References

1. Lioe TFEH, Allen DC, Spence RA (1999) The role of fine needle aspiration cytology (FNAC) in the investigation of superficial lymphadenopathy; uses and limitations of the technique. Cytopathology 10:291–297.
2. Kocjan G (1997) The role of FNAC in diagnosis of lymph node enlargements. Cytopathology 8 (suppl):2–3.
3. Liu ES, Bernstein JM, Sculerati N et al (2001) Fine needle aspiration biopsy of pediatric head and neck masses. Int J Pediatr Otorhinolaryngol 60:135–140.
4. Das DK (1999) Value and limitations of fine-needle aspiration cytology in diagnosis and classification of lymphomas: a review. Diagn Cytopathol 21:240–249.
5. Hehn ST, Grogan TM, Miller TP (2004) Utility of fine-needle aspiration as a diagnostic technique in lymphoma. J Clin Oncol 22:3046–3052.
6. Dong HY, Harris NL, Preffer FI et al (2001) Fine-needle aspiration biopsy in the diagnosis and classification of primary and recurrent lymphoma: a retrospective analysis of the utility of cytomorphology and flow cytometry. Mod Pathol 14:472–481.
7. Daskalopoulou D, Harhalakis N, Maouni N et al (1995) Fine needle aspiration cytology of non-Hodgkin's lymphomas. A morphologic and immunophenotypic study. Acta Cytol 39:180–186.
8. Katz R (1997) Pitfalls in the diagnosis of fine-needle aspiration of lymph nodes. Monogr Pathol 39:118–33.
9. Liu K, Mann KP, Vitellas KM et al (1999) Fine-needle aspiration with flow cytometric immunophenotyping for primary diagnosis of intra-abdominal lymphomas. Diagn Cytopathol 21:98–104.
10. Henrique RM, Sousa ME, Godinho MI et al (1999) Immunophenotyping by flow cytometry of fine needle aspirates in the diagnosis of lymphoproliferative disorders: a retrospective study. J Clin Lab Anal 13:224–228.
11. Meda BA, Buss DH, Woodruff RD et al (2000) Diagnosis and subclassification of primary and recurrent lymphoma. The usefulness and limitations of combined fine-needle aspiration cytomorphology and flow cytometry. Am J Clin Pathol 113:688–699.
12. Young NA, Al-Saleem T (1999) Diagnosis of lymphoma by fine-needle aspiration cytology using the revised European–American classification of lymphoid neoplasms. Cancer 87:325–345.
13. Mourad WA, Tulbah A, Shoukri M et al (2003) Primary diagnosis and REAL/WHO classification of non-Hodgkin's lymphoma by fine-needle aspiration: cytomorphologic and immunophenotypic approach. Diagn Cytopathol 28: 191–195.
14. Landgren O, Porwit MacDonald A, Tani E et al (2004) A prospective comparison of fine-needle aspiration cytology and histopathology in the diagnosis and classification of lymphomas. Hematol J 5:69–76.
15. Mayall F, Johnson S (2007) Immunoflow cytometry compared with PCR for the identification of clonality in FNAs of T-cell-rich B-cell lymphomas. Cytopathology 18:117–119.
16. Caraway NP, Gu J, Lin P, Romaguera J et al (2005) The utility of interphase fluorescence in situ hybridization for the detection of the translocation t(11;14)(q13;q32) in the diagnosis of mantle cell lymphoma on fine-needle aspiration specimens. Cancer 105:110–118.
17. Safley AM, Buckley PJ, Creager AJ et al (2004) The value of fluorescence in situ hybridization and polymerase chain reaction in the diagnosis of B-cell non-Hodgkin lymphoma by fine-needle aspiration. Arch Pathol Lab Med 128:1395-1403.
18. Jeffers MDMJ, Farquharson MA, Stewart CJ et al (1997) Analysis of clonality in cytologic material using the polymerase chain reaction (PCR). Cytopathology 8:114–121.
19. Alkan SLC, Sarago C, Sidawy MK et al (1995) Polymerase chain reaction detection of immunoglobulin gene rearrangement and bcl-2 translocation in archival glass slides of cytologic material. Diagn Mol Pathol 4:25–31.
20. Aiello ADD, Giardini R, Alasio L et al (1997) PCR analysis of IgH and BCL2 gene rearrangement in the diagnosis of follicular lymphoma in lymph node fine-needle aspiration. A critical appraisal. Diagn Mol Pathol 6:154–160.
21. Jiang F, Katz RL (2002) Use of interphase fluorescence in situ hybridization as a powerful diagnostic tool in cytology. Diagn Mol Pathol 11:47–57.
22. Haralambieva E, Banham AH, Bastard C et al (2003) Detection by the fluorescence in situ hybridization technique of MYC translocations in paraffin-embedded lymphoma biopsy samples. Br J Haematol 121:49–56.
23. Gong JZ, Snyder MJ, Lagoo AS et al (2004) Diagnostic impact of core-needle biopsy on fine-needle aspiration of non-Hodgkin lymphoma. Diagn Cytopathol 31:23–30.
24. Swerdlow SH, Campo E, Harris NL et al (eds) (2008) World Health Organization Classification of Tumours of Haematopoietic and Lymphoid Tissues. IARC Press, Lyon.
25. Chen L, Kuriakose P, Hawley RC et al (2005). Hematologic malignancies with primary retroperitoneal presentation: clinicopathologic study of 32 cases. Arch Pathol Lab Med 129:655–660.
26. Flanders E, Kornstein MJ, Wakely PE Jr et al (1993) Lymphoglandular bodies in fine-needle aspiration cytology smears. Am J Clin Pathol. 5:566–569.
27. Khurana KK, Stanley MW, Powers CN, Pitman MB (1998) Aspiration cytology of malignant neoplasms associated with granulomas and granuloma-like features: diagnostic dilemmas. Cancer 84:84–91.
28. Pilotti S, Di Palma S, Alasio L et al (1993) Diagnostic assessment of enlarged superficial lymph nodes by fine needle aspiration. Acta Cytol 37:853–866.
29. Sudilovsky D, Cha I (1998) Fine needle aspiration cytology of dermatopathic lymphadenitis. Acta Cytol 42:1341–1346.
30. Das DK, Gulati A, Bhatt NC (2001) Sinus histiocytosis with massive lymphadenopathy (Rosai-Dorfman disease): report of two cases with fine-needle aspiration cytology. Diagn Cytopathol 24:42-45.
31. Kardos TF, Kornstein MJ, Frable WJ (1988) Cytology and immunocytology of infectious mononucleosis in fine needle aspirates of lymph nodes. Acta Cytol 32:722–726.
32. Stanley MW, Steeper TA, Horwitz CA et al (1990). Fine-needle aspiration of lymph nodes in patients with acute infectious mononucleosis. Diagn Cytopathol 6:323–329.
33. Reid AJ, Miller RF, Kocjan GI (1998) Diagnostic utility of fine needle aspiration cytology in HIV-infected patients with lymphadenopathy. Cytopathology 9:230–239.

34. Lowe SM, Kocjan GI, Edwards SG, Miller RF (2008) Diagnostic yield of fine-needle aspiration cytology in HIV-infected patients with lymphadenopathy in the era of highly active antiretroviral therapy. Int J STD AIDS 19:553–556.
35. Kucukardali Y, Solmazgul E, Kunter E et al (2007) Kikuchi-Fujimoto Disease: analysis of 244 cases. Clin Rheumatol 26:50–54.
36. Tong TR, Chan OW, Lee KC (2001) Diagnosing Kikuchi disease on fine needle aspiration biopsy: a retrospective study of 44 cases diagnosed by cytology and 8 by histopathology. Acta Cytol 45:953–957.
37. Tsang WY, Chan JK (1994) Fine-needle aspiration cytologic diagnosis of Kikuchi's lymphadenitis. A report of 27 cases. Am J Clin Pathol 102:454–458.
38. Hsueh EJ, Ko WS, Hwang WS, Yam LT (1993) Fine-needle aspiration of histiocytic necrotizing lymphadenitis (Kikuchi's disease). Diagn Cytopathol 19:448–452.
39. Pileri SA, Ascani S, Leoncini L et al (2002) Hodgkin's lymphoma: the pathologist's viewpoint. J Clin Pathol 55:162–176.
40. Zhang JR, Raza AS, Greaves TS, Cobb CJ (2006) Fine-needle aspiration diagnosis of Hodgkin lymphoma using current WHO classification–re-evaluation of cases from 1999-2004 with new proposals. Diagn Cytopathol 34: 397–402.
41. Gatter KC, Warnke (2001) Diffuse large B-cell lymphoma. In: Jaffe ES, Harris NL, Stein H, Vardiman JW (eds) Pathology and Genetics of Tumours of Hematopoietic and Lymphoid Tissues. World Health Organization Classification of Tumours. IARC Press, Lyon, pp 171–176.
42. de Leval L, Harris NL (2003) Variability in immunophenotype in diffuse large B-cell lymphoma and its clinical relevance. Histopathology 43:509–528.
43. Rosenwald A, Wright G, Chan WC et al (2002) The use of molecular profiling to predict survival after chemotherapy for diffuse large-B-cell lymphoma. N Engl J Med 346:1937–1947.
44. Boleti E, Johnson PW (2007) Primary mediastinal B-cell lymphoma. Hematol Oncol 25:157–163.
45. Silverman JF, Raab SS, Park HK (1993) Fine-needle aspiration cytology of primary large-cell lymphoma of the mediastinum: cytomorphologic findings with potential pitfalls in diagnosis. Diagn Cytopathol 9:209–214.
46. Wright DH (1999) What is Burkitt's lymphoma and when is it endemic? Blood 93:758.
47. Knowles DM (1996) Etiology and pathogenesis of AIDS-related non–Hodgkin's lymphoma. Hematol Oncol Clin North Am. 10:1081–1109.
48. Das DK, Gupta SK, Pathak IC et al (1987) Burkitt-type lymphoma. Diagnosis by fine needle aspiration cytology. Acta Cytol 31:1–7.
49. Powers CN, Wakely PE Jr, Silverman JF et al (1990) Fine needle aspiration biopsy of extramedullary plasma cell tumors. Mod Pathol 3:648–653.
50. Pai RR, Raghuveer CV (1996) Extramedullary plasmacytoma diagnosed by fine needle aspiration cytology. A report of four cases. Acta Cytol 40:963–966.
51. Das DK, Francis IM, Sharma PN et al (2009) Hodgkin's lymphoma: Diagnostic difficulties in fine-needle aspiration cytology. Diagn Cytopathol 16. [Epub ahead of print]
52. Mourad WA, al Nazer M, Tulbah A (2003) Cytomorphologic differentiation of Hodgkin's lymphoma and Ki-1+ anaplastic large cell lymphoma in fine needle aspirates. Acta Cytol 47:744–748.
53. Harris NL (1999) Hodgkin's disease: classification and differential diagnosis. Mod Pathol 12:159–175.
54. McCune RC, Syrbu SI, Vasef MA (2006) Expression profiling of transcription factors Pax-5, Oct-1, Oct-2, BOB.1, and PU.1 in Hodgkin's and non-Hodgkin's lymphomas: a comparative study using high throughput tissue microarrays. Mod Pathol 19:1010-1018.
55. Pangalis GA, Angelopoulou MK, Vassilakopoulos TP (1999) B-chronic lymphocytic leukemia, small lymphocytic lymphoma, and lymphoplasmacytic lymphoma, including Waldenström's macroglobulinemia: a clinical, morphologic, and biologic spectrum of similar disorders. Semin Hematol 36:104–114.
56. Berger F, Muller-Hermelink HK, Isaacson PG et al (2001) Lymphoplasmacytic lymphoma / Waldenstrom macroglobulinemia. In: Jaffe ES, Harris NL, Stein H, Vardiman JW (eds) Pathology and Genetics of Tumours of Hematopoietic and Lymphoid Tissues. World Health Organization Classification of Tumours. IARC Press, Lyon, pp 132–134.
57. O'Connell FP, Pinkus JL, Pinkus GS (2004) CD138 (syndecan-1), a plasma cell marker immunohistochemical profile in hematopoietic and nonhematopoietic neoplasms. Am J Clin Pathol 121:254–263.
58. Banks PM, Chan J, Cleary ML et al (1992) Mantle cell lymphoma. A proposal for unification of morphologic, immunologic, and molecular data. Am J Surg Pathol 16:637–640.
59. Rassidakis GZ, Tani E, Svedmyr E et al (1999) Diagnosis and subclassification of follicle center and mantle cell lymphomas on fine-needle aspirates: A cytologic and immunocytochemical approach based on the Revised European-American Lymphoma (REAL) classification. Cancer 87:216–223.
60. Nathwani BN, Pirls MA, Harris NL et al (2001) Follicular lymphoma. In: Jaffe ES, Harris NL, Stein H, Vardiman JW (eds) Pathology and Genetics of Tumours of Hematopoietic and Lymphoid Tissues. World Health Organization Classification of Tumours. IARC Press, Lyon, pp 162–167.
61. Gong Y, Caraway N, Gu J et al (2003) Evaluation of interphase fluorescence in situ hybridization for the t(14;18)(q32;q21) translocation in the diagnosis of follicular lymphoma on fine-needle aspirates: a comparison with flow cytometry immunophenotyping. Cancer 99:385–393.
62. Sun W, Caraway NP, Zhang HZ et al (2004) Grading follicular lymphoma on fine needle aspiration specimens. Comparison with proliferative index by DNA image analysis and Ki 67 labeling index. Acta Cytol 48:119–126.
63. Isaacson PG, Harris NL, Nathwani BN et al (2001) Nodal marginal zone B-cell lymphoma. In: Jaffe ES, Harris NL, Stein H, Vardiman JW (eds) Pathology and Genetics of Tumours of Hematopoietic and Lymphoid Tissues. World Health Organization Classification of Tumours. IARC Press, Lyon, p 161.
64. Campo E, Miquel R, Krenacs L et al (1999) Primary nodal marginal zone lymphomas of splenic and MALT type. Am J Surg Pathol 23:59–68.
65. Isaacson PG, Du MQ (2004) MALT lymphoma: from morphology to molecules. Nat Rev Cancer 4:644–653.

66. Pinkus GS, O'Hara CJ, Said JW (1990). Peripheral/post-thymic T-cell lymphomas: a spectrum of disease. Clinical, pathologic, and immunologic features of 78 cases. Cancer 65:971–998.
67. Mayall F, Darlington A, Harrison B (2003) Fine needle aspiration cytology in the diagnosis of uncommon types of lymphoma. J Clin Pathol 56:821–825.
68. Manosca F, Ariga R, Bengana C et al (2004) Fine-needle aspiration of subcutaneous panniculitis-like T-cell lymphoma. Diagn Cytopathol 31:338–339.
69. Delsol G, Ralfkiaer E, Stein H et al (2001) Anaplastic large cell lymphoma. In: Jaffe ES, Harris NL, Stein H, Vardiman JW (eds) Pathology and Genetics of Tumours of Hematopoietic and Lymphoid Tissues. World Health Organization Classification of Tumours. IARC Press, Lyon, pp 230–235.
70. Ng WK, Ip P, Choy C, Collins RJ (2003) Cytologic and immunocytochemical findings of anaplastic large cell lymphoma: analysis of ten fine-needle aspiration specimens over a 9-year period. Cancer 99:33–43.
71. Rapkiewicz A, Wen H, Sen F, Das K (2007) Cytomorphologic examination of anaplastic large cell lymphoma by fine-needle aspiration cytology. Cancer 111:499–507.
72. McCluggage WG, Anderson N, Herron B, Caughley L (1996) Fine needle aspiration cytology, histology and immunohistochemistry of anaplastic large cell Ki-1-positive lymphoma. A report of three cases. Acta Cytol 40:779–785.
73. Kim SE, Kim SH, Lim BJ et al (2004) Fine needle aspiration cytology of small cell variant of anaplastic large cell lymphoma. A case report. Acta Cytol 48:254–258.
74. Bernard A, Boumsell L, Patte C, Lemerie J (1986) Leukemia versus lymphoma in children: a worthless question? Med Pediatr Oncol 14:148–157.
75. Soslow RA, Baergen RN, Warnke RA (1999) B-lineage lymphoblastic lymphoma is a clinicopathologic entity distinct from other histologically similar aggressive lymphomas with blastic morphology. Cancer 85:2648–2654.
76. Sheibani K, Nathwani BN, Winberg CD et al (1987) Antigenically defined subgroups of lymphoblastic lymphoma. Relationship to clinical presentation and biologic behavior. Cancer 60:183–190.
77. Hughes JH, Caraway NP, Katz RL (1998) Blastic variant of mantle-cell lymphoma: cytomorphologic, immunocytochemical, and molecular genetic features of tissue obtained by fine-needle aspiration biopsy. Diagn Cytopathol 19:59–62.

5 Cytological Pattern Profiling of Tumors from Different Visceral Sites

5.1 Preliminary Remarks

The cytological findings in FNB samples from the large majority of primary and secondary tumors detected in visceral sites, as well as those of metastatic tumors appearing in lymph nodes or soft tissues, can be classified according to the principles of pattern analysis. In the given case, this approach first requires identifying the specific category that the constituent cells belong to and then, if possible, classifying the set of observed morphological changes according to distinctive cytological patterns. The description of cytological features should be reproducibly standardized. At least nine major cytomorphological cell types can be identified. These are listed in Table 5.1. Each category includes a variable number of possible distinctive patterns. Once the major pattern has been identified, the diagnostic possibilities are dramatically reduced. The next step is to reach a conclusive diagnosis by prudent deductive reasoning based on additional ancillary data and/or clinical findings. Although a definitive diagnosis is not always possible, the identification of a specific pattern is nonetheless of importance for further clinical management of the case.

Table 5.1 Major categories of cell morphology in FNB smears (excluding lymphoid lesions)

- glandular
- squamous or squamoid basaloid
- transitional
- small
- large
- clear
- oxyphil/oncocytic or oncocytoid
- epithelioid and spindle

5.2 Glandular-Cell Morphology

Definition. Glandular epithelium is made up of cells with a cylindrical or cuboid morphology that are endowed with several functional properties, including the synthesis, secretion, and accumulation of mucin. Tumors of glandular epithelium are supported by a variable component of vascular or fibrous stroma, which strongly influences the morphological picture and the number of epithelial cells in the cytological sample. The cytological appearance of the harvest varies according to the degree of differentiation. In FNB samples from well-differentiated tumors, epithelial glandular cells tend to cluster in tubular, acinar, or papillary aggregates, and their cylindrical or cuboid morphology is well-preserved. By contrast, in the cells of poorly differentiated tumors they tend to lose their organized pattern and their growth is often "solid" and structureless, or they appear partially or totally non-cohesive.

Moreover, they frequently lose their functional properties, as manifested by a loss of the original cylindrical or cuboid morphology, by a reduced amount of cytoplasm and, eventually, by an increase in nuclear size and a significant change in nuclear morphology. Five cytological patterns involving a glandular epithelial morphology are recognized and discussed in the following.

5.2.1 *Tubulo-Acinar Pattern*

- Clean background with the presence of stromal fragments, isolated fibrocytes, and histiocytes.
- Variable cellularity of the sample, more often abundant.
- Prevailing tendency to cellular aggregation.

- Two-dimensional sheets with little or no nuclear overlap.
- Tubular cords and variably large three-dimensional aggregates.
- Minimal molding and possible "streaming" of nuclei within the aggregates.
- Frequent peripheral nuclear palisading.
- Luminal spaces within the aggregates variably present.
- Well-evident external membrane with a variable amount of cytoplasm.
- Small and uniform nuclei with minimal variability in size.
- Nuclear membrane well-outlined.
- Finely granular chromatin with small nucleoli.

Cytomorphology. The main feature of the tubulo-acinar pattern is well-evident at low-power view and is represented by a tendency of cells to form two- or three-dimensional aggregates. The latter may be in the form of elongated cords, trabeculae, or syncytia. Nuclear palisading is prominent at the periphery of the aggregates. At higher magnification, it is evident that the cells retain a cylindrical or cuboid appearance. Nuclear morphology is monotonous (Fig. 5.1). The background is clear and shows the

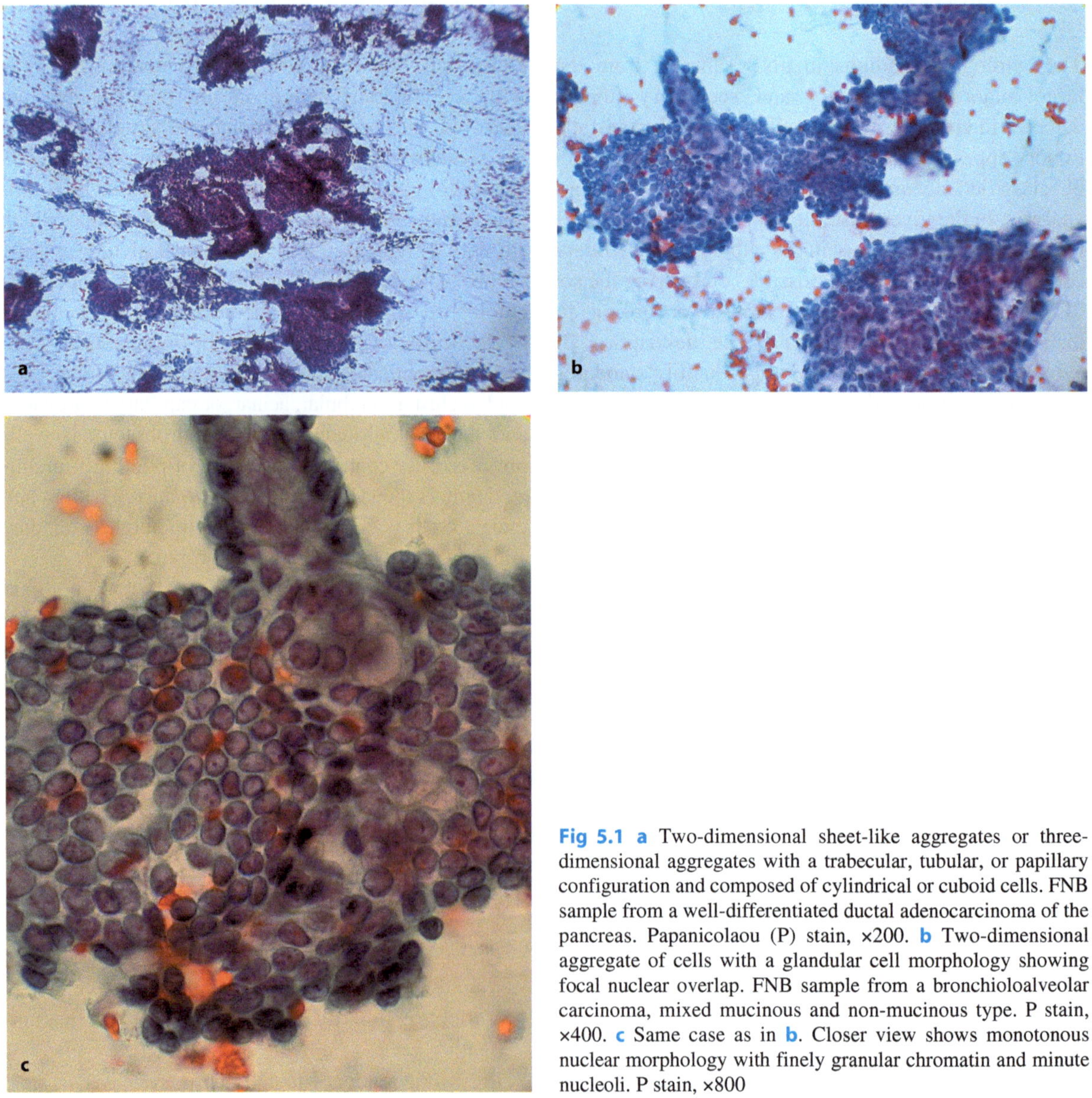

Fig 5.1 a Two-dimensional sheet-like aggregates or three-dimensional aggregates with a trabecular, tubular, or papillary configuration and composed of cylindrical or cuboid cells. FNB sample from a well-differentiated ductal adenocarcinoma of the pancreas. Papanicolaou (P) stain, ×200. b Two-dimensional aggregate of cells with a glandular cell morphology showing focal nuclear overlap. FNB sample from a bronchioloalveolar carcinoma, mixed mucinous and non-mucinous type. P stain, ×400. c Same case as in b. Closer view shows monotonous nuclear morphology with finely granular chromatin and minute nucleoli. P stain, ×800

presence of fibrocytes, stromal fragments, and histiocytes.

Interpretation. The tubulo-acinar pattern is typically seen in well-differentiated epithelial tumors, both in primary and in metastatic sites. In some cases, the chance of a tumor-like lesion, a benign tumor, or a tumor with borderline malignancy should be taken into account, for example in the liver (bile duct adenoma) or ovary (serous or mucinous tumors).

5.2.2 Tubulo-Papillary Pattern

- Papillary or morular aggregates composed of cylindrical cells with nuclear overlap.
- Minor component of two-dimensional sheets.
- Elongated cylindrical cells (especially as isolated elements).
- Elongated nuclei with variable chromatin pattern.
- Nuclear inclusions, pseudoinclusions, or nuclear grooves.
- Small nucleoli.
- Amphophilic pale cytoplasm or eosinophilic cytoplasm (thyroid, kidney).

Cytomorphology. The tubulo-papillary pattern of aggregation is mainly or mostly papillary, with well-evident nuclear overlap (Fig. 5.2a–d). The nuclei may appear elongated and pseudostratified. True papillary aggregates, when present, show a definite connective-tissue core (Fig. 5.2a,d). More frequently,

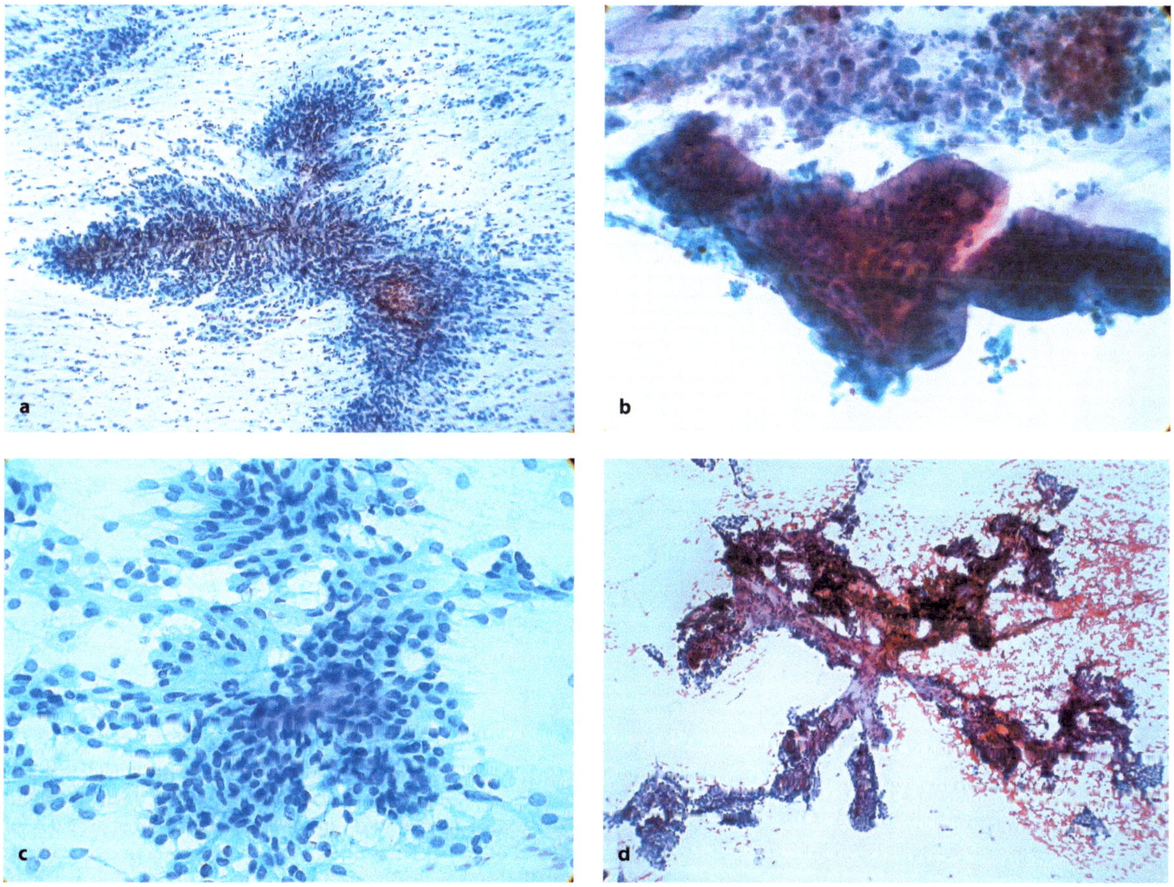

Fig 5.2 a Large papillary aggregate showing a connective-tissue stalk. The tumor cells are cylindrical and elongated, appear to radiate from the stalk, and show a tendency to loose cohesion; isolated cells are seen in the background. FNB sample from a poorly differentiated duct carcinoma of the pancreas. P stain, ×200. **b** Pseudopapillary aggregate of mucin-secreting cylindrical cells. Note that the cells are clustered as palisades and radiate from a central core; necrotic cells are seen in the background. FNB sample from a metastatic adenocarcinoma of the colon into the liver. P stain, ×400. **c** Elongated cells are aggregated in micropapillary structures lacking a connective-tissue stalk. FNB sample from a papillary renal cell carcinoma. P stain, ×400. **d** Large and ramified papillary aggregate showing a well defined connective-tissue stalk. FNB sample from a papillary carcinoma of the thyroid. P stain, ×200

the aggregates are three-dimensional, with a peripheral palisade of nuclei (pseudopapillae), and lack a connective-tissue stalk (Fig 5.2b). Sometimes, the papillae are composed of only a few cells (micropapillae) and are intimately admixed with one another (Fig 5.2c).

Interpretation. The tubulo-papillary pattern is typically seen in well-differentiated epithelial tumors arising in sites including the pancreas, ovary, kidney, lung, and thyroid. The amount of true papillary aggregates is variable and may even be completely lacking (as seen in papillary carcinoma of the thyroid). The micropapillary pattern is mainly seen in papillary renal cell carcinoma and in the micropapillary variant of breast carcinoma. Close examination of the cellular features is of help to possibly demonstrate eosinophilic *nuclear inclusion bodies* (bronchoalveolar carcinoma), *pseudoinclusions* due to endonuclear cytoplasmic invagination (serous papillary carcinoma of the ovary, papillary carcinoma of the kidney and thyroid), *nuclear grooves* (serous papillary carcinoma of the ovary and pancreas, papillary carcinoma of the thyroid), or *cilia* (bronchoalveolar carcinoma, serous papillary carcinoma of the ovary and pancreas).

5.2.3 Mucinous Pattern

- Mucoid substance in the background, with histiocytes and inflammatory infiltrate.
- Cellularity variable.
- Two-dimensional aggregates with a sharp outline.
- Three-dimensional aggregates sometimes in the form of cords, trabeculae, papillae, or pseudopapillae.
- Amphophilic cytoplasm of cells with possible vacuoles of mucin accumulation.
- Isolated cells with or without a signet-ring-cell morphology variably present.

Cytomorphology. The presence of a variable amount of mucoid substance in the background is the main feature of the mucinous pattern (Fig. 5.3). The aggre-

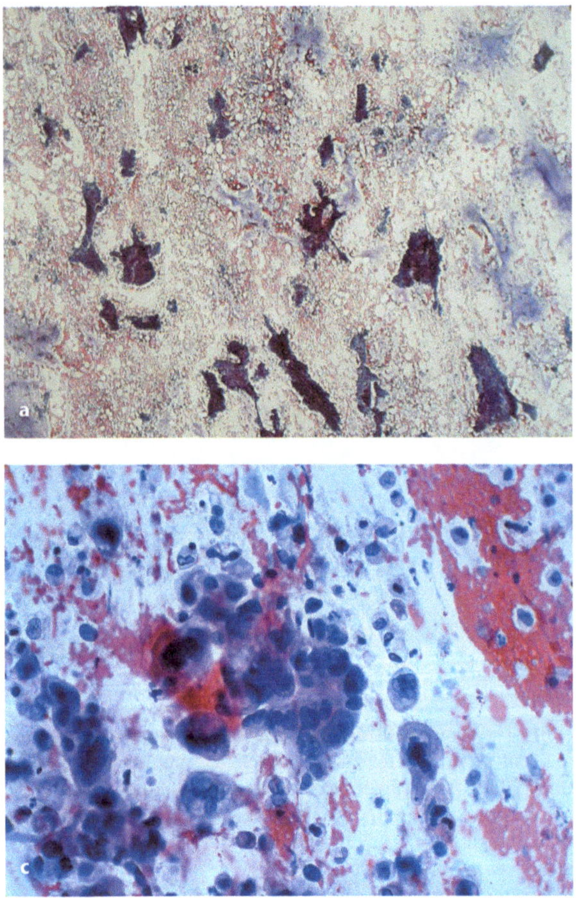

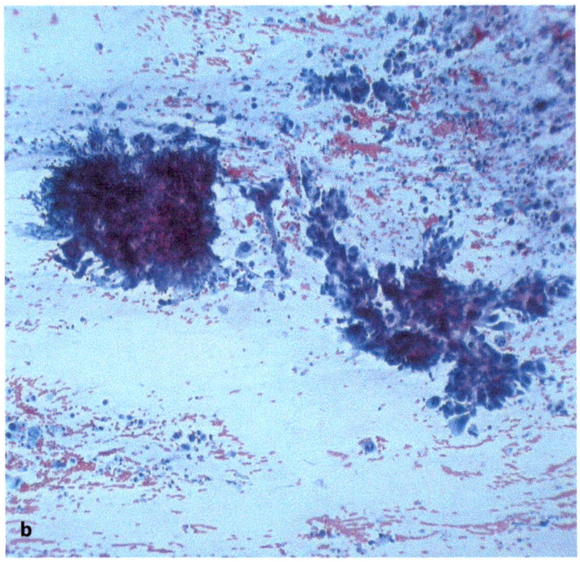

Fig 5.3 **a** Low-power view of a smear, showing abundant mucinous ground substance in the background and abundant cellularity consisting of two- and three-dimensional aggregates of cuboid or cylindrical cells. FNB sample from a liver metastasis of colorectal mucinous adenocarcinoma. P stain, ×200. **b** Tumor cells are found as isolated elements or are clustered in large three-dimensional aggregates. They have a variable amount of cytoplasm, which appears optically clear. Same case as in **a**. P stain, ×480. **c** Tumor cells are non-cohesive or loosely cohesive and display a moderate amount of cytoplasm containing multiple mucin vacuoles. FNB smear from a poorly differentiated mucinous carcinoma of the ovary. P stain, ×1000

gation pattern tends to be two- or three-dimensional, respectively, in well-differentiated and poorly differentiated tumors. The number of non-cohesive cells increases in the latter.

Interpretation. The mucinous pattern is typically seen in metastatic deposits of adenocarcinoma of colorectal and gastric origin; in tumors of the pancreas, ovary, and lung; and in cholangiocarcinoma in primary and metastatic sites. Detection of this pattern in a sample collected from an intra-abdominal or peri-intestinal tumor mass strongly suggests pseudomyxoma peritonei secondary to a mucinous carcinoma of the appendix or ovary.

5.2.4 Solid, Three-Dimensional (Structureless) Pattern

- Variably necrotic, hemorrhagic, or mucoid background with granulocytes and histiocytes.
- Three-dimensional aggregation prevalent.
- Solid structureless aggregates, or cords and/or branching trabeculae with a "peritheliomatous" appearance.
- Prominent nuclear molding, with possible peripheral nuclear palisading.
- Cellular dissociation variably expressed, with small cellular aggregates.
- Anisonucleosis, with prominent nucleoli.
- Grossly granular chromatin.
- Fragile cytoplasm often with indistinct cellular borders.

Cytomorphology. The cells in a structureless sample tend to form three- rather than two-dimensional aggregates. The background often contains necrotic cellular debris and/or red blood cells. Nuclei are highly variable in size and shape, with prominent nucleoli and a grossly granular chromatin texture. Larger aggregates are composed of several nuclear layers and appear structureless or as cords or trabeculae (Fig. 5.4). Smaller aggregates consisting of less than ten cells are often detected. Cellular dissociation and necrosis may be prominent; sometimes the cells are attached to branching blood vessels in a peritheliomatous pattern, with necrosis and/or dissociation of tumor cells farther away from the vessels.

Interpretation. The solid, three-dimensional pattern is seen in samples collected from poorly differentiated adenocarcinomas originating in different sites. The primary tumor site may be identified in some patients on the basis of immunocytochemical data and proper correlation with clinical findings and imaging data. The differential diagnosis encompasses other tumors with a non-glandular phenotype, such as poorly differentiated urothelial carcinoma, neuroendocrine carcinoma, and poorly differentiated squamous cell carcinoma.

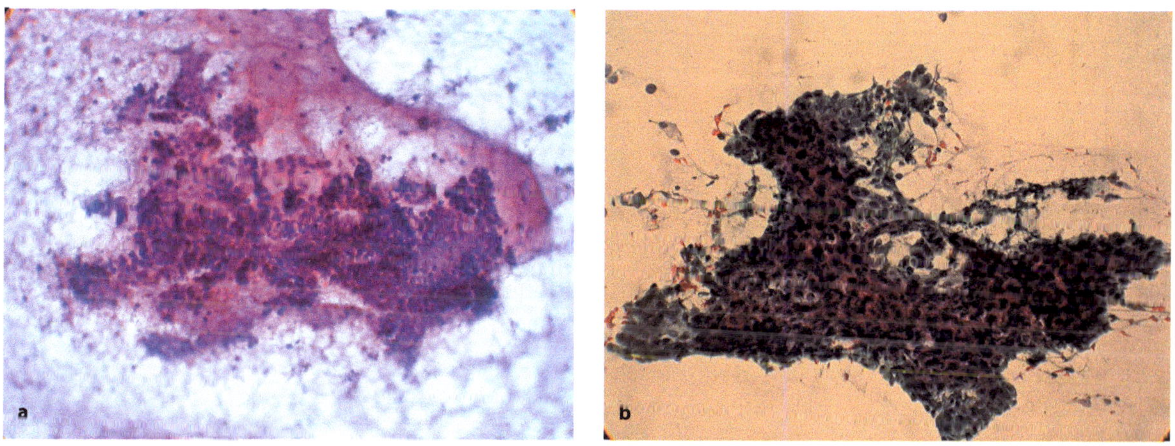

Fig 5.4 **a** A large aggregate of cells with a glandular cell morphology, composed of several nuclear layers, and appearing practically structureless. FNB smear from pancreatic duct carcinoma. P stain, ×400. **b** A large trabecular aggregate of cells with a glandular cell morphology showing focal peripheral palisading of cells. Same case as in **a**. P stain, ×400.

5.2.5 Non-Cohesive Cell Pattern

- Variably necrotic, hemorrhagic, or mucoid background with granulocytes and histiocytes.
- Mostly or exclusively non-cohesive cells.
- Possible signet-ring-like cellular changes.
- Anisonucleosis, with prominent nucleoli.
- Grossly granular chromatin.
- Fragile cytoplasm often with indistinct cellular borders.

Cytomorphology. The non-cohesive pattern is, as the name implies, dominated by the tendency of cells to non-cohesiveness (Fig. 5.5a). Tumor cells can have a signet-ring appearance, which is characterized by a voluminous intracytoplasmic vacuole that displaces the nucleus to the periphery (Fig. 5.5b).

Interpretation. The non-cohesive pattern is characteristically seen in metastatic adenocarcinoma of gastric origin; in peculiar variants of adenocarcinomas of the breast, urinary bladder, and pancreas; and in cholangiocarcinoma. In general, a signet-ring appearance (due to the accumulation of mucin) is characteristic of a gastric primary tumor, while a targetoid appearance of the vacuole (due to the presence of a centrally located inclusion body) is a strong indication of a primary breast tumor.

5.2.6 Immunohistochemical Identification of the Primary Tumor Site

The epithelial glandular-cell morphology is rather frequently encountered in FNB samples of superficial and deep tumor masses in adult patients. In such patients, it is necessary to differentiate between a primary and a metastatic tumor at the site of needle sampling, or to identify the site of the primary when confronted with a clearly metastatic lesion. The former situation occurs, for example, in the liver, lung, or ovary because primary and metastatic tumors in these organs can share the morphology of epithelial tumors of glandular origin. The latter situation occurs when, for example, an enlarged lymph node in a superficial or deep location is sampled and the cytological picture indicates an epithelial tumor with features of glandular origin. In this case, the site of the primary tumor should be identified with reasonable certainty.

Since morphological data are unlikely to provide specific hints as to the tumor primary, an additional immunohistochemical evaluation of the specimen is required along with judicious correlation with clinical data. To confront this task, a wide armamentarium of immunohistochemical reagents has traditionally been employed, including hormone products (thyroglobulin, calcitonin, parathyroid hormone), hormonal

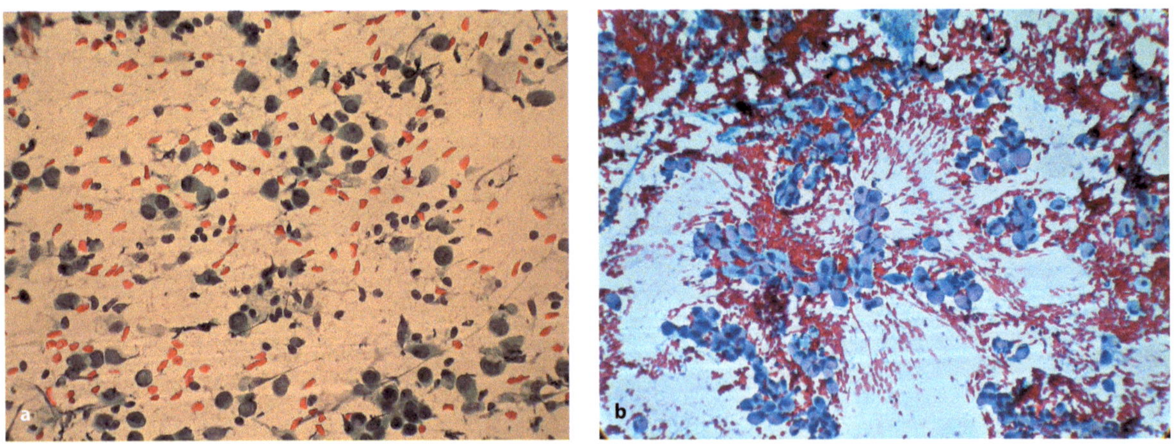

Fig 5.5 **a** Round to polygonal cells that appear totally non-cohesive. FNB sample from a breast carcinoma metastatic into a supraclavicular lymph node. P stain, ×400. **b** Loosely cohesive or non-cohesive cells containing a voluminous intracytoplasmic mucin vacuole that displaces the nucleus (signet-ring cell appearance). FNB sample from a pulmonary metastasis of gastric carcinoma. P stain, ×400

Table 5.2 CK7, CK20, CDX-2, and TTF-1 immunohistochemical reactivity in adenocarcinoma cells according to the site of origin

Tumor primary site	Combined CK7/CK20 profile			CDX-2 (%)	TTF-1 (%)
	More frequent	Less frequent	Occasional		
Stomach	CK7+/CK20+	CK7+/CK20-	CK7-/CK20+	70	0
Small intestine	CK7+/CK20+	CK7+/CK20-	CK7-/CK20-	60	0
Large intestine	CK7-/CK20+	CK7+/CK20+	CK7-/CK20-	95	10
Rectum	CK7+/CK20+	CK7-/CK20+	CK7+/CK20-	95	0
Pancreatic-biliary tree	CK7+/CK20-	CK7+/CK20+	CK7-/CK20+	30	0
Lung	CK7+/CK20-	CK7+/CK20+	CK7-/CK20-	15	90
Breast	CK7+/CK20-	CK7+/CK20+	CK7-/CK20-	0	0
Ovary, mucinous	CK7+/CK20+	CK7+/CK20-	CK7-/CK20+	80	0
Ovary, non-mucinous	CK7+/CK20-	CK7+/CK20-	CK7-/CK20-	< 5	20
Endocervix	CK7+/CK20+	CK7+/CK20-	CK7-/CK20+	0	< 5
Endometrium	CK7+/CK20-	CK7+/CK20+	CK7-/CK20-	0	20
Prostate, acinar	CK7-/CK20-	CK7+/CK20-	CK7+/CK20+	< 5	0

receptors (estrogen, progesterone, androgens), organ-specific markers (PSA for prostatic carcinoma or GCDFP-15 for breast carcinoma). More recently, an approach based on the combined investigation of cytokeratin 7 (CK7) and cytokeratin 20 (CK20) expression in tumor cells has gained considerable popularity [1–10]. Epithelia from different viscera or from different segments of the gastrointestinal tract differ in their expression of these cytokeratins and a sort of "site-specific" CK7/CK20 profile can be delineated [1,2]. Many published studies have been aimed at establishing whether tumors originating in these different sites retain the same site-specific CK7/CK20 immunohistochemical profile in metastatic sites. Despite early enthusiasm, a general consensus has never been reached mainly due to different methodologies (for review see Tot, 2002 [1]). It is possible, however, to identify two main categories: a constant and strong expression of CK20, and poor or absent expression of CK7 [1]. Tumors belonging to the first category include adenocarcinoma of the large intestine and stomach as well as urothelial carcinoma. The second category includes carcinomas arising in the prostate, kidney, and large intestine. Moreover, there are tumors that show a predictably different CK7/CK20 profile in their primary location compared to in their metastatic sites. In particular, adenocarcinomas of the stomach, biliary tract, or endometrium show a tendency to lose CK20 expression at metastatic sites, while carcinomas of the prostate and lung tend to gain CK20 expression in metastatic sites [1]. Finally, the strong expression of CK7, characteristic of adenocarcinoma of the pancreas and breast as well as of non-mucinous ovarian carcinoma in primary sites, inevitably disappears at metastatic sites.

If one takes the above limitations into account, evaluating the CK7/CK20 profile turns out to be useful in the identification of *groups* of possible primary sites. Table 5.2 illustrates the immunoreactivity profiles of each primary tumor according to frequency. Three different profiles can thus be delineated [1–10]: a more frequent one (50–60% of patients), a less frequent one (30–40% of patients), and one that is only occasionally seen (<10% of patients). Some of the tumors on the list (non-mucinous ovarian carcinoma and endometrial carcinoma) tend to retain their profile more than others but significant exceptions do occur. Consequently, different groups of possible primaries can be identified according to a probabilistic approach.

The immunohistochemical armamentarium has been expanded recently by two additional markers, thyroid transcription factor 1 (TTF-1) and CDX-2, which can provide useful discriminating criteria [11–23]. Both of them show nuclear positivity. The former is preferentially expressed in tumors of the thyroid and lower respiratory tract, but there are a few exceptions, i.e., some ovarian carcinomas [16] and some colorectal carcinomas that metastasize to the lung [18]. The cytoplasmic expression of TTF-1 has been described in hepatocellular carcinoma and, occasionally, in cholangiocellular carcinoma [19]. CDX-2 is expressed in tumors with enteric differentiation and is thus also detected at sites other than the gastrointestinal tract, e.g., in some ovarian and endocervical tumors and in tumors of the nasal mucosa [13,15,20,21]. Finally, "aberrant" expression of CDX-2 has been detected in acinar carcinoma of the prostate [22] and in carcinoma of the lung [23]. If these limitations are considered, testing for CK7, CK20, TTF-1, and CDX-2 in a combined approach (Table 5.2) is potentially useful to increase the predictive value of immunohistochemistry in identifying the primary tumor site in many patients [24].

5.3 Squamous or Squamoid Cell Morphology

Definition. Tumors recapitulating the morphology of squamous cell epithelium are widespread in the body and differ from one another according to the degree of cellular differentiation and the presence of concomitant intracellular and/or extracellular keratinization. Two cytological patterns are observed.

5.3.1 Keratinizing Pattern

- Amorphous eosinophilic or orangeophilic material in the background with necrotic detritus, inflammatory cells, and histiocytes.
- Three-dimensional aggregates alternate with non-cohesive cells or small cellular aggregates.
- Triangular-shaped, oval, or elongated cells sometimes with long prolongations.
- Round, oval, or elongated hyperchromatic nuclei.
- Dense chromatin with occasional small nucleoli.
- Single-cell keratinization demonstrated by cytoplasmic orangeophilia.

Cytomorphology. The main peculiarity of the keratinizing pattern is the presence of amorphous masses of eosinophilic or orangeophilic material in the background (Fig. 5.6a). The latter may contain parakeratotic cells with hyperchromatic nuclei having an oval, elongated, or angulated profile. While three-dimen-

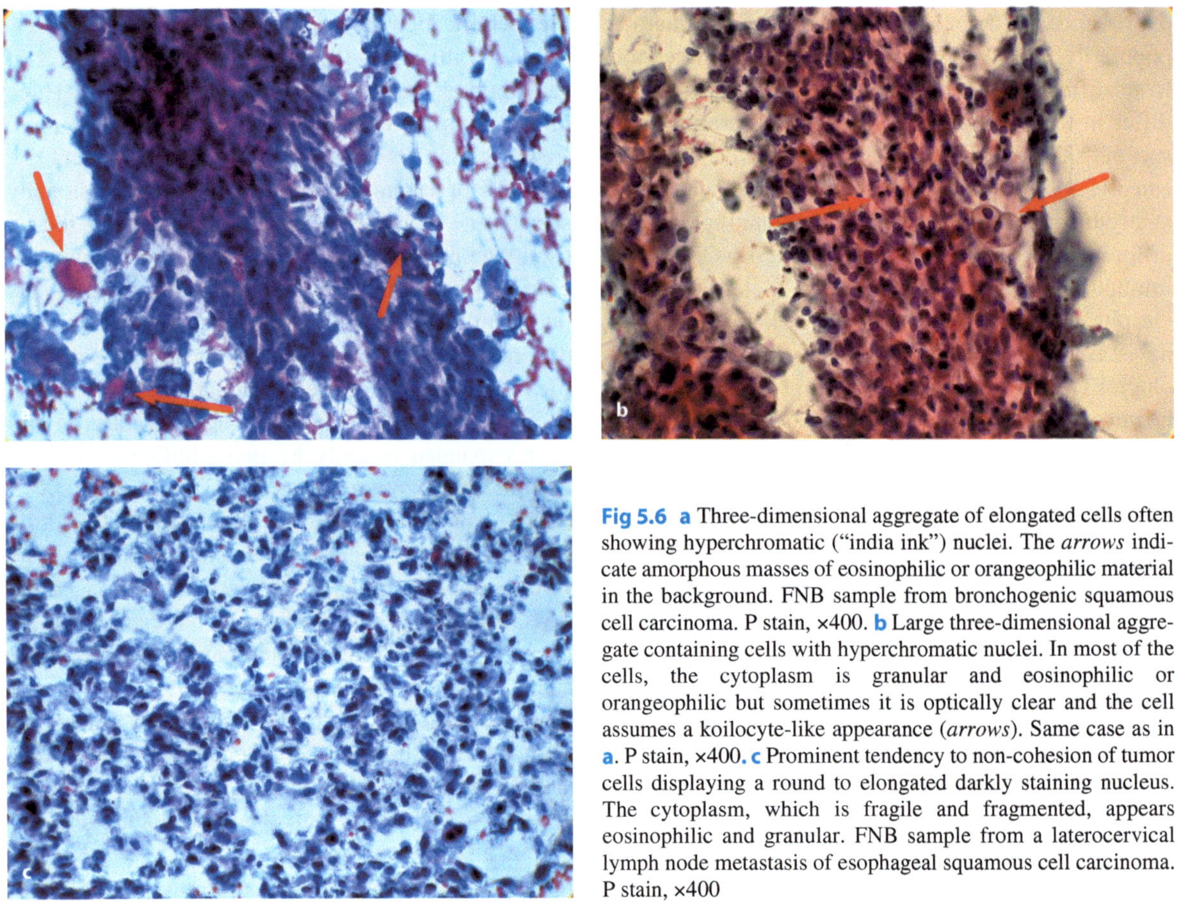

Fig 5.6 **a** Three-dimensional aggregate of elongated cells often showing hyperchromatic ("india ink") nuclei. The *arrows* indicate amorphous masses of eosinophilic or orangeophilic material in the background. FNB sample from bronchogenic squamous cell carcinoma. P stain, ×400. **b** Large three-dimensional aggregate containing cells with hyperchromatic nuclei. In most of the cells, the cytoplasm is granular and eosinophilic or orangeophilic but sometimes it is optically clear and the cell assumes a koilocyte-like appearance (*arrows*). Same case as in **a**. P stain, ×400. **c** Prominent tendency to non-cohesion of tumor cells displaying a round to elongated darkly staining nucleus. The cytoplasm, which is fragile and fragmented, appears eosinophilic and granular. FNB sample from a laterocervical lymph node metastasis of esophageal squamous cell carcinoma. P stain, ×400

sional aggregates are present, the cells tend to be non-cohesive or grouped in small aggregates. Squamous cells characteristically have a dense hyperchromatic nucleus of variable shape and size and a variable amount of cytoplasm. Sometimes, a definite perinuclear clear halo is seen and the cells assume a koilocyte-like appearance (Fig. 5.6b).

Interpretation. The keratinizing pattern is typically seen in samples from keratinizing squamous cell carcinoma. The upper aerodigestive tract, lower respiratory tract, and the skin are the most common primary sites. The lymph nodes of the head and neck and mediastinum are most frequently involved by metastatic disease.

5.3.2 Non-Keratinizing Pattern

- Necrotic detritus or abundant blood, inflammatory cells, and histiocytes in the background.
- Three-dimensional aggregation prevalent.
- Intermediate to large cells with an ovoid, elongated, or spindle shape.
- Round, oval, or elongated vesicular nuclei.
- Coarsely granular chromatin texture with small nucleoli.
- Well-defined outer cytoplasmic borders.

Cytomorphology. The non-keratinizing pattern is dominated by three-dimensional aggregates (cords and trabeculae) that are never large but rather variably branch and interconnect with one another. The nuclei may be polarized or in pseudopalisades. They are characterized by a coarsely granular chromatin while prominent nucleoli are practically never seen (Fig. 5.7a,b). In a distinct variant, tumor cells are of intermediate to small size, due to sparse cytoplasm; their nuclei may show a variable extent of crushing artifacts, thus simulating small-cell carcinoma (Fig. 5.7c). The differentiation from this variant is obtained morphologically only when it is possible to detect the distinct intercellular bridges typical of squamous cell

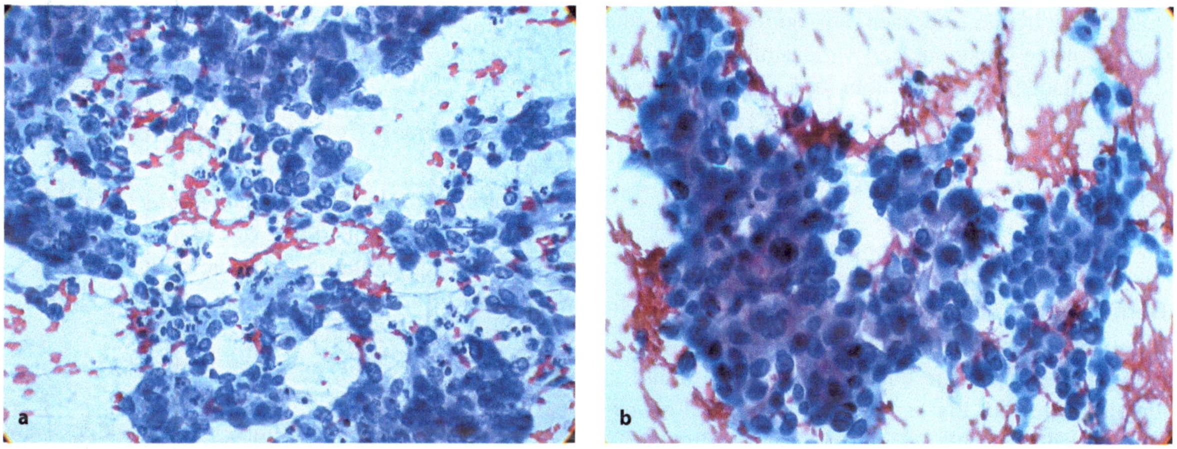

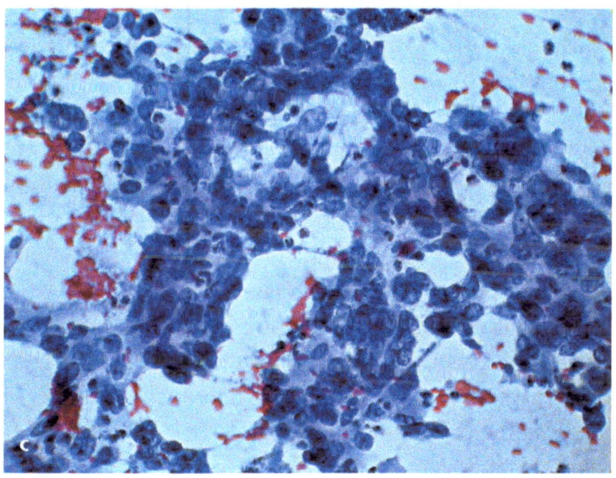

Fig 5.7 a Branching cords of medium-sized cells with large nuclei and moderate amounts of cytoplasm. The chromatin texture is coarsely granular and nucleoli are lacking; the cytoplasm is amphophilic and occasionally infiltrated by granulocytes. FNB sample from a bronchogenic non-keratinizing squamous cell carcinoma. P stain, ×400. **b** In this three-dimensional and trabecular-type aggregate, tumor cells are round to polygonal. Their nuclei are rather variable in size and shape and occasionally contain small nucleoli. Same case as in **a**. P stain, ×400. **c** Tumor cells display a coarsely granular chromatin with focal "crushing" artifacts. Same case as in **a**. P stain, ×400

carcinoma. Immunohistochemically, the detection of neuroendocrine markers and/or CD56 favors small-cell carcinoma [25] while positivity for CK5 and p63 indicates a diagnosis of squamous cell carcinoma [26].

Interpretation. The detection of a squamous cell carcinoma is frequent in endothoracic tumor masses due to a high incidence of bronchogenic malignancies showing this phenotype. This pattern can also be seen in tumors metastatic to the lung or mediastinal lymph nodes but originating from a large number of possible primary sites, mainly, the superior aerodigestive tract, skin, female genital tract, and urinary tract. Anaplastic carcinoma of the thyroid can present as a squamous cell carcinoma especially in metastatic sites. In the abdomen, this pattern can be detected in tumors metastatic to the liver, adrenal gland, and retroperitoneal lymph nodes. The primary sites of these malignancies are the same as those listed above, with the addition of bronchogenic carcinoma, which shows a peculiar propensity to early localization in the adrenal gland. Primary tumors with a squamous cell pattern that occur in the abdomen are quite unusual and consist of the squamous cell variant of carcinoma of the gallbladder and squamous cell carcinoma originating in ovarian teratoma. Squamous cell carcinoma in metastatic sites is almost never well-differentiated.

5.4 Basaloid-Cell Morphology

Definition. Basaloid cells are similar to the basal cells of squamous cell epithelium. They are small due to their poor cytoplasmic content and have a round to angulated nucleus that is hyperchromatic and always lacks a well-evident nucleolus. Basaloid cells are the integral component of the basaloid variant of squamous cell carcinoma and adenoid cystic carcinoma. These tumors differ widely with respect to their natural history and histogenesis but are included in this category due to their possible morphological similarities in FNB samples.

5.4.1 *Basaloid Squamous Cell Carcinoma Pattern*

- Erythrocytes and necrotic debris in the background with stromal fragments.
- Cellular aggregation definitely prevalent.
- Three-dimensional aggregates that form cords and trabeculae.
- Small cells with a narrow cytoplasmic rim and round to oval hyperchromatic nuclei.
- Rather marked nuclear pleomorphism with frequent mitotic figures and apoptosis.
- Elongated or spindle cells occasionally seen.

Cytomorphology. In the basaloid squamous cell carcinoma pattern, cellular aggregation prevails over dissociation, and nuclei appear atypical to the extent that small-cell carcinoma can enter the differential diagnosis. The presence of elongated or spindle cells, frequent necrotic cells, and a necrotic debris background is highly characteristic (Fig. 5.8).

Interpretation. The basaloid variant of squamous cell carcinoma is an aggressive malignancy that originates mostly in the upper respiratory tract, oral cavity, esophagus, and trachea [27–29]. It affects middle-aged and elderly people. Early metastases occur in regional lymph nodes, the lung, and liver.

5.4.2 *Adenoid Cystic Carcinoma Pattern*

- Clear background with stromal fragments and variable number of round bare nuclei.
- Globoid accumulations of mucin-like material in the background.
- Cellular dissociation prevalent.
- Three-dimensional aggregates that form cords, trabeculae, acini, sometimes rosette-like.
- Aggregation of cells around globoid deposits of mucin-like material.
- Small cells with a narrow cytoplasmic rim and round to oval vesicular nuclei.

Cytomorphology. In adenoid cystic carcinoma, at least in the non-anaplastic variant, cellular dissociation is characteristically prevalent. Cell nuclei appear more regular in size and shape as well as vesicular and monomorphous. The background contains a variable amount of globoid accumulations of mucin-like material. Cells clustering around these globules in a grape-like fashion are a typical and diagnostic feature of adenoid cystic carcinoma (Fig. 5.9).

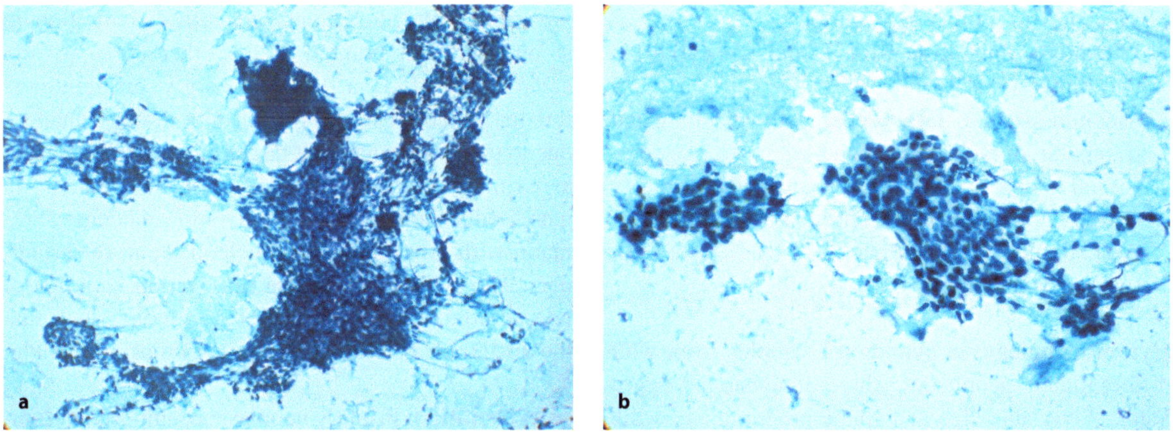

Fig 5.8 **a** Three-dimensional aggregate of elongated or spindle cells of small size with darkly staining elongated nuclei and a small amount of cytoplasm. Crushing artifacts of nuclei are seen. FNB sample from a lymph node metastasis of a basaloid carcinoma of the oral floor. P stain, ×400. **b** Same case as in **a**. Closer view of the characteristic darkly staining and homogeneous nuclei. P stain, ×600

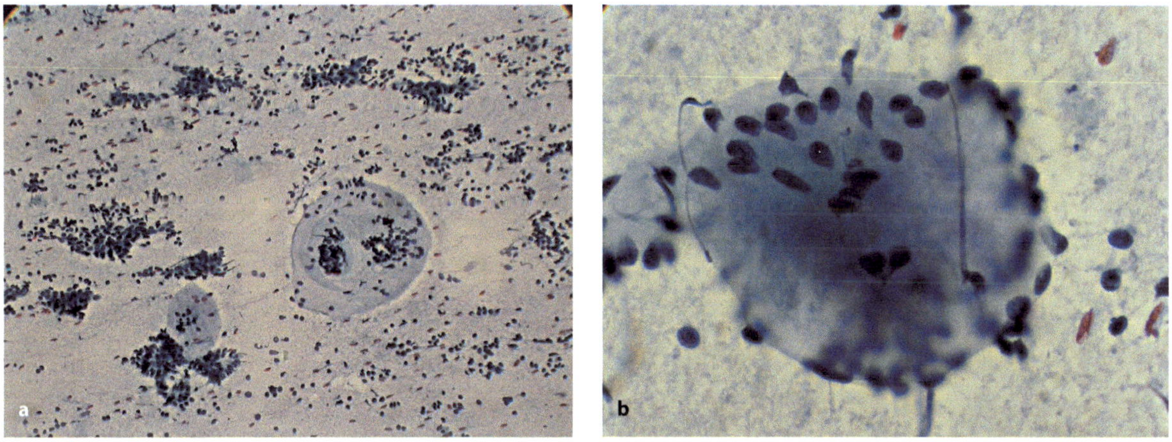

Fig 5.9 **a** In adenoid cystic carcinoma, the smear typically contains small cells, with darkly staining nuclei, dispersed in the background or clustered in tubulo-acinar aggregates. Peculiar globular structures of mucoid substance are also seen in the background. P stain, ×400. **b** High-power view of a globular mucinous structure that appears to be enveloped by cells with barely discernible cytoplasm and darkly staining nuclei. P stain, ×1000

Interpretation. Adenoid cystic carcinoma can be observed in a wide age group, including young adults, and is a rather ubiquitous tumor as it can originate in major and minor salivary glands, nasal cavities, breast, lung, prostate, and uterine cervix. The tumor is most frequently sampled by FNB in the salivary glands [30] and breast [31]. Metastatic dissemination occurs via blood vessels; thus, lymph node metastases are rarely seen. These tumors sometimes present in the liver or lung as a metastatic malignancy with an unknown primary.

5.5 Transitional-Cell Morphology

Definition. Transitional epithelium is a pseudostratified epithelium containing cells that appear elongated, cuboidal, squamoid, or flat—hence the name "transitional." Tumors with a transitional cell histogenesis display a peculiar cytological pattern that is easily demonstrated by FNB; but in poorly differentiated variants there is a significant morphological overlap with tumors of glandular- or squamous-cell morphology.

- Tendency to cellular aggregation.
- Prevailing three-dimensional and syncytial-like two-dimensional aggregates.
- Medium-sized to large cells, with an elongated, triangular, or racket-like shape.
- Round to oval nuclei, often eccentrically placed.
- Grossly granular to dense chromatin.
- Amphophilic, basophilic, or "clear" cytoplasm (never eosinophilic or orangeophilic).

Cytomorphology. In cytological samples from well-differentiated neoplasms, three-dimensional aggregates of variable size and shape predominate, while cellular dissociation is minimal or absent. The cells within the aggregates are round to elongated, with distinct cytoplasmic borders. The cytoplasm is well-evident, homogeneous, amphophilic, and never eosinophilic. Nuclei are round to oval or elongated with possible lobation. Chromatin texture is grossly granular; prominent nucleoli are never seen (Fig. 5.10a,b). At the periphery of the aggregates, or present as isolated elements, are cells that are globoid at one end and pointed at the other ("cercariform cells") [32] (Fig. 5.10c). In poorly differentiated tumors, by contrast, the overall morphology changes due to the appearance of a larger number of elongated and spindle-shaped cells, with elongated nuclei, an increased nuclear to cytoplasmic ratio, and dense chromatin with gross granules. Nucleoli are never prominent. The cytological picture can overlap with that of non-keratinizing squamous cell carcinoma such that the distinction between the two is at times impossible.

Interpretation. Primary neoplasms composed of transitional cells can be encountered in the abdomen, urinary tract (urothelial carcinoma), or ovary (Brenner's tumor). Not unusually, urothelial carcinoma of the renal pelvis expands, simulating a tumor mass of the renal parenchyma. Transitional-cell carcinoma typically occurs in the nasal cavity and paranasal sinuses, and is frequently associated with early metastasis to the lymph nodes of the neck. Tumors composed of

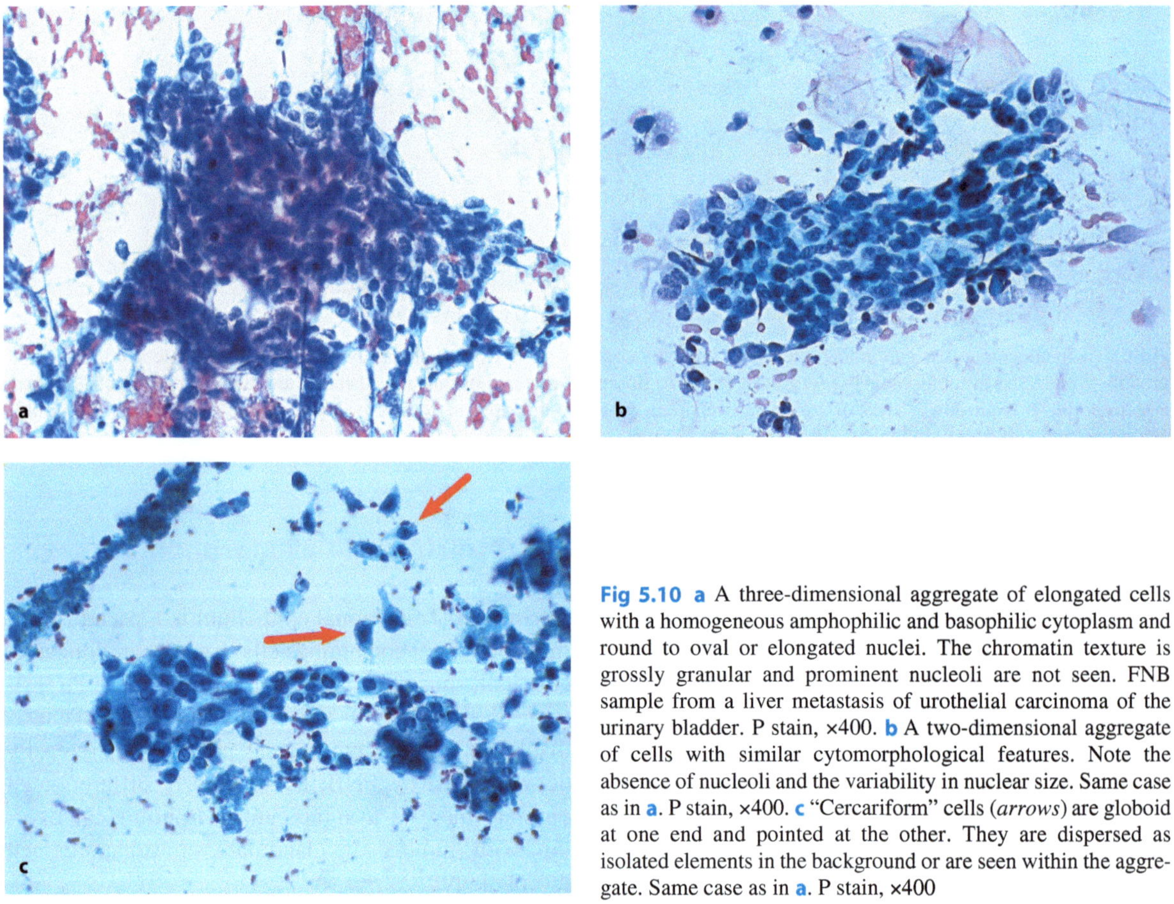

Fig 5.10 **a** A three-dimensional aggregate of elongated cells with a homogeneous amphophilic and basophilic cytoplasm and round to oval or elongated nuclei. The chromatin texture is grossly granular and prominent nucleoli are not seen. FNB sample from a liver metastasis of urothelial carcinoma of the urinary bladder. P stain, ×400. **b** A two-dimensional aggregate of cells with similar cytomorphological features. Note the absence of nucleoli and the variability in nuclear size. Same case as in **a**. P stain, ×400. **c** "Cercariform" cells (*arrows*) are globoid at one end and pointed at the other. They are dispersed as isolated elements in the background or are seen within the aggregate. Same case as in **a**. P stain, ×400

transitional cells are much more commonly sampled by FNB at metastatic sites than at the primary tumor site. Typically, the liver and the lung are common sites of metastatic spread of urothelial carcinoma. The coexpression of CK20 and CD10 is helpful in identifying the tumor [33,34]

5.6 Small-Cell Morphology

Definition. A large variety of tumors show a solid and trabecular growth of cells that appear to be small in size. The small appearance of the cells is due to the barely perceptible amount of cytoplasm whereas the longer axis of the nuclei of these cells can exceed 2×RBC. Thus, the cellular size is roughly equal to that of the nucleus. Additional features are a peculiar chromatin texture that is variably granular, the lack of a prominent nucleolus, and a variable tendency to chromatin degradation. Tumors composed of small cells display different cytological patterns on FNB; these are classified according to the degree of cellular pleomorphism, the extent of cellular non-cohesion, and nuclear atypia.

5.6.1 Monomorphous Cell Pattern with Tendency to Aggregation and Mild Nuclear Atypia

- Aggregation of cells highly prevalent, with a tendency to form large aggregates.
- Small nuclei (<2×RBC) (Fig. 5.11a).
- Round to oval nuclei.
- Finely granular chromatin texture ("salt and pepper" appearance) (Fig. 5.11b).
- Small nucleoli, single or multiple (2–3).
- Significant amount of cytoplasm, with frequent eccentric displacement of the nucleus (Fig. 5.11b).

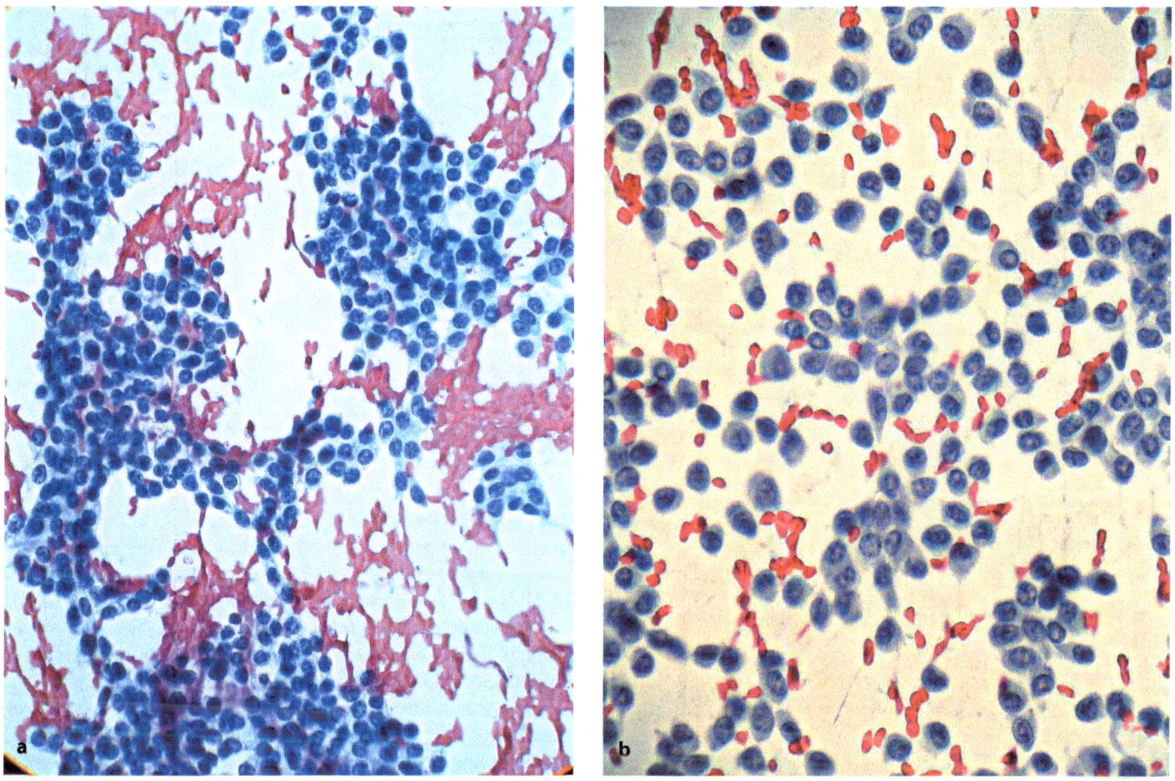

Fig 5.11 **a** Sheets of small to medium-sized cells with scanty cytoplasm and round and monotonous nuclei. The chromatin is finely granular and no nucleoli are visible. FNB sample from a liver metastasis of small intestinal carcinoid tumor. P stain, ×800. **b** Small to medium-sized cells with a moderate amount of cytoplasm, round nuclei, and a slight tendency to non-cohesion; sometimes the nucleus is displaced at the periphery. The chromatin texture is characteristically finely and slightly coarsely granular ("salt and pepper" appearance), with occasional small nucleoli. FNB sample from a well differentiated endocrine carcinoma of the pancreas. P stain, ×1200

- Possible "button-like" cytoplasmic inclusions (better seen in smears stained according to the May Grünwald Giemsa method).

Cytomorphology. Cellularity in samples showing a monomorphous pattern is generally abundant. The cells are clustered in large two-dimensional aggregates that show little tendency to nuclear overlap, or in microacini, tubules, Indian files, or pseudorosettes. The cytoplasm is generally moderate in amount and finely granular. The small, round nucleus is eccentrically displaced, giving the cell a plasma-cell-like morphology (Fig. 5.11b). Nucleoli are only occasionally seen and are small (Fig. 5.11a,b). The cell is round to oval or sometimes has an elongated end. In paraffin sections from cell blocks, the nuclei appear to be of uniform size and equidistant from one another; the cytoplasmic borders are indistinct. In addition, the nuclei may polarize as palisades at the periphery of the aggregates.

Interpretation. The monomorphous pattern is typically observed in well-differentiated neuroendocrine tumors (typical carcinoid) of the gut and lower respiratory tract, as well as in endocrine tumors of the pancreas, both in primary and metastatic sites. The aggregation pattern and cellular morphology are quite characteristic and the diagnosis is readily made. Immunohistochemical demonstration of neuroendocrine markers in tumor cells is of help in confirming the diagnosis (see below).

5.6.2 Pleomorphic Cell Pattern with Tendency to Aggregation and Marked Nuclear Atypia

- Aggregation of cells prevalent, with a tendency to form small aggregates (Fig. 5.12a).
- Nuclear size variable, usually ranging mostly between 2× and 3×RBC.

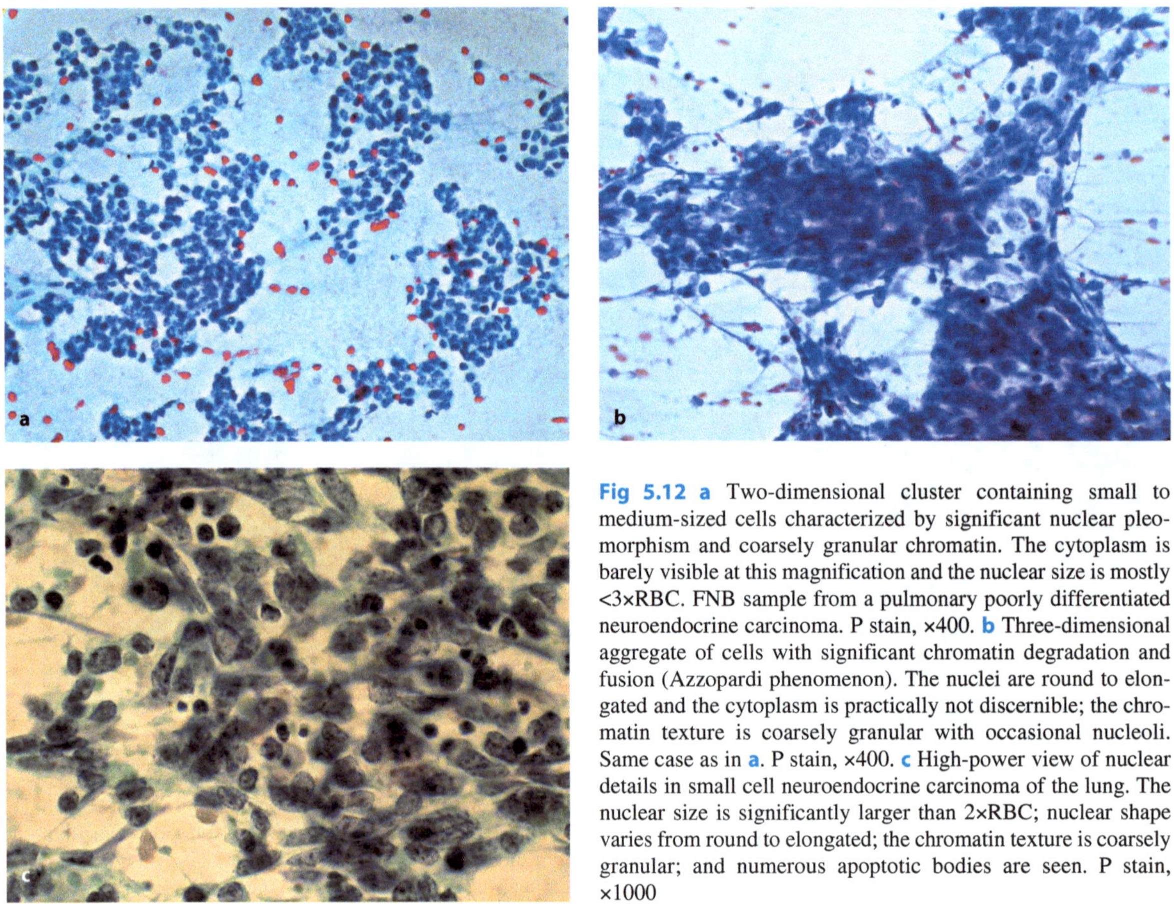

Fig 5.12 a Two-dimensional cluster containing small to medium-sized cells characterized by significant nuclear pleomorphism and coarsely granular chromatin. The cytoplasm is barely visible at this magnification and the nuclear size is mostly <3×RBC. FNB sample from a pulmonary poorly differentiated neuroendocrine carcinoma. P stain, ×400. **b** Three-dimensional aggregate of cells with significant chromatin degradation and fusion (Azzopardi phenomenon). The nuclei are round to elongated and the cytoplasm is practically not discernible; the chromatin texture is coarsely granular with occasional nucleoli. Same case as in **a**. P stain, ×400. **c** High-power view of nuclear details in small cell neuroendocrine carcinoma of the lung. The nuclear size is significantly larger than 2×RBC; nuclear shape varies from round to elongated; the chromatin texture is coarsely granular; and numerous apoptotic bodies are seen. P stain, ×1000

- Elongated nuclei, with possible lobation and clefts.
- Nuclear fragility with variable degree of crushing artifact (Azzopardi's [35] phenomenon) (Fig. 5.12b).
- Chromatin texture granular with a tendency to coarse granules (Fig. 5.12a).
- Presence of small single or multiple nucleoli (Fig. 5.12a,c).
- Possible detection of mitotic figures.
- Barely perceptible cytoplasm, forming a narrow perinuclear rim (Fig. 5.12a–c).
- Possible detection of perinuclear "button-like" cytoplasmic inclusion bodies (better seen in smears stained according to the May Grünwald Giemsa method).

Cytomorphology. The pleomorphic pattern is typically seen in poorly differentiated and small-cell neuroendocrine carcinomas but is less pronounced in the former than in the latter. In poorly differentiated neuroendocrine carcinoma, there is a greater tendency to cellular aggregation, the nuclei are less fragile, and a small amount of cytoplasm is retained (Fig. 5.12a). Conversely, in small-cell carcinoma, there is a marked tendency to necrosis and a less cellularity. The nuclei are very fragile and often resemble filaments of highly basophilic material (Fig. 5.12b). Cellular aggregates may be replaced by accumulations of amorphous highly basophilic material, which is derived from massive nuclear disintegration and fusion (Azzopardi phenomenon [35]). In addition, blood vessels dispersed in the background appear to be "encrusted" with this peculiar necrotic material. In aggregates containing viable cells, the nuclear profile is irregular due to the presence of clefts or partial lobation; the cytoplasm is practically absent, the chromatin texture is grossly granular, and small nucleoli are seen. Nuclear size in most cells is >2×RBC (Fig. 5.12c).

Interpretation. While poorly differentiated and small-cell neuroendocrine carcinomas are practically ubiquitous, the main sites of the primary tumor are the lower respiratory tract, urinary bladder, gallbladder, and skin (Merkel cell carcinoma). Immunohistochemical demonstration of neuroendocrine markers in tumor cells is of paramount importance to confirm the diagnosis. Chromogranin is easily demonstrated in well-differentiated neuroendocrine tumors but its expression may be completely lacking in poorly differentiated and small-cell carcinomas. Instead, synaptophysin and protein gene product 9.5 are more sensitive markers. In addition, small-cell carcinoma expresses CD56 [25] and CK8/18, at least focally. Testing for the combined expression of CDX-2 and TTF-1 allows primary tumors of the intestine (CDX-2+/TTF-1-) to be distinguished from those of the lung (CDX-2-/TTF-1+) and other possible primary sites (CDX-2-/TTF-1-) [36,37]. Of note, TTF-1 is expressed in 25% of neuroendocrine carcinomas of the urinary bladder and occasionally those of endocervical origin [38,39]. Merkel cell neuroendocrine carcinoma shows a characteristic globular or button-like immunopositivity for CK20 and EMA and is TTF-1 negative [40]. The differential diagnosis of small-cell carcinoma mainly includes poorly differentiated nonkeratinizing squamous cell carcinoma composed of small elements. Immunohistochemistry is of help in this distinction (see above). Finally, the tendency of cells to aggregate is a useful criterion to rule out a highly pleomorphic malignant lymphoma.

5.6.3 Pleomorphic Cell Pattern with Marked Cellular Dissociation

- Necrotic, hemorrhagic, or myxoid background.
- Abundant cellularity.
- Cells are semi-cohesive with focal pseudoaggregation (Indian files, rosettes).
- Small to intermediate-sized cells.
- Sparse cytoplasm (occasionally, more abundant), with nuclear displacement.
- Round to oval nuclei, with possible marked nuclear pleomorphism.
- Coarsely granular chromatin texture and no nucleoli (constant).
- Occasional mitotic figures.
- Occasional large bizarre cells or multinucleated or spindle cells.

Cytomorphology. This pleomorphic pattern is dominated by the presence of small to medium-sized cells (up to 3×RBC in diameter) having sparse or no cytoplasm and a characteristic coarsely granular chromatin texture with no nucleoli. The cells show little tendency to aggregation and often form semi-cohesive clusters. In contrast to the monotony of the chromatin texture and cytoplasmic features, there is a rather marked variation in cellular shape (round to oval to spindle-like)

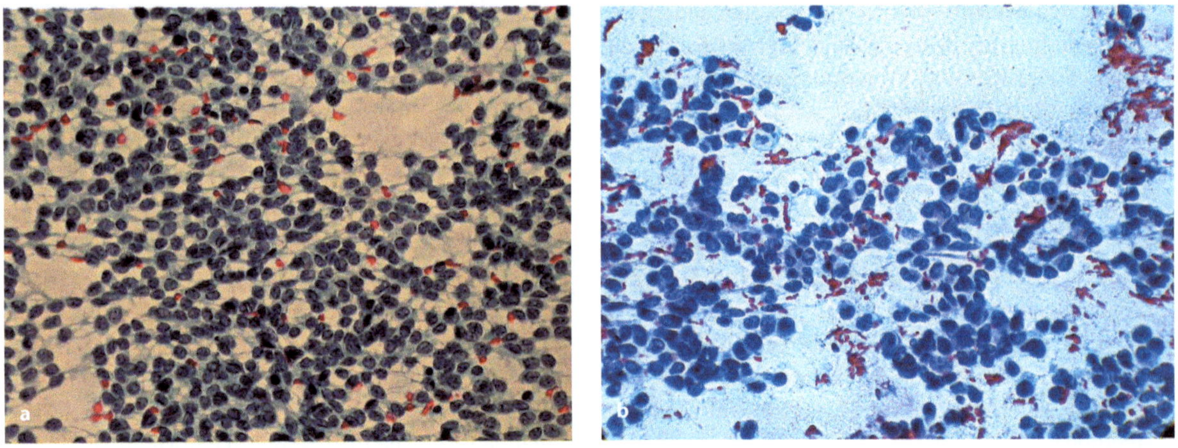

Fig 5.13 a Loosely cohesive or non-cohesive round cells with scant cytoplasm and pleomorphic nuclei with coarsely granular chromatin and no prominent nucleoli. Nuclear size is ≥2×RBC. FNB sample from a peripheral neuroectodermal tumor (PNET) primary in the kidney. P stain, ×400. b Medium-sized cells with pleomorphic nuclei and focal tendency to pseudoaggregation; the cytoplasm is sometimes well-evident and responsible for nuclear displacement to the periphery. The chromatin texture is coarsely granular and there is frequent nuclear lobation. The background contains necrotic debris. FNB sample from a patient with alveolar rhabdomyosarcoma. P stain, ×400

and size (mostly small and intermediate, but with possible large elements) that accounts for the pleomorphic appearance of the cellular harvest (Fig. 5.13).

Interpretation. This type of pleomorphism is typically seen in small- and round-cell sarcomas, e.g., Ewing's sarcoma/primitive neuroectodermal tumor (ES/PNET), rhabdomyosarcoma, some malignant peripheral nerve sheath tumors, and sometimes in malignant melanoma, especially in metastatic sites. The tendency to form semi-cohesive clusters is of help to rule out lymphoblastic lymphoma or the blastoid variant of mantle cell lymphoma, both of which share many morphological features with pleomorphic-type tumors but are generally characterized by a non-cohesive cell pattern. The correct interpretation of such samples is based not only on a proper clinicopathological correlation but also on immunohistochemical and molecular studies of the cell population. Tumor cells belonging to the ES/PNET group are characterized by membrane positivity for CD99, with variable expression of NSE, PGP 9.5, neurofilaments, Leu-7, synaptophysin, and cytokeratins [41]. CD99 positivity is also encountered in lymphoblastic lymphomas, synovial sarcoma, mesothelioma, neuroendocrine carcinoma, and rhabdomyosarcoma; thus, its expression is not sufficient to allow a diagnosis of ES/PNET tumors. For this reason, demonstration of the fusion product of the t(11;22)(q24;q12) translocation represents the gold standard for a reliable diagnosis [42]. The diagnosis of rhabdomyosarcoma is obtained by immunohistochemistry, specifically, by demonstrating cell positivity for desmin, muscle-specific actin, MyoD1, and myogenin [43]. Malignant melanoma can be ruled out by the determination of cellular expression of S100P, HMB45, and Melan-A.

5.7 Large-Cell Morphology

Definition. Cells are defined as "large" if their largest diameter is ≥4×RBC. Tumor cells appear large due to the presence of a voluminous nucleus and an abundant cytoplasm. The latter is homogeneous or microvacuolated and, by definition, should neither be clear nor intensely eosinophilic. A predominance of large cells in the harvest is generally indicative of the monophasic pattern; the biphasic pattern is associated with a spindle cell component.

5.7.1 *Monophasic Pattern*

- Necrotic or hemorrhagic background.
- Marked tendency to cellular non-cohesion and prevalence of isolated elements.
- Prevalence of large cells (always >4–5×RBC) (Fig. 5.14a,b).

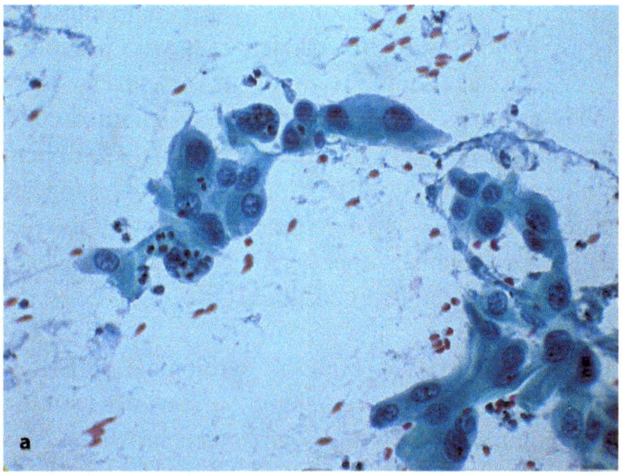

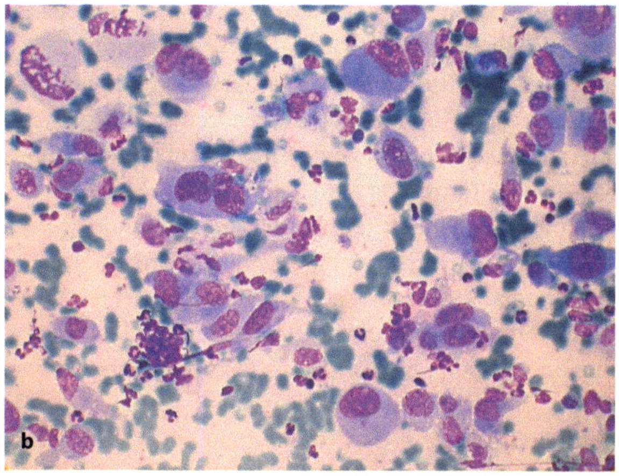

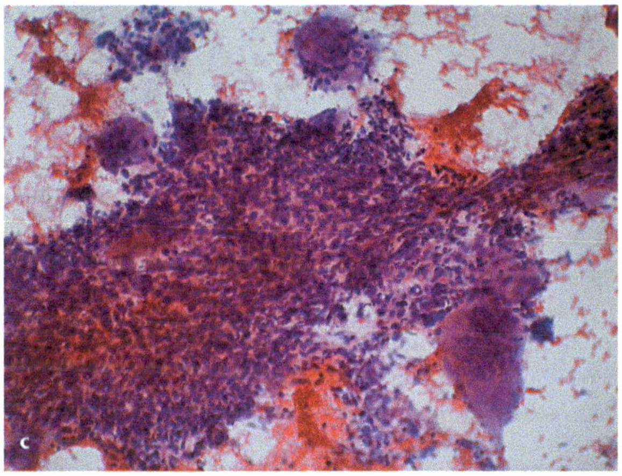

Fig 5.14 **a** Large polygonal cells with large nuclei, abundant cytoplasm, and distinct cell borders. In some cases, the greatest cellular diameter is about ten-fold the diameter of a RBC. One cell contains granulocytes in its cytoplasm. FNB smear from a large cell bronchogenic carcinoma. P stain, ×400. **b** In smears stained using the May Grünwald Giemsa method, the cytoplasm of large cells is gray to green and nuclear pleomorphism is well-evident. ×600. **c** Spindle cells and large giant and multinucleated cells coexist in the biphasic pattern. FNB sample from an anaplastic carcinoma of the thyroid gland. P stain, ×400

- Polygonal, or oval, round, or elongated shape.
- Intermediate-sized to large nuclei that may be eccentric (Fig. 5.14a,b).
- Pleomorphic chromatin texture, i.e., homogeneous, dense, alternating to coarsely granular or "band-like" (Fig. 5.14b).
- Prominent single or multiple nucleoli, sometimes of bizarre shape.
- Atypical mitoses.
- Amphophilic, rarely basophilic, and abundant, not fragile, cytoplasm (Fig. 5.14a).
- Cytoplasmic vacuoles with lymphophagocytosis or erythrophagocytosis (Fig. 5.14a).

Cytomorphology. Large cells may represent the only component of the sample or they may be mixed with a minor component (<20%) of poorly differentiated adenocarcinoma or squamous cell carcinoma. In both cases, cellular atypia markedly stands out. The cells are highly variable in size and shape, with more than occasional bizarre elements including large and pleomorphic nuclei as well as large and/or multiple nucleoli. The cytoplasm is abundant and frequently appears vacuolated. Phagocytosis of small lymphocytes or erythrocytes (cell-in-cell phenomenon) is seen. When a component of more typical adenocarcinoma or squamous cell carcinoma fails to be recognized, the differential diagnosis includes highly pleomorphic malignancies such as melanoma, high-grade peripheral T-cell lymphoma, or pleomorphic sarcoma. Generally, large-cell carcinoma cells show the characteristic cytoplasmic lymphophagocytosis (emperipolesis), which is useful in their distinction from other pleomorphic tumors. Amelanotic malignant melanoma may retain at least focal melanin pigment granules, which helps in correct identification of the tumor. It is noteworthy that both carcinoma and melanoma may be characterized by large cells having a rhabdoid appearance and accumulations of large eosinophilic cytoplasmic inclusions. The distinction between the two can be made only on the basis of immunohistochemical data.

Interpretation. Typical examples of large-cell carcinoma occur primarily in the lower respiratory tract, pancreas, and thyroid. Less frequently, this pattern is seen in renal cell carcinoma, adrenal cortical carcinoma, hepatocellular carcinoma, and choriocarcinoma (in its pure form or in association with other germ cell tumors). As already pointed out, these tumors generally enter the differential diagnosis with malignant melanoma, pleomorphic sarcoma, and large-cell lymphomas. Immunohistochemistry is almost always the only option in a difficult differential diagnosis, but large cells may not express any lineage-specific markers, probably due to a virtual intracytoplasmic "dilution" of these substances. For this reason, the sensitivity of some immunohistochemical tests may be reduced and a conclusive result thereby precluded. Vimentin immunopositivity is generally well preserved and it serves at least as a demonstration that the negativity for all other markers is not due to poor fixation or other artifacts. The first approach is to test for the wide-spectrum cytokeratins (CK), S100P, and CD45 together. The CK+/CD45- profile suggests a carcinoma irrespective of possible positivity for S100P; the CK-/S100P+/CD45- profile is indicative of a malignant melanoma, and CK-/S100P-/CD45+ of malignant lymphoma. A vimentin+/CK-/S100P-/CD45- profile suggests a sarcoma but it is important to point out that this result is frequently encountered in large-cell carcinoma. Moreover, actin positivity in this setting does not rule out carcinoma, as sarcomatoid carcinomas may express actin rather than cytokeratin.

5.7.2 Biphasic Pattern

- Necrotic or hemorrhagic background with variable cellularity.
- Concomitant large multinucleated cells and aggregates of spindle cells (in variable proportion) (Fig. 5.14c).
- Some or most large cells showing a large number of clustered, overlapping, bland-appearing nuclei containing prominent nucleoli, consistent with an osteoclast-type multinucleated giant cell.
- Spindle cells of small to intermediate size and tightly clustered in large three-dimensional aggregates.

Cytomorphology. The biphasic pattern is referred to as such because of the presence of two apparently unrelated cellular components: one comprising very large, frequently multinucleated cells with a definite "osteoclast-like" appearance (Fig. 5.14c), and the other made up of medium-sized, definitely spindled cells. The latter are found in large and thick three-dimensional aggregates and have a fibrocyte-like appearance. There is no apparent transition between the two cell types, which appear to proliferate together although in variable proportions.

Interpretation. The biphasic cytological pattern is mainly seen in the sarcomatoid variant of anaplastic carcinoma of the thyroid with "osteoclast-like" cells and in a peculiar variant of pancreatic carcinoma of undifferentiated type.

5.8 Clear-Cell Morphology

Definition. Primary tumors may be partly or entirely composed of intermediate to large cells that in paraffin sections of tissue samples processed for histological examination contain a clear empty-looking cytoplasm. In ethanol-fixed and Papanicolaou-stained cytological smears, the cytoplasm of these "clear" cells is, instead, pale and amphophilic, due to the presence of finely granular material. Moreover, in aggregates with multiple layers of cells, the cytoplasm may even become eosinophilic. In air-dried smears stained with Romanowsky stain, the otherwise clear cytoplasm contains a finely granular gray material. By definition, the term "clear-cell morphology" is reserved for cytological samples in which the clear-cell component is ≥80%.

- Clear and proteinaceous to hemorrhagic background, with necrotic debris (Fig. 5.15a).
- Tendency to cellular aggregation (wide variability in the number of cells per aggregate).
- Polygonal, oval, round, or elongated shape or partially spindled.
- Abundant and homogeneous cytoplasm, pale and amphophilic with peripheral vacuolization (Fig. 5.15b).
- Well-defined peripheral outline (Fig. 5.15 a,b)
- Nuclear size variable, from small (1–2×RBC) to large (>2×RBC).
- Dense or vesicular and peripherally marginated chromatin.
- Nucleoli evident only in high-grade tumors.

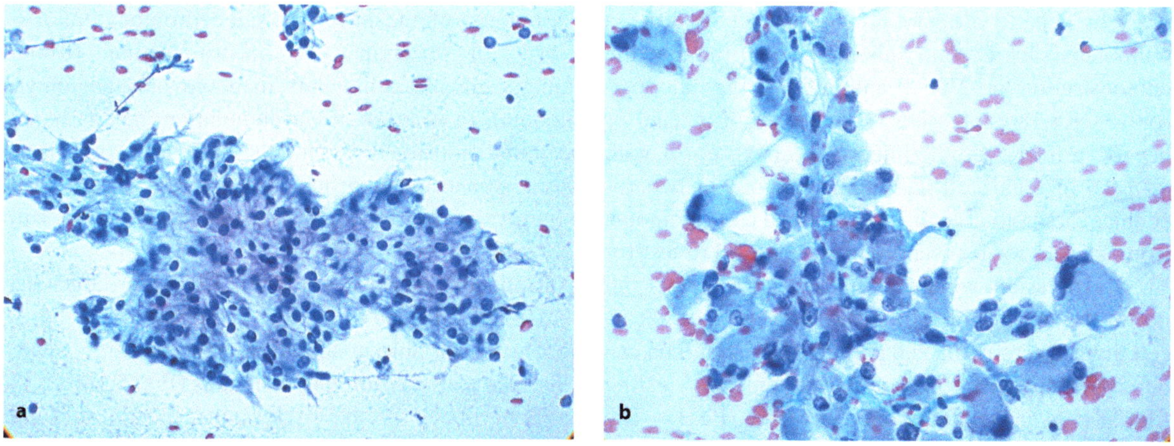

Fig 5.15 **a** A syncytial cluster of large polygonal cells with clear cytoplasm and distinct cell borders. FNB sample from a clear cell renal carcinoma. P stain, ×400. **b** In P-stained smears, the cytoplasm of "clear" cells is sometimes amphophilic and finely granular, with only peripheral microvacuolization. Same case as in **a**. ×400

Cytomorphology. Tumors with a clear-cell morphology can be graded as well-differentiated or poorly differentiated. Nuclear size is a reliable indicator of the grade of tumor differentiation, as it varies from small (diameter <2×RBC) in well-differentiated tumors to large (diameter >3×RBC) in poorly differentiated tumors. Similarly, in the former, the chromatin texture is finely granular and nucleoli are absent or difficult to demonstrate, while in the latter the chromatin is coarsely granular, dense, or fragile. Nucleoli are prominent and possibly of bizarre shape. The aggregation pattern is variable. The tendency to cell clustering is more common in well-differentiated tumors while the cells in poorly differentiated tumors tend to non-cohesion (Fig. 5.15a,b). In addition, the cells often appear to be peripherally anchored to the wall of dissociated blood vessels.

Interpretation. Tumors composed of clear cells are ubiquitous and may be epithelial or non-epithelial in origin. Clear-cell carcinoma primarily arises in the kidney, lung, thyroid, adrenal cortex, or ovary. These tumors show a somewhat predictable and peculiar pattern of metastatic seeding as they localize in organs that are sites of primary clear-cell tumors themselves. Thus, clear-cell renal cell carcinoma frequently metastasizes into the liver, adrenal cortex, or the thyroid, posing difficult problems in the differential diagnosis—as it will thus include primary clear-cell tumors in these sites. Similarly, early metastasis of clear-cell hepatocellular carcinoma may often occur within the adrenal cortex, and clear-cell carcinoma of the ovary may frequently metastasize to the liver. The retroperitoneal lymph nodes are the site of early metastatic involvement by both renal and adrenal cortical clear-cell carcinomas, and both malignancies rapidly progress, with pulmonary metastases. Finally, the liver, adrenal cortex, and mediastinal and retroperitoneal lymph nodes are preferential sites of metastatic seeding for clear-cell carcinomas arising in the lung, thyroid, and parathyroid glands. Malignant melanoma and its soft-tissue counterpart, i.e., clear-cell sarcoma of the tendon sheath, should also be added to the list of metastatic malignancies possibly having a clear-cell morphology.

5.8.1 Immunohistochemistry of Clear-Cell Tumors

Immunohistochemistry is of help in determining the lineage of clear-cell tumors (epithelial vs. non-epithelial) and, sometimes, their site of origin. Carcinoma can be distinguished from melanoma by investigating the immunoreactivity for cytokeratin and melanoma markers. It is important, however, to point out that in roughly 10% of cases metastatic melanoma is positive for CK8,18 [44] and CEA [45]. The site of origin of a clear-cell carcinoma can be determined by testing for CK8,18, the high molecular weight cytokeratin CK34βe12, monoclonal CEA (mCEA), and TTF-1 expression [46]. Positivity for CK34βe12 excludes a renal or hepatic primary tumor, instead favoring a pulmonary site of origin; this can be confirmed by the demonstration of TTF-1 and mCEA immunopositivity. CK8,18 expression is indicative of a renal or hepatic primary only. Vimentin is coexpressed with CK8,18 in renal cell carcinoma but not in hepatocellular carcinoma. To distinguish renal cell carcinoma from adrenal cortical carcinoma it is useful to test for EMA expression, which is detected in the former but not in the latter [47]. The distinction between clear-cell thyroid carcinoma and parathyroid carcinoma can be accomplished by immunohistochemically testing for TTF-1 and parathyroid hormone (PTH). The former is expressed in thyroid carcinoma and the latter in parathyroid carcinoma; their positivities are mutually exclusive. The detection of increased serum levels of PTH obviously provides additional evidence of a parathyroid carcinoma. Germ cell tumors, in particular seminoma and yolk-sac tumor, can include a cellular component with clear-cell features. Both metastasize to the retroperitoneal lymph nodes, liver, and lung, or they can occur as an extragonadal primary tumor mass in the retroperitoneum and mediastinum.

5.9 Oxyphil/Oncocytic- or Oncocytoid-Cell Morphology

Definition. Oxyphil or oncocytic cells (or Hurthle cells in the thyroid) comprise a peculiar cell type that in hematoxylin and eosin (H&E) routinely stained paraffin sections is characterized by an abundant eosinophilic cytoplasm. These cells are typically round-oval or polygonal in shape, and intermediate to large in size. In cytological preparations, they retain their abundant cytoplasm, which stains eosinophilic in Papanicolaou-stained smears or pink to gray-blue in Romanowsky-stained smears. The designation "oxyphil morphology" requires that at least 80% of the cytological sample is composed of such cells. Oxyphil cells are rarely encountered in normal tissues but may represent a significant component of several tumoral and pseudotumoral proliferations. The increase in cytoplasmic content and the peculiar granular appearance of the cytoplasm reflect the accumulation of mitochondria (oncocytic tumors of the thyroid, parathyroid, salivary glands, kidney, adrenal cortex, and gonadal stroma), neuroendocrine granules (medullary carcinoma of the thyroid, neuroendocrine carcinoma of the pancreas, pheochromocytoma), or fibrils of different type (gastrointestinal stromal tumors, granular cell tumors, rhabdomyoma, angiomyolipoma). In addition, the accumulation may assume a globular appearance, with the formation of a large intracytoplasmic inclusion (rhabdoid appearance) [48].

- Prevalence of aggregates made up of few cells, with tendency to cellular dissociation.
- Cells of intermediate (Fig. 5.16a) to large size (Fig. 5.16b) due to abundant cytoplasm.
- Nuclei variable in size, from small to large, sometimes with a prominent nucleolus (Fig. 5.16b).
- Bare nuclei in the background mostly in small chains, often characterized by dense chromatin.
- Possible intranuclear cytoplasmic inclusions (pseudonucleoli).
- Oxyphil cells frequently admixed with endothelial cells or anchored to isolated blood vessels.

Cytomorphology. The main cytomorphological features of this type of sample is the diverse aggregation pattern, since cells in the same sample may present as trabeculae, cords, or follicles (Hürthle cell tumors). Nuclear pleomorphism may be prominent but is not a marker of malignancy. Similarly, large nucleoli can be seen more than occasionally in benign tumors. Nuclear pseudoinclusions are a characteristic finding in Hürthle cell tumors of the thyroid and in pheochromocytoma. Necrotic cells or bare isolated nuclei are rather common (Fig. 5.16a,b).

Interpretation. Oxyphil cells represent a major component of several tumors originating primarily in the abdomen, such as hepatocellular carcinoma, renal oncocytoma, some tumors of the pancreas, pheochromocytoma and paraganglioma, yolk-sac tumor, and sex cord-stromal tumors of the ovary. In addition, tumors entirely composed of oxyphil cells (oncocytomas) occur primarily in the thyroid, salivary glands, and parathyroid glands. Apocrine carcinoma of the skin and breast also belong to this category. Tumors exhibiting oncocytic features and most frequently arising within the chest are bronchogenic carcinoid tumors and salivary-gland-type tumors. Finally, it is worth mentioning the occurrence of a peculiar variant of carcinoma, composed of oncocytoid cells closely resembling hepatocytes and designated "hepatoid carcinoma." This tumor variant can develop in the stomach [49], ovary, pancreas, or lung,

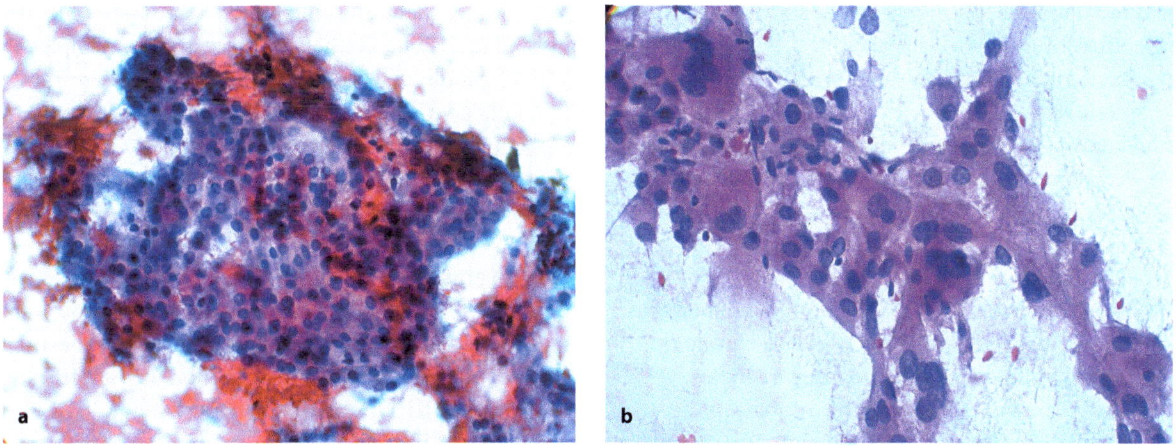

Fig 5.16 a A cluster of medium-sized oncocytic cells displaying abundant and granular cytoplasm that stains pink to red in P-stained smears. The nuclei are round and look somewhat monotonous. FNB sample from a renal oncocytoma. ×400. b Pleomorphic oncocytic cells showing nuclei of variable size and shape with a granular and eosinophilic cytoplasm. FNB sample from pulmonary metastasis of oncocytic carcinoma primary in the thyroid gland. P stain, ×400

and may be associated with the secretion of α-fetoprotein (AFP). In general, an oncocytic or oncocytoid cell tumor in typical sites does not pose any diagnostic problems, especially when a correct correlation with clinical findings and imaging data is available. The distinction of benign vs. malignant oncocytic tumor, particularly in the thyroid, parathyroid, and salivary glands, cannot be accomplished solely by FNB. Similarly, oncocytomas of the kidney are generally benign tumors but the partial sampling of FNB cannot determine whether the oncocytic cells in the sample merely represent a component of an otherwise typical clear-cell carcinoma, papillary carcinoma, or chromophobe-cell carcinoma. Therefore, any judgment regarding malignancy should be deferred to histological examination of the entire lesion. Immunohistochemistry can be used in the differential diagnosis of primary vs. metastatic tumor, especially in the liver. EMA positivity of the tumor cells favors the diagnosis of a renal malignancy [47]. Tumor cell expression of Hepar 1 and AFP supports a diagnosis of hepatocellular carcinoma. The lack of any of these markers would indicate an adrenal cortical origin of the tumor [48]. In the salivary glands, primary oncocytoma can be distinguished from metastatic renal cell carcinoma with oncocytoid features by testing for CK20 and CD10 expression. The former is frequently CK20+/CD10- while the latter shows the opposite profile [50].

5.10 Epithelioid- and Spindle-Cell Morphology

Definition. Epithelioid cells are non-epithelial cells but have a distinct epithelial-like appearance. They are oval to elongated in shape, intermediate to large in size, and have well-demarcated external outlines. The nucleus is centrally or eccentrically placed, the chromatin is generally vesicular, and a nucleolus of variable size is regularly present. The cytoplasm is homogeneous or granular in but not vacuolated. In cytological smears, these cells tend to be non-cohesive. Epithelioid cells should be distinguished from epithelioid histiocytes, which have a similar size and shape but lack nucleoli and frequently contain cytoplasmic vacuoles. Moreover, the features of typical epithelioid cells merge with those of elongated and definitely spindle-shaped cells, having an elongated nucleus and a similarly granular or homogeneous appearing cytoplasm. By contrast, epithelioid histiocytes are always mixed with small lymphocytes, plasma cells, and multinucleated giant cells. Epithelioid cells are important constituents in several types of mesenchymal, melanocytic, and mesothelial tumor proliferations and almost always merge morphologically with spindle cells. Since epithelioid and spindle-shaped cells always coexist in such tumors, although in rather variable proportions, the definition of this morphological pattern includes both cell types and covers a large spectrum of lesions.

- Background clear to hemorrhagic, with stromal fragments.
- Variable amount of cellularity.
- Prevalence of non-cohesive cells with a tendency to form aggregates of few cells.
- Elongated ovoid, sometimes polygonal cells with a centrally placed nucleus.
- Large nucleus with possible prominent nucleolus.
- Finely or coarsely granular or dense chromatin.
- Possible intranuclear cytoplasmic vacuoles.
- Finely granular amphophilic or basophilic cytoplasm and a distinct cellular membrane.
- Possible melanin pigment granules within the cytoplasm (malignant melanoma and related tumors).
- Large pleomorphic cells possibly present.

Cytomorphology. In samples in which the epithelioid-cell morphology prevails, the most salient cytological findings are the prevalent cellular non-cohesion and a variable degree of cell pleomorphism as opposed to the rather monomorphic nuclei, which are mostly oval to elongated in shape (Fig. 5.17). In such samples, one should diligently search for intranuclear cytoplasmic inclusions, which are frequent morphological indicators of malignant melanoma. Melanin granules in the cytoplasm may assist in confirming this diagnosis but it is important to stress that intranuclear cytoplasmic inclusions are seen in tumors other than melanoma, including medullary carcinoma of the thyroid and some epithelioid sarcomas. In samples in which spindle cells are prevalent, the cells are rarely non-cohesive and tend to cluster around capillary vessels (Fig. 5.18a). The cytoplasm can be moderately abundant (Fig. 5.18b) or sparse to the extent that it is practically not discernible (Fig. 5.18a).

Interpretation. The prototypes of neoplasms presenting with an epithelioid-cell morphology are metastatic malignant melanoma and gastrointestinal stromal tumors. Immunohistochemically, melanoma cells express S100P, HMB-45, and Melan-A. S100P is a very sensitive marker but its reactivity in metastatic tumors may be reduced in up to 50% of cases and/or patchily distributed within the lesion [51]. Conversely, HMB-45 and Melan-A are less sensitive but more specific, and more frequently expressed in metastatic sites. Therefore, S100P expression should be tested along with that of HMB-45 and Melan-A to warrant a reliable sensitivity of these markers. Gastrointestinal stromal tumors typically coexpress CD34 and CD117 (see Chapter 6) [49]. *Synovial sarcoma* is another example of a mesenchymal tumor with an epithelioid-cell morphology. This ubiquitous tumor can originate primarily in the soft tissues of the trunk or it may induce metastatic deposits in the retroperitoneal or mediastinal lymph nodes, the liver, or the lung. Synovial sarcoma cells are typically reactive for CD99, EMA, and bcl-2, and 50–80% of these tumors

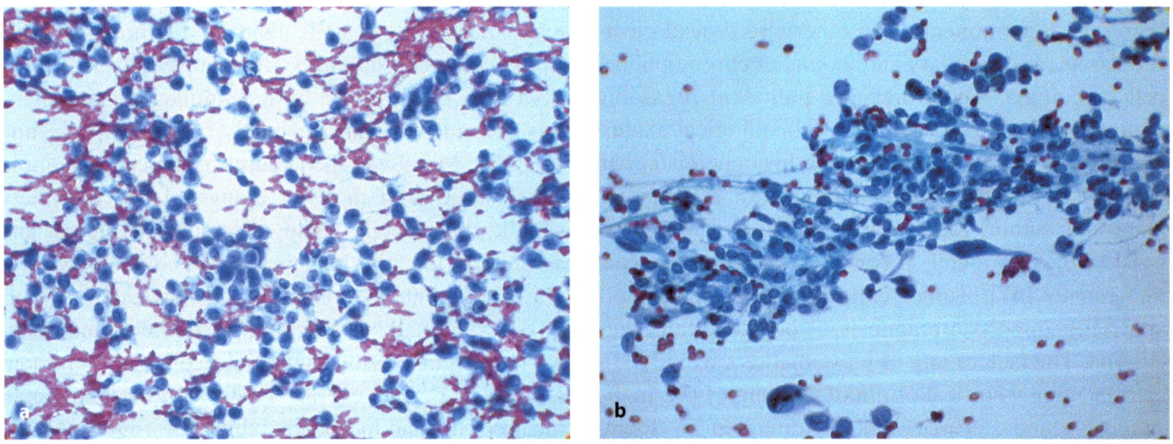

Fig 5.17 **a** Epithelioid cells are ovoid or elongated, sometimes polygonal, cells with a centrally placed nucleus and a distinct nucleolus. FNB sample from a patient with amelanotic malignant melanoma. P stain, ×400. **b** Epithelioid and spindle cells coexist in this field; while the elements share a common nuclear morphology, their shape varies from ovoid or elongated to definitely spindle-like. FNB sample from a patient with renal cell sarcomatoid carcinoma. P stain, ×400.

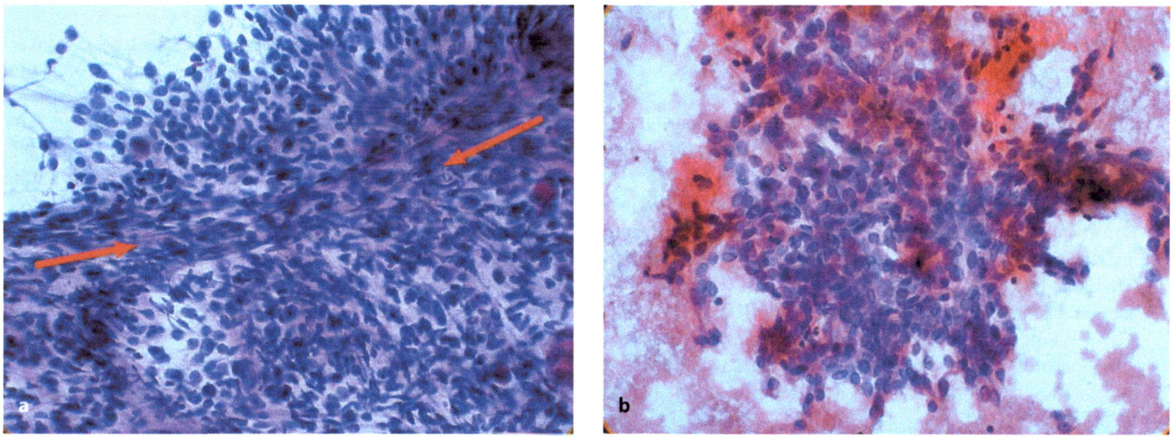

Fig 5.18 a A three-dimensional cluster of spindle cells that seem to radiate from a capillary vessel (indicated by the *arrows*). The cytoplasm of spindle cells is practically not visible. FNB sample from a case of spindle cell leiomyosarcoma. P stain, ×400. **b** A three-dimensional cluster of spindle and epithelioid cells showing a moderate amount of cytoplasm. The nuclei appear monotonous, with a finely granular chromatin. FNB sample from a patient with monophasic synovial sarcoma. P stain, ×400

coexpress a wide spectrum of cytokeratins [52]. The spindle cell tumor most frequently detected in visceral sites is *sarcomatoid carcinoma*. Due to its morphology, this tumor must be differentiated from true sarcomas of high-grade malignancy. In this setting, the demonstration of EMA or cytokeratin is of little diagnostic help due to the reduced expression of these markers in sarcomatoid carcinoma. Instead, the investigation of p63 expression provides a more reliable and sensitive approach [53].

References

1. Tot T (2002) Cytokeratins 20 and 7 as biomarkers: usefulness in discriminating primary from metastatic adenocarcinoma. Eur J Cancer 38:758–763.
2. Tot T (1999) Adenocarcinomas metastatic to the liver: the value of cytokeratins 20 and 7 in the search for unknown primary tumors. 85:171–177.
3. Moll R, Löwe A, Laufer J, Franke WW (1992) Cytokeratin 20 in human carcinomas. A new histodiagnostic marker detected by monoclonal antibodies. Am J Pathol 140:427–447.
4. Loy TS, Calaluce RD (1994) Utility of cytokeratin immunostaining in separating pulmonary adenocarcinomas from colonic adenocarcinomas. Am J Clin Pathol 102.764–767.
5. Lagendijk JH, Mullink H, Van Diest PJ et al (1998) Tracing the origin of adenocarcinomas with unknown primary using immunohistochemistry: differential diagnosis between colonic and ovarian carcinomas as primary sites. Hum Pathol 29:491–497.
6. Loy TS, Calaluce RD, Keeney GL (1996) Cytokeratin immunostaining in differentiating primary ovarian carcinoma from metastatic colonic adenocarcinoma. Mod Pathol 9:1040–1044.
7. Lagendijk JH, Mullink H, Van Diest PJ et al (1998) Tracing the origin of adenocarcinomas with unknown primary using immunohistochemistry: differential diagnosis between colonic and ovarian carcinomas as primary sites. Hum Pathol 29:491–497.
8. Tan J, Sidhu G, Greco MA et al (1998) Villin, cytokeratin 7, and cytokeratin 20 expression in pulmonary adenocarcinoma with ultrastructural evidence of microvilli with rootlets. Hum Pathol 29:390–396.
9. Chu P, Wu E, Weiss LM (2000) Cytokeratin 7 and cytokeratin 20 expression in epithelial neoplasms: a survey of 435 cases. Mod Pathol 13:962–972.
10. Wauters CC, Smedts F, Gerrits LG et al (1995) Keratins 7 and 20 as diagnostic markers of carcinomas metastatic to the ovary. Hum Pathol 26:852–855.
11. Chuang WY, Yeh CJ, Chu PH (2008) Expression of thyroid transcription factor-1 in brain metastases: A useful indicator of pulmonary origin. J Clin Neurosci 15:643–646.
12. Strickland-Marmol LB, Khoor A, Livingston SK, Rojiani A (2007) Utility of tissue-specific transcription factors thyroid transcription factor 1 and Cdx2 in determining the primary site of metastatic adenocarcinomas to the brain. Arch Pathol Lab Med 131:1686–1690.
13. Tanaka S, Saito K, Ito T et al (2007) CDX2 as a useful marker of colorectal adenocarcinoma metastases to lung in pre-operative biopsy specimens. Oncol Rep 18:87–92.
14. Zhang MQ, Lin F, Hui P et al (2007) Expression of mucins, SIMA, villin, and CDX2 in small-intestinal adenocarcinoma. Am J Clin Pathol 128:808–816.
15. Hong SM, Cho H, Moskaluk CA et al (2005) CDX2 and MUC2 protein expression in extrahepatic bile duct carcinoma. Am J Clin Pathol 124:361–370.

16. Kubba LA, McCluggage WG, Liu J et al (2008) Thyroid transcription factor-1 expression in ovarian epithelial neoplasms. Mod Pathol 21:485–490.
17. Siami K, McCluggage WG, Ordonez NG et al (2007) Thyroid transcription factor-1 expression in endometrial and endocervical adenocarcinomas. Am J Surg Pathol 31: 1759–1763.
18. Compérat E, Zhang F, Perrotin C et al (2005) Variable sensitivity and specificity of TTF-1 antibodies in lung metastatic adenocarcinoma of colorectal origin. Mod Pathol 18:1371–1376.
19. Lei JY, Bourne PA, diSant'Agnese PA, Huang J (2006) Cytoplasmic staining of TTF-1 in the differential diagnosis of hepatocellular carcinoma vs cholangiocarcinoma and metastatic carcinoma of the liver. Am J Clin Pathol 125:519–525.
20. McCluggage WG, Shah R, Connolly LE, McBride HA (2008) Intestinal-type cervical adenocarcinoma in situ and adenocarcinoma exhibit a partial enteric immunophenotype with consistent expression of CDX2. Int J Gynecol Pathol 27:92–100.
21. Ortiz-Rey JA, Alvarez C, San Miguel P et al (2005) Expression of CDX2, cytokeratins 7 and 20 in sinonasal intestinal-type adenocarcinoma. Appl Immunohistochem Mol Morphol 13:142–146.
22. Herawi M, De Marzo AM, Kristiansen G, Epstein JI (2006) Expression of CDX2 in benign tissue and adenocarcinoma of the prostate. Hum Pathol 38:72–78.
23. Mazziotta RM, Borczuk AC, Powell CA, Mansukhani M (2005) CDX2 immunostaining as a gastrointestinal marker: expression in lung carcinomas is a potential pitfall. Appl Immunohistochem Mol Morphol 13:55–60.
24. Park S-Y, Kim BH, Kim JH et al (2007) Panels of immunohistochemical markers help determine primary sites of metastatic adenocarcinoma. Arch Pathol Lab Med 131:1561–1567.
25. Kontogianni K, Nicholson AG, Butcher D, Sheppard MN (2005) CD56: a useful tool for the diagnosis of small cell lung carcinomas on biopsies with extensive crush artefact. J Clin Pathol 58:978–980.
26. Kaufmann O, Fietze E, Mengs J, Dietel M (2001) Value of p63 and cytokeratin 5/6 as immunohistochemical markers for the differential diagnosis of poorly differentiated and undifferentiated carcinomas. Am J Clin Pathol 116:823–830.
27. Tsang WY, Chan JK, Lee KC et al (1991) Basaloid-squamous carcinoma of the upper aerodigestive tract and so-called adenoid cystic carcinoma of the oesophagus: the same tumour type? Histopathology 19:35–46.
28. Banks ER, Frierson HF Jr, Mills SE et al (1992) Basaloid squamous cell carcinoma of the head and neck. A clinicopathologic and immunohistochemical study of 40 cases. Am J Surg Pathol 16:939–946.
29. Wan SK, Chan JK, Tse KC (1992) Basaloid-squamous carcinoma of the nasal cavity. J Laryngol Otol 106:370–371.
30. Nagel H, Hotze HJ, Laskawi R et al (1999) Cytologic diagnosis of adenoid cystic carcinoma of salivary glands. Diagn Cytopathol 20:358–366.
31. Gupta RK, Green C, Naran S et al (1999) Fine-needle aspiration cytology of adenoid cystic carcinoma of the breast. Diagn Cytopathol 20:82–84.
32. Hida CA, Gupta PK (1999) Cercariform cells: are they specific for transitional cell carcinoma? Cancer 87:69–74.
33 Southgate J, Harnden P, Trejdosiewicz LK (1999) Cytokeratin expression patterns in normal and malignant urothelium: a review of the biological and diagnostic implications. Histol Histopathol 14:657–664.
34. Murali R, Delprado W (2005) CD10 immunohistochemical staining in urothelial neoplasms. Am J Clin Pathol 124:371–379.
35. Azzopardi JG (1959) Oat-cell carcinoma of the bronchus. J Pathol Bacteriol 78:513–519.
36. Jaffee IM, Rahmani M, Singhal MG, Younes M (2006) Expression of the intestinal transcription factor CDX2 in carcinoid tumors is a marker of midgut origin. Arch Pathol Lab Med 130:1522–1526.
37. Lin X, Saad RS, Luckasevic TM et al (2007) Diagnostic value of CDX-2 and TTF-1 expressions in separating metastatic neuroendocrine neoplasms of unknown origin. Appl Immunohistochem Mol Morphol 15:407–414.
38. Alijo Serrano F, Sánchez-Mora N, Angel Arranz J et al (2007) Large cell and small cell neuroendocrine bladder carcinoma: immunohistochemical and outcome study in a single institution. Am J Clin Pathol 128:733–739.
39. Carlson JW, Nucci MR, Brodsky J (2007) Biomarker-assisted diagnosis of ovarian, cervical and pulmonary small cell carcinomas: the role of TTF-1, WT-1 and HPV analysis. Histopathology 51:305–312.
40. Pulitzer MP, Amin BD, Busam KJ (2009) Merkel cell carcinoma: review. Adv Anat Pathol 16:135–144.
41. Folpe AL, Goldblum JR, Rubin BP et al (2005) Morphologic and immunophenotypic diversity in Ewing family tumors: a study of 66 genetically confirmed cases. Am J Surg Pathol 29:1025–1033.
42. Delattre O, Zucman J, Melot T et al (1994) The Ewing family of tumors—a subgroup of small-round-cell tumors defined by specific chimeric transcripts. N Engl J Med 331:294–299.
43. Parham DM, Webber B, Holt H et al (1991) Immunohistochemical study of childhood rhabdomyosarcomas and related neoplasms. Results of an Intergroup Rhabdomyosarcoma study project. Cancer 67:3072–3080.
44. Mooi WJ, Deenik W, Peterse JL, Hogendoorn PCW (1995) Keratin immunoreactivity in melanoma of soft parts (clear cell sarcoma). Histopathology 27:61–65
45. Selby WL, Nance KV, Park HK (1992) CEA immunoreactivity in metastatic malignant melanoma. Mod Pathol 5:415–419.
46. Miller RT (2005) Immunohistochemistry in the differential diagnosis of clear cell carcinoma from the kidney, liver, and lung. Propath Immunohistochemistry Newsletter http://www.propathlab.com/pdf/2005-04_clear_cell_ca.pdf.
47. Kumar D and Kumar S (1993) Adrenal cortical adenoma and adrenal metastasis of renal cell carcinoma: immunohistochemical and DNA ploidy analysis. Mod Pathol 6:36–40.
48. Nappi O, Ferrara G, Wick MR (1999) Neoplasms composed of eosinophilic polygonal cells: an overview with consideration of different cytomorphologic patterns. Semin Diagn Pathol 16:82–90.
49. Kumashiro Y, Yao T, Aishima S et al (2007) Hepatoid adenocarcinoma of the stomach: histogenesis and progression in association with intestinal phenotype. Hum Pathol 38:857–863.

50. Ozolek JA, Bastacky SI, Myers EN, Hunt JL (2005) Immunophenotypic comparison of salivary gland oncocytoma and metastatic renal cell carcinoma. Laryngoscope 115:1097–1100.
51. Zubovits J, Buzney E, Yu L, Duncan LM (2004) HMB-45, S-100, NK1/C3, and MART-1 in metastatic melanoma. Hum Pathol 35:217–223.
52. Pelmus M, Guillou L, Hostein I (2002) Monophasic fibrous and poorly differentiated synovial sarcoma: immunohistochemical reassessment of 60 t(X;18)(SYT-SSX)-positive cases. Am J Surg Pathol 26:1434–1440.
53. Lewis JS, Ritter JH, El-Mofty S (2005) Alternative epithelial markers in sarcomatoid carcinomas of the head and neck, lung, and bladder-p63, MOC-31, and TTF-1. Mod Pathol 18:1471–1481.

Abdomen

6

6.1 Focal Liver Lesions

6.1.1 Hepatocellular Carcinoma

6.1.1.1 Clinicopathological Correlates

Hepatocellular carcinoma (HCC) is associated with cirrhosis in the large majority of patients [1]. The tumor can present in nodular, multinodular, or diffuse forms. Clinically, the serum α-fetoprotein (AFP) titer is increased and the value correlates with the size of the tumor mass. Histologically, the tumor consists of a proliferation of cells variably resembling normal hepatocytes, according to the degree of differentiation. Diverse growth patterns are recognized, including trabecular, acinar, pseudoglandular or adenoid, and scirrhous [1]. Tumor cells in well-differentiated malignancies typically are usually made up of oxyphil-type cells but a significant proportion of tumors assume a clear-cell morphology. The fibrolamellar and sclerosing variants of HCC are two important tumor entities, both occurring in young age groups and in the non-cirrhotic liver. The latter variant is often associated clinically with hypercalcemia [1].

6.1.1.2 Cytomorphology

- Moderate to abundant cellularity (Fig. 6.1).
- Concomitant aggregated and non-cohesive cells (Fig. 6.2).
- Laminar, trabecular, or acinar pattern of aggregation (Fig. 6.2).
- Non-cohesive cells admixed with bare and atypical nuclei (Fig. 6.3).
- Hepatocyte-like morphology in well-differentiated tumors with abnormally increased nuclear/cytoplasmic ratio and intermediate to large nuclei containing a single prominent nucleolus (Fig. 6.4)
- Eosinophilic and granular (oxyphil) cytoplasm with variable content of pigment granules (Fig. 6.5).
- Possible clear-cell change in a variable proportion of elements (Fig. 6.6).
- Presence of a crowded network of capillary lumina within aggregates (Fig. 6.7a) delimited by endothelial cells (Fig. 6.7b).
- Integration with core-needle biopsy (CNB) histology required to possibly detect: (a) architectural changes, such as nuclear crowding, increased cell thickness of hepatocyte plates, or acinar structures (Fig. 6.8); (b) biliary thrombi (Fig. 6.9);

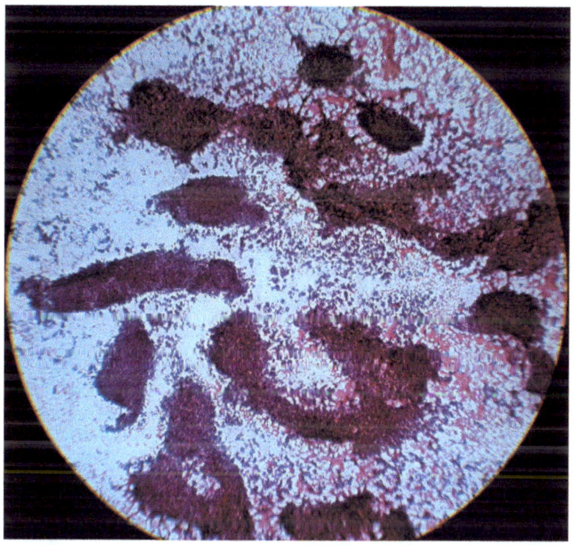

Fig. 6.1 Low-power view of a FNB sample collected from a well-differentiated hepatocellular carcinoma, showing abundant cellularity. Papanicolaou (P) stain, ×40

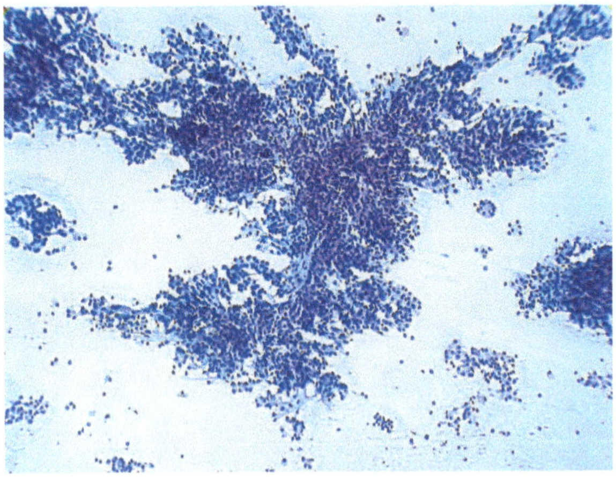

Fig. 6.2 Cohesive cells form laminar or trabecular clusters and are associated with dissociated cells. P stain, ×200

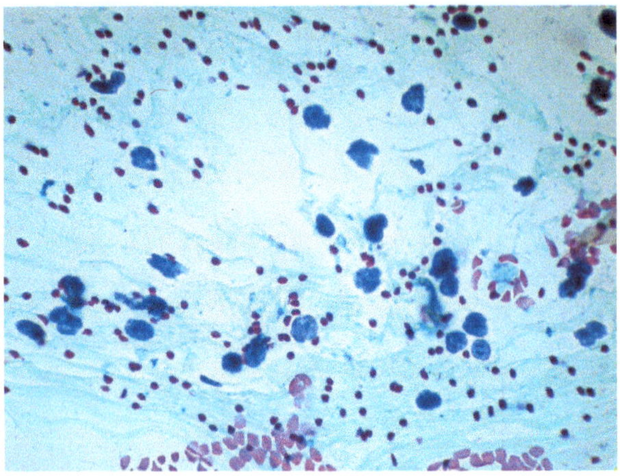

Fig. 6.3 Bare and naked atypical nuclei are seen in the background. Compare their size with that of red blood cells. P stain, ×400

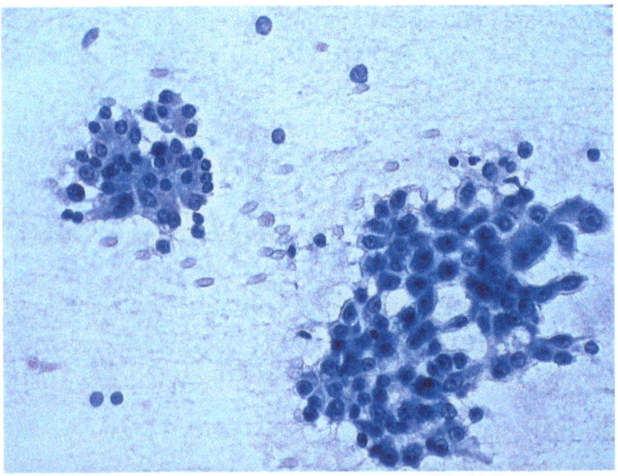

Fig. 6.4 Well-differentiated hepatocellular carcinoma tumor cells assume a distinct hepatocyte-like morphology; their nuclei are large and contain a single prominent nucleolus. P stain, ×400

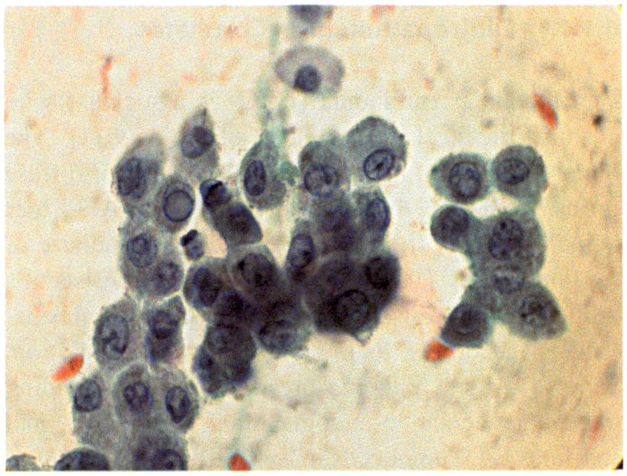

Fig. 6.5 At high magnification, hepatocellular carcinoma cells may have an eosinophilic and granular (oxyphilic) cytoplasm with a variable content of pigment granules; in this case, a distinct nuclear vacuole is seen. P stain, ×100

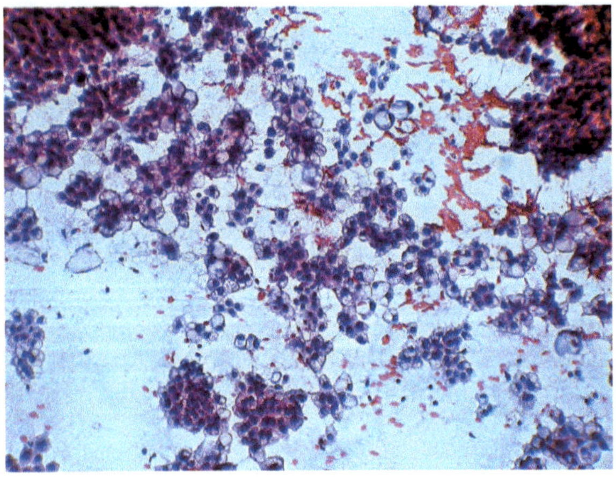

Fig. 6.6 Clear cell change is seen in the cytoplasm of most of these cells. P stain, ×400

(c) immunohistochemical evidence of sinusoidal capillarization (CD34 and CD31 immunopositivity) (Fig. 6.10); or (d) bile canalicular pattern (CEA and/or CD10 positivity) (Fig. 6.11); and (e) histochemical evidence of stromal rarefaction, as seen by silver impregnation (Fig. 6.12).

The cytopathological diagnosis of well-differentiated HCC is very often very problematic [2–6], such that an examination that combines smears and cell-block histological material will potentially provide more informative and conclusive data [4]. In fact, the sensitivity of the cytopathological evaluation alone is rather poor, 75–80%, even in highly experienced hands, whereas a combined examination of smear and

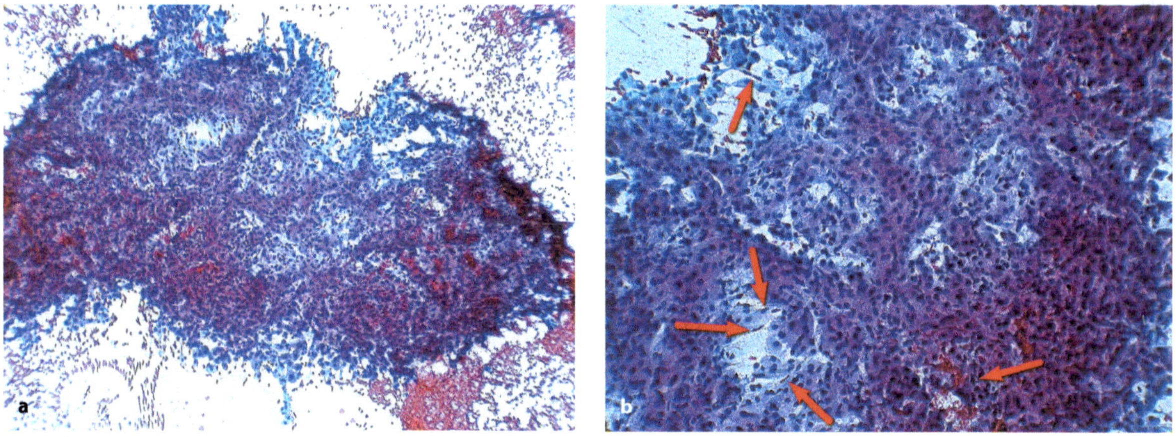

Fig. 6.7 **a** A large three-dimensional aggregate containing a crowded network of capillary lumina which are easily discerned due to their content of red blood cells. P stain, ×200. **b** Endothelial cells having elongated and hyperchromatic nuclei (*arrows*) are admixed with hepatocytes and sometimes appear to delimit capillary lumina. P stain, ×400

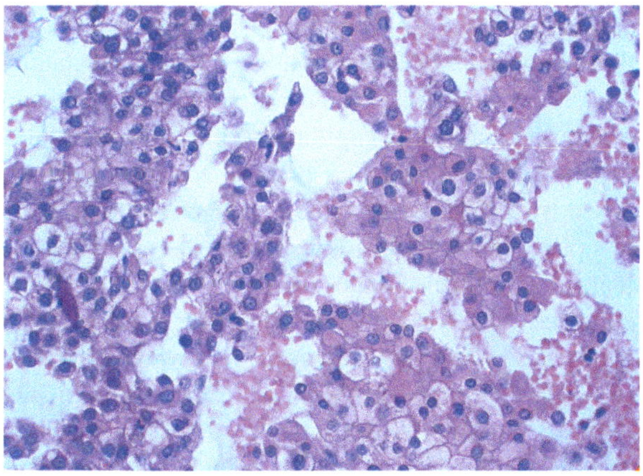

Fig. 6.8 Microhistological view of a needle-rinse sample showing increased cell thickness of hepatocyte plates and focal clear cell change. Hematoxylin and eosin (H&E) stain, ×400

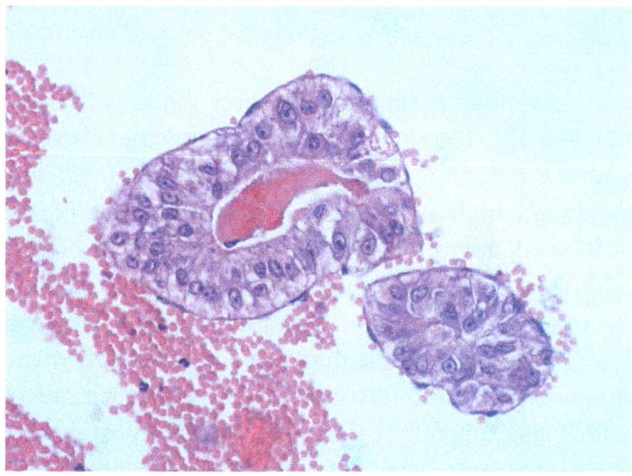

Fig. 6.9 A pseudoglandular aggregate of hepatocytes (on the *left*) contains a biliary thrombus; the other aggregate has an acinar configuration. Note that both aggregates are surrounded by endothelial cells. Paraffin section stained with H&E, ×400

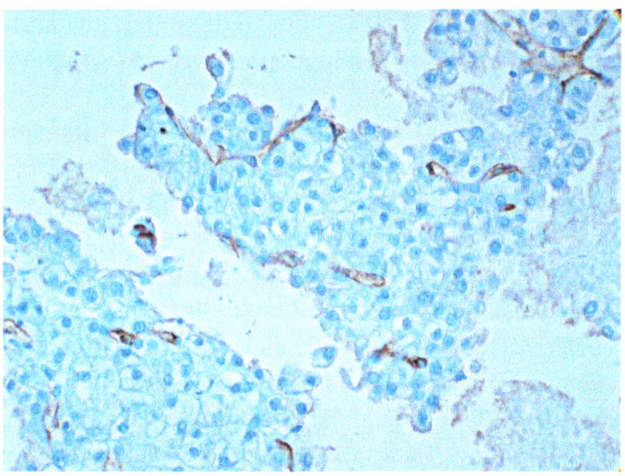

Fig. 6.10 CD34 immunopositivity is seen in endothelial cells. This finding is a marker of the "capillarization" of sinusoids. Paraffin section counterstained with hematoxylin, ×400

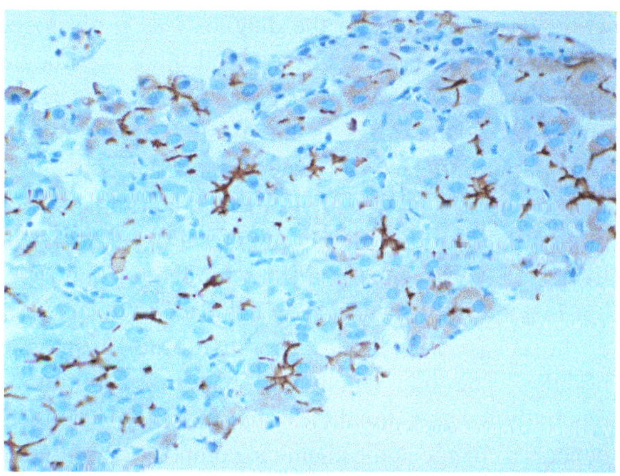

Fig. 6.11 CD10 immunostaining discloses a peculiar "bile canalicular" pattern of positivity on the membrane of neoplastic hepatocytes. Paraffin section counterstained with hematoxylin, ×400

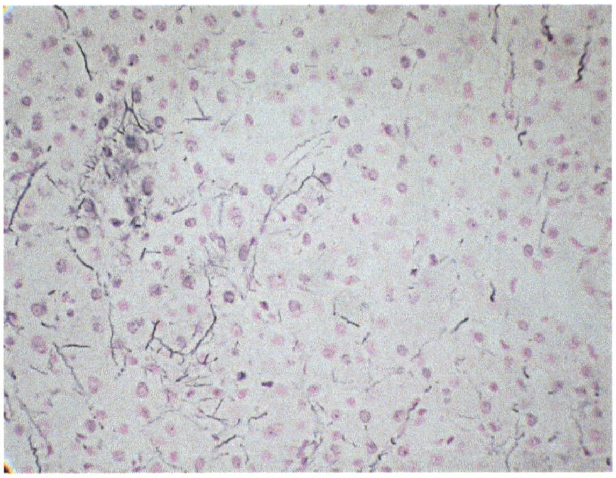

Fig. 6.12 Silver impregnation stain documents a rarefaction in argentophilic fibrils within the interstitium of well-differentiated hepatocellular carcinoma. Paraffin section counterstained with nuclear fast red, ×400

microhistological samples increases the sensitivity to 85–90% [2]. The specificity of morphological investigation is not influenced by the combined approach and is always high (about 98%) [2,4]. The aim of the combined microhistological evaluation is to collect additional data concerning structural atypia, changes in the microcirculation, the immunohistochemical reactivity of the cell membrane, and the histochemical properties of the interstitial ground substance, all of which may support the diagnosis. Finally, most experts recommend also acquiring an adequate core-needle sample of the extralesional parenchyma [7–9].

Early and well-differentiated HCC is a hypercellular nodule made up of acini, thin trabeculae, and remodeling of the cord structure [9]. Microhistological evaluation is of help in the diagnosis as it discloses nuclear crowding, three or more cell-thick hepatocyte plates, and a trabecular arrangement [7–9]. The capillarization of sinusoids is manifested by the linear CD34 immunoreactivity detected on the sinusoidal surface in HCC [10], in contrast with a complete lack of reactivity for this marker in normal or hyperplastic liver (Fig. 6.10). This is a sensitive feature for HCC but is not totally specific as it also can be detected in cirrhosis as well as regenerative and dysplastic nodules. The bile canalicular pattern of immunoreactivity for polyclonal CEA and CD10 of HCC cells denotes a change in the chemical composition of tumor cell membranes on the pole opposite the sinusoidal surface, as evidenced by a linear reactivity (Fig. 6.11). This finding is a poorly sensitive but highly specific change in HCC [11–13]. Rarefaction occurs in the argentophilic fibrils within the interstitium of well-differentiated HCC, a feature easily detected by common silver impregnation stains (Fig. 6.12). Combined with the disappearance of portal tracts, this provides a rather sensitive but not optimally specific criterion for the diagnosis [7,8]. Finally, positive immunostaining of tumor cells for glypican-3, a heparan sulfate proteoglycan, is the latest and most promising tool in the differential diagnosis of HCC as the marker is expressed in HCC but not in hepatocellular adenoma, regenerative nodules, or dysplastic nodules. Conflicting data have been reported, however, on the sensitivity of glypican-3 in fine-needle biopsy (FNB) material [14–16].

HCC can be differentiated from a *high-grade dysplastic nodule* based mainly on the detection of three or more cell-thick hepatocyte plates, substantial nuclear crowding, the formation of pseudoglands, and a diffuse (not focal) capillarization of the sinusoids [7,17]. *Large regenerative nodules* are properly diagnosed by a very effective diagnostic criterion, i.e., the complete similarity in architectural pattern and cellular features between intra- and extralesional tissue collected by CNB [7]. *Hepatocellular adenoma* also enters the differential diagnosis with well-differentiated HCC [7,9]. This benign tumor is typically unifocal, does not develop in a cirrhotic background, and mostly occurs in female patients of reproductive age or in male patients undergoing hormone medication (anabolizing drugs) [1]. In general, cytopathological or histopathological observations in needle-biopsy samples do not assist in the differential diagnosis of well-differentiated HCC; thus, a definitive diagnosis of benignancy in ambiguous cases is generally discouraged.

The diagnosis of intermediately to poorly differentiated HCC in smear cytology is facilitated by the detection of a high tendency to cellular non-cohesion, the presence of three-dimensional aggregates of variable size formed by the complex ramification of trabeculae or plates of hepatocyte-like cells with a high nuclear/cytoplasmic ratio, and significant nuclear changes (Fig. 6.13). The aggregation pattern can include tubular structures, acini, and pseudopapillae, thus imitating poorly differentiated adenocarcinoma. This is particularly true for the pseudoglandular variant of HCC, which poses a challenging problem in a

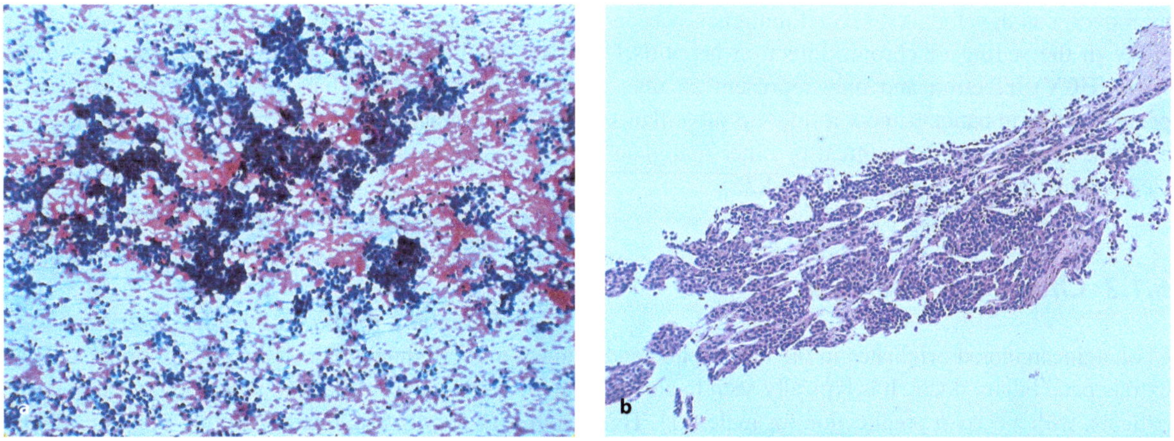

Fig. 6.13 **a** In FNB smears from poorly differentiated hepatocellular carcinoma, the tumor cells may assume a small cell morphology. P stain, ×400. **b** A core-needle sample showing a peculiar tubular or trabecular configuration of neoplastic hepatocytes. Paraffin section stained with hematoxylin and eosin, ×400

differential diagnosis that includes cholangiocarcinoma. In addition, tumor cells can display an overt clear-cell change, or even a "signet ring" appearance, or assume an Indian file arrangement. Clear-cell HCC can enter the differential diagnosis with a metastatic carcinoma primary located in the kidney, adrenal cortex, ovary, lung, or thyroid, or with other non-epithelial tumors made up of clear cells (malignant melanoma, sarcoma, gastrointestinal stromal tumors) [1]. In some cases, the tumor cells are large and pleomorphic with abundant cytoplasm and bizarre nuclei (pleomorphic variant); in others, the cells are small, contain sparse cytoplasm, and have a great tendency to non-cohesion, thus imitating a metastatic small-cell carcinoma. In all these cases, proper diagnosis of HCC relies upon the results of immunohistochemical studies of microhistological samples. It is worth noting that HCC cells in well-differentiated tumors are poorly reactive for cytokeratins, as they may express CK8,18 but usually not CK7 or CK20 [18]. TTF-1, Hep-Par, and AFP positivity of the cytoplasm is seen in, respectively, 70–90%, 70–80% and <50% of cases [12,19,20]. Furthermore, poorly differentiated tumors may show positivity for CK7 and CK19 as well [21].

6.1.1.3 Diagnosis of Hepatocellular Carcinoma

Nowadays, FNB is used to diagnose HCC only in a minority of cases. Instead, imaging techniques are the gold standard procedure for diagnosing lesions of small size that appear in the cirrhotic liver [3,7,8,12]. Imaging diagnosis of HCC in cirrhosis is based on the detection of abnormal arterial vascularization, especially by contrast techniques such as CT, MRI, or contrast ultrasound (US). Pathognomonic findings include early enhancement in the arterial phase and subsequent washout. Progression of such to the extent that the nodule becomes hypovascular (or isovascular) compared to the surrounding parenchyma is the most specific finding. If it is detected in a nodule >2 cm, then HCC can be diagnosed with confidence [3,22]. In addition, even a single imaging technique showing typical findings in a nodule ≥1 cm that newly appeared during a surveillance program is sufficient for a reliable diagnosis of HCC [22]. Imaging techniques allow a confident and conclusive diagnosis of HCC in about 70% of patients, with a 2.5% false-positive rate [22]. In the remaining patients, a tissue diagnosis is required and should be accomplished by US-guided fine-needle and core-needle biopsy samplings of the nodular lesion [7,8]. US-guided biopsy of HCC has only few false-negative results, which can be minimized by a repeat biopsy. In fact, FNB provides the only possibility to diagnose HCC in hospitals or clinics lacking the above-mentioned diagnostic imaging facilities and when the tumor is unexpectedly encountered in a patient with a non-cirrhotic liver. The latter situation seems to be more frequent in patients with hepatitis B virus (HBV)-related chronic hepatitis and is typically observed in those residing in less-developed countries, where HBV infection is endemic [23]. HCC, moreover, can develop as a second malignancy especially in the setting of chronic infection hepatitis C virus (HCV) infection and may represent an unexpected finding in patients under follow-up surveillance after the diagnosis and treatment of other malignancies (mainly malignant lymphoma) [24,25].

6.1.2 Cholangiocarcinoma

Cholangiocarcinoma originates in the intrahepatic and extrahepatic biliary ducts. It is typically seen in elderly patients, with a certain predilection for males [1]. The clinical onset is mainly characterized by symptoms caused by obstructive jaundice. In the liver, the tumor presents as a single mass or as multiple confluent nodules localized close to the hilar region (central cholangiocarcinoma) or in the subcapsular parenchyma (peripheral cholangiocarcinoma). There is also a diffuse form of the tumor that involves multiple adjacent segments. "Klatskin's tumor" refers to a variant of cholangiocarcinoma originating in the large perihilar extrahepatic biliary ducts; it secondarily and retrogressively involves the hilar liver parenchyma and forms a space-occupying tumor mass [1]. Histologically, cholangiocarcinoma is an adenocarcinoma of the usual type, with intracellular mucin synthesis and a tubular, trabecular, or cord-like pattern of invasive growth that elicits a generally intense desmoplastic reaction. The latter is probably the only morphological peculiarity of the tumor, as an intense stromal reaction is less frequently seen in metastatic adenocarcinoma. In a minority of cases, the tumor cells may also assume a clear-cell or signet-ring morphology. Finally, cholangiocarcinoma also may assume an adenosquamous or lymphoepithelioma-like appearance [1]. On FNB, the cytological sample demonstrates a glandular-cell morphology. Since there are no specific features distinguishing a primary from a secondary metastatic adenocarcinoma, the term "adenocarcinoma, uncertain if primary or metastatic" should be used in the pathological report. Immunohistochemically, well-differentiated forms of cholangiocarcinoma cells are CK7+/CK20- while poorly differentiated tumors may express CK20 [18]. No specific marker demonstrating a biliary-tract origin of the tumor is available; rather, cholangiocarcinoma cells share the same immunohistochemical profile as tumors of the pancreatic ducts [1]. The diagnosis of cholangiocarcinoma is often made by exclusion if the patient presents with huge liver involvement by a sclerosing and mucinous adenocarcinoma but has no evidence of an extrahepatic primary tumor.

6.1.3 Carcinoma of the Gallbladder Involving the Liver

Adenocarcinoma of the gallbladder anterior wall is much more frequent than cholangiocarcinoma and can involve the adjacent hepatic parenchyma early in the course of the disease, thus presenting as a tumor mass in the liver. Histologically, the tumor's appearance is typical of adenocarcinoma but in about 15–20% of patients it may assume the morphology of squamous cell carcinoma, or mucinous, clear-cell, or small-cell carcinoma. The latter is often combined with an otherwise typical adenocarcinoma or a typical carcinoid [1]. Consequently, the FNB sample recapitulates a glandular-cell morphology or that of a squamous cell carcinoma, etc., with no distinct features allowing a clear-cut distinction from cholangiocarcinoma or metastatic adenocarcinoma. Involvement of hepatic hilar lymph nodes is an early event. Adenocarcinoma arising from the posterior wall of the gallbladder may infiltrate the duodenal wall, transverse mesocolon, or gastric wall and may grow as a retroperitoneal mass. Tumor relapse following surgical excision of the gallbladder occurs within the anterior abdominal wall close to the surgical scar; this site is therefore frequently used as a target of FNB (see below).

6.2 Pancreatic Tumors

6.2.1 Ductal Adenocarcinoma

6.2.1.1 Clinicopathological Correlates

Ductal adenocarcinoma is the most frequent malignancy of the pancreas and occurs mainly in individuals older than 40 years. In about two-thirds of such patients, the tumor is located in the pancreatic head, while in the remaining one-third it is in the body and tail of the pancreas [26]. At clinical onset, patients with the tumors of the former type typically have a rapidly progressive obstructive jaundice, while the symptomatology is much more attenuated and

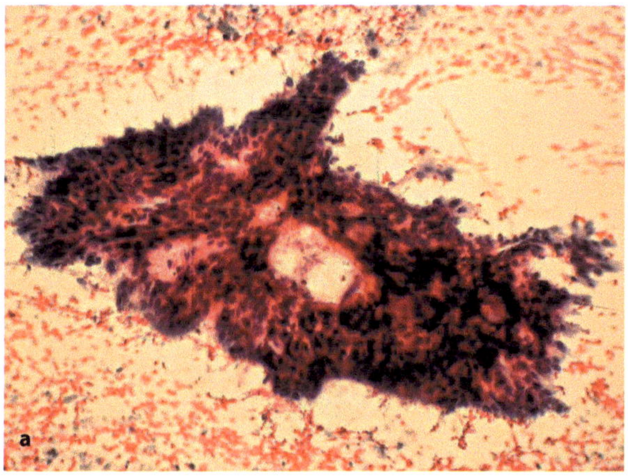

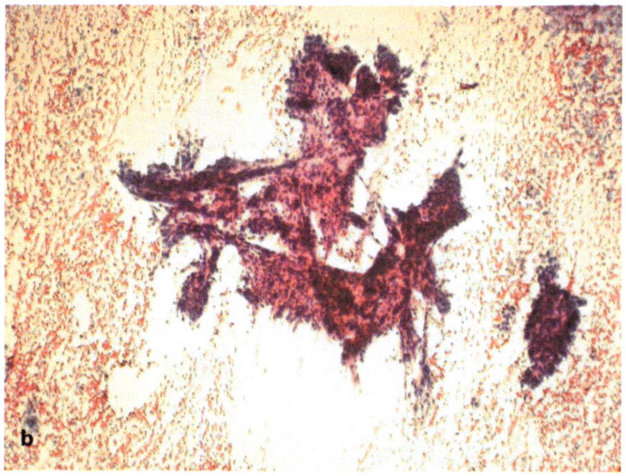

Fig. 6.14 **a** A large three-dimensional aggregate of epithelial glandular cells showing secondary lumina within the cluster and a marked tendency to nuclear overlapping. P stain, ×400. **b** A large three-dimensional aggregate of epithelial glandular cells showing a bizarre configuration with focal pseudopapillae or acinar structures at the periphery. P stain, ×200

non-specific for patients with tumors in the latter site. There is early metastatic involvement of the regional and hilar hepatic lymph nodes. Early metastasis within the liver from an occult pancreatic tumor is generally induced by an adenocarcinoma arising in the body and the tail of the organ. Histologically, ductal carcinoma presents as an otherwise typical adenocarcinoma and is composed of tubular structures of variable shape and size that are lined by cylindrical cells that accumulate mucin intracellularly. Less frequently, the tumor presents either as an adenosquamous carcinoma, as a mixed ductal-type and endocrine carcinoma, or as a ductal-type and acinar carcinoma [26].

6.2.1.2 Cytomorphology

The diagnosis of pancreatic tumors by FNB can be accomplished percutaneously and through echo-endoscopy [27–34]. In samples collected from these tumors, the cells display a glandular-cell morphology but a wide repertoire of cytological patterns can be seen. The diagnosis of moderately to poorly differentiated adenocarcinoma is sufficiently easy due to abundant cellularity, well-evident cellular atypia, the tendency to cellular non-cohesion, and the detection of necrotic debris in the background. Recognition of well-differentiated tumors is, by contrast, made difficult by the possible overlap in cellular changes between bland-looking malignant cells and the hyperplastic ductal or acinar cells induced by chronic pancreatitis, especially sclerosing pancreatitis. In fact, the exclusive evaluation of tissue sections prepared from microhistological samples may be of little or no help in the differential diagnosis; instead, a definitive diagnosis may be obtained by confirming the presence of characteristic patterns of aggregation and cytological changes seen in smears. The following observations support a diagnosis of a well-differentiated ductal adenocarcinoma: (a) marked tendency of nuclear overlapping in aggregates (Fig. 6.14); (b) a marked variability in nuclear size, with nuclei two- to four-fold larger than others in the same aggregate (Fig. 6.15);

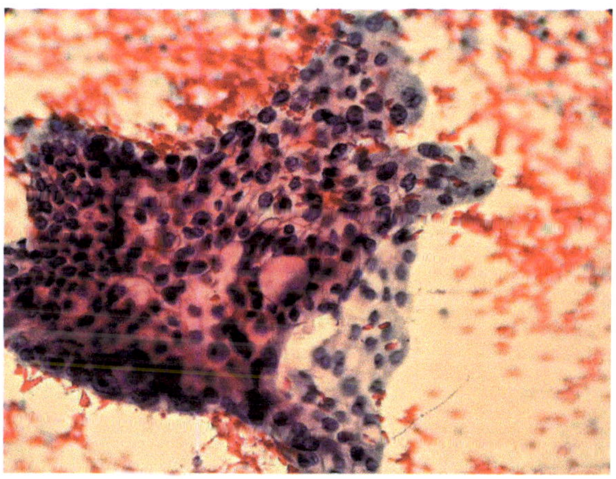

Fig. 6.15 High-power view discloses a marked variation in nuclear size and shape within the same aggregate. P stain, ×400

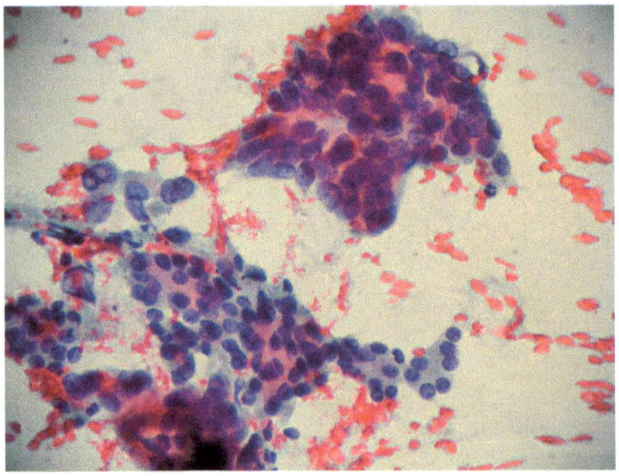

Fig. 6.16 Nuclear molding is obvious in these clusters of epithelial glandular cells. Note also marked variation in nuclear size. P stain, ×400

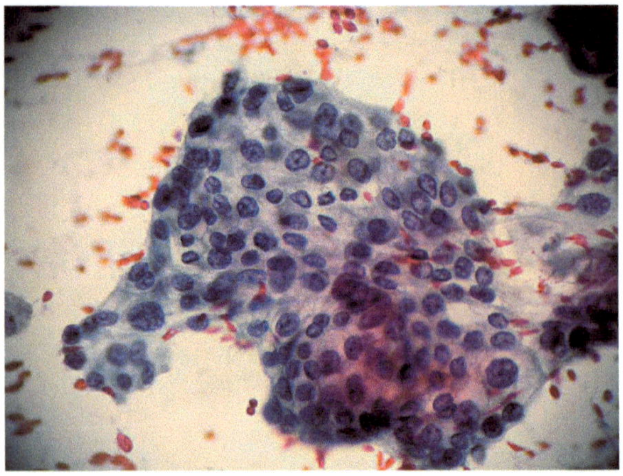

Fig. 6.17 Marked irregularity of the nuclear profile, with nuclear folds and notching, is particularly evident in this aggregate. P stain, ×1000

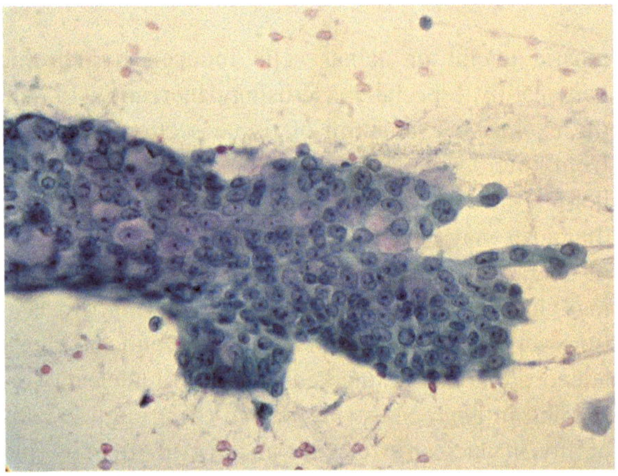

Fig. 6.18 Prominent nucleoli are seen in this aggregate of epithelial glandular cells. Note that nuclear size variation is not prominent in this particular field. P stain, ×400

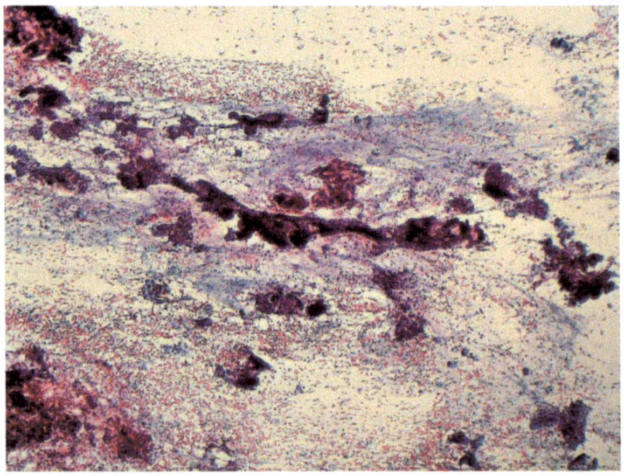

Fig. 6.19 Large and irregular three-dimensional aggregates are seen in a mucinous background. P stain, ×200

(c) the presence of significant nuclear molding (Fig. 6.16); (d) marked irregularity of the nuclear profile, with nuclear folds and notching (Fig. 6.17); (e) the detection of prominent eosinophilic nucleoli together with a coarsely granular chromatin and parachromatin clearing (Fig. 6.18) [27–34]. Additional findings favoring the diagnosis of adenocarcinoma include the presence of necrotic debris and/or inflammatory cells and/or mucin in the background (Fig. 6.19), or the presence of bare nuclei. In many cases of well-differentiated tumors, however, a conclusive diagnosis cannot be reached and the case should be reported as "suspicious" for carcinoma.

6.2.2 Acinar Cell Carcinoma

Acinar cell carcinoma of the pancreas is a rare malignancy occurring in individuals at any age, including those in the first and second decades of life. This aggressive tumor can develop in any segment of the pancreas [26,35]. Nonetheless, if diagnosed early, it is amenable to surgical resection. Accordingly, overall survival and disease-free survival are significantly higher than for patients with ductal-type adenocarcinoma. Histologically, pancreatic acinar cell carcinoma comprises a solid and trabecular growth of medium to large cells with a characteristic oncocytoid appearance: abundant granular cytoplasm with a monomorphous and regular polarized nucleus containing a well-evident nucleolus. Acinar tumor cells are immunoreactive for lipase, trypsin, and chymotrypsin and may have an otherwise typical ductal-type and/or endocrine cellular component. There is very little reported experience regarding FNB sampling and subsequent diagnosis of acinar cell carcinoma; less than ten cases have been reported in the literature [36,37]. The cytological yield has been generally described as made up of cells with an oncocytic/oncocytoid morphology and nuclei characterized by a prominent nucleolus. Cytoplasmic immunohistochemical reactivity for lipase is diagnostic [26].

6.2.3 Mucinous Cystic Neoplasms

6.2.3.1 Clinicopathological Correlates

Mucinous cystic neoplasms are almost exclusively encountered in middle-aged women. The tumor can be located in the body or the tail of the pancreas and generally consists of a cystic component with a minor solid portion [26]. Cystic tumors can be uniloculated or multiloculated, their size varying between 2 and 30 cm in the largest diameter. Benign (mucinous cystoadenoma) and malignant (cystoadenocarcinoma) tumors are recognized. In the former, the cyst wall is covered by a mucinous epithelium lacking any atypical features while in the latter the epithelial cells show frankly atypical features and a papillary or pseudopapillary growth pattern. The differential diagnosis should include intraductal papillary tumors involving the large pancreatic ducts.

6.2.3.2 Cytomorphology

Percutaneous or endoscopic-ultrasound FNB sampling can provide valuable diagnostic information but the procedure may be poorly sensitive [38,39]. When the FNB yield is richly cellular, a reliable diagnosis of cystic mucinous tumor is easily made if the sample shows the features of glandular-cell morphology and a papillary growth pattern (Fig. 6.20). In some cases, the mucinous epithelial cells look more atypical and pleomorphic (Fig. 6.21). If the sample is poorly cellular, then any diagnostic hypothesis should be considered only with great caution due to the high false-negative rate of the procedure. In tumors >3 cm, FNB exclusion of malignancy is not reliable and strongly discouraged [39]. Hemosiderin-laden macrophages are characteristically found in benign tumors but this is not a specific feature.

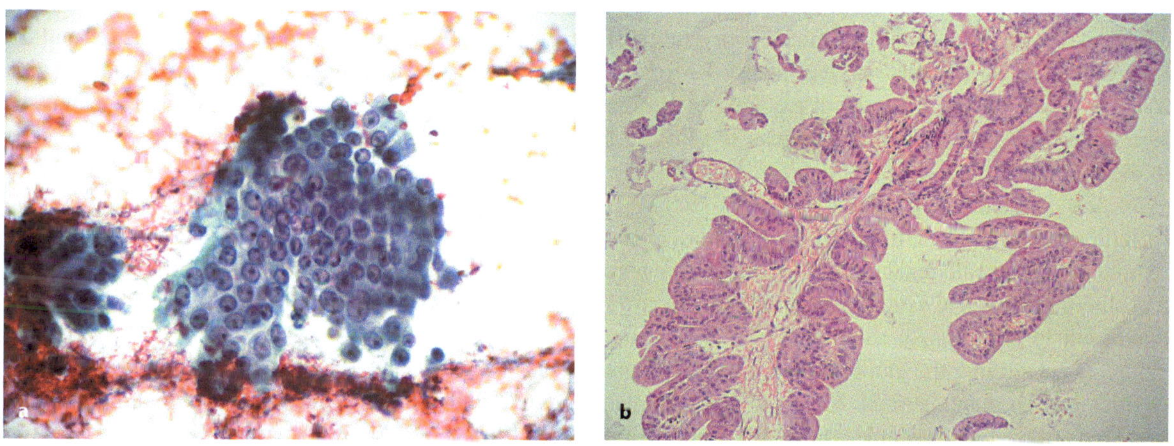

Fig. 6.20 a A papillary aggregate of epithelial glandular cells showing well-evident nucleoli. P stain, ×100. b Microhistological view of a papillary aggregate showing a connective-tissue stalk. Paraffin section from cell-block material collected by needle rinse, stained with H&E, ×200

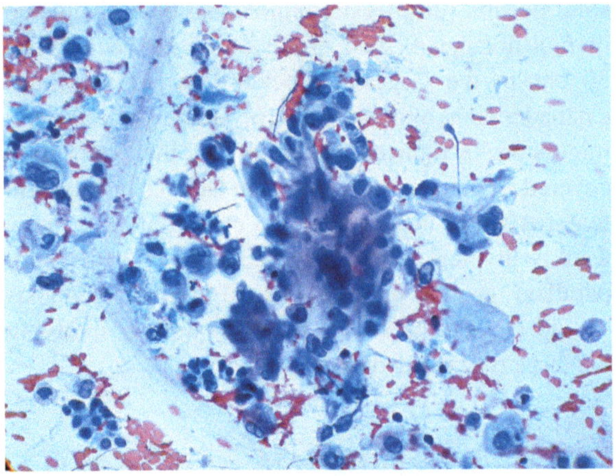

Fig. 6.21 Marked variation in nuclear size and nuclear hyperchromasia are occasionally found in FNB samples of mucinous cystic tumors of the pancreas. P stain, ×400

6.2.4 Serous Cystic Neoplasms

Serous cystic neoplasms of the pancreas are benign tumors made up of confluent cysts of variable size lined by a monolayered epithelium of cylindrical cells containing a non-mucinous, glycogen-rich cytoplasm [26,40,41]. Epithelial cells are typically monomorphous and lack any atypia; sometimes and focally, they cover small papillary vegetations. The aspirated fluid is typically clear and often acellular. In cytological preparations, epithelial cells, when detected, form loose aggregates, appear cylindrical or polygonal, and have a round to oval and vesicular nucleus. CNB sampling is useful to document the multiple microcystic nature of the lesion and can demonstrate the intense PAS positivity of epithelial cells. A typical example of benign serous cystic neoplasm of the pancreas is illustrated in the internet at the *Foro de Diagnostico por Imagen (Foropat)* website [42]. The differential diagnosis includes mucinous cystic tumor of the pancreas, cystic lymphangioma, cystic renal tumor [43] and multicystic mesothelioma [44]. Cystic lymphangioma is easily diagnosed in core-biopsy samples if the endothelial nature of cells lining the empty-looking and confluent cavities can be demonstrated. In cytological samples prepared from the aspirated fluid, the endothelial cells are very sparse and the diagnosis is generally made by exclusion due to the lack of cylindrical and/or cuboid cells.

6.2.5 Tumors of the Endocrine Pancreas

6.2.5.1 Clinicopathological Correlates

Endocrine tumors of the pancreas are rare but all are potentially malignant. Endocrine symptoms are noted in 60–80% of these patients. The tumors are typically localized in the body and tail of the pancreas and their largest size at diagnosis is about 1–5 cm [45]. Due to their preferential site of origin, these tumors do not generally induce obstruction of the main pancreatic ducts, thus, if not functional, these tumors are discovered only at a relatively late stage. In fact, the chance of identifying a tumor of the endocrine pancreas is directly proportional to its ability to induce a clinically relevant endocrine syndrome. Histologically, the tumor consists of a solid trabecular, ribbon-like, gyriform, or solid patternless "medullary" growth of essentially cuboid and uniform cells with a round nucleus and a well-evident nucleolus. The cytoplasm is finely granular and eosinophilic. Large cells with a clear cytoplasm or a rhabdoid appearance are occasionally evident.

6.2.5.2 Cytomorphology

The cytological picture is of a small-cell pattern, with marked cellular monomorphism and little tendency to cellular dissociation (see Chapter 5 and Fig. 6.22a,b) [46,47]. The immunohistochemical evaluation in CNB tissue sections or cell-block preparations obtained by needle rinse discloses positive reactivity for neuroendocrine markers (Fig. 6.22c) and for Leu-7(CD15). The cells do not generally stain positive for CK7 or CK20, but CK8, 18 and CK19 may be expressed and expression seems to bear prognostic significance [48].

6.2.6 Undifferentiated and Spindle Cell Carcinoma

This rare variant of carcinoma of the pancreas has a definite pleomorphic and/or sarcomatoid morphology [26]. In addition, these tumors show similarities with anaplastic carcinoma of the thyroid. The FNB sample may appear highly necrotic, with a variable number of aggregates of pleomorphic cells

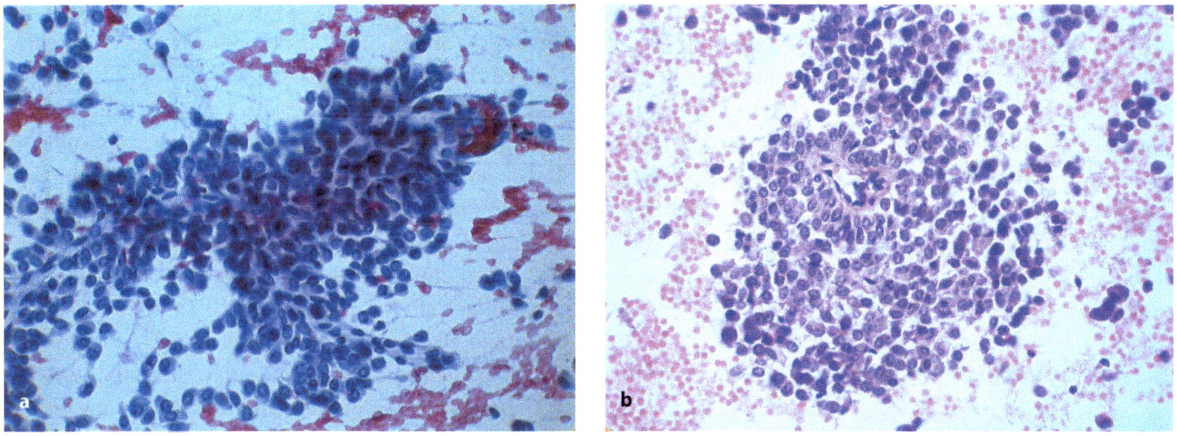

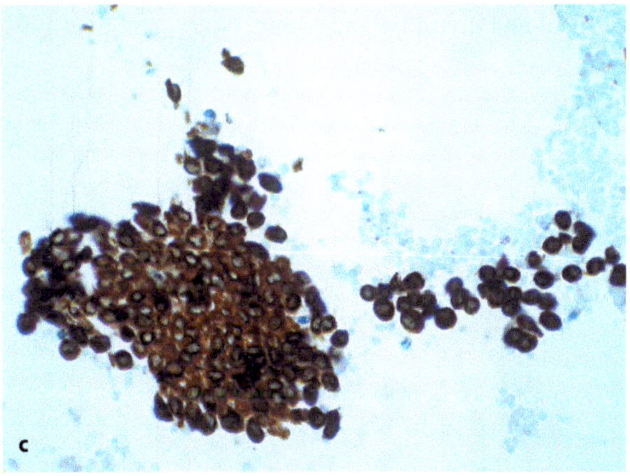

Fig. 6.22 **a** A three-dimensional aggregate of cells showing monotonous nuclei and a small amount of cytoplasm; at the periphery, there is a tendency to loss of cellular cohesion. P stain, ×400. **b** Cell-block paraffin section shows small cells with round nuclei and the characteristic "salt and pepper" appearance of chromatin; there is a small amount of eosinophilic, somewhat granular cytoplasm. H&E stain, ×400. **c** Immunostaining for chromogranin decorates the cytoplasm of tumor cells. Paraffin section from cell-block material, counterstained with hematoxylin, ×400

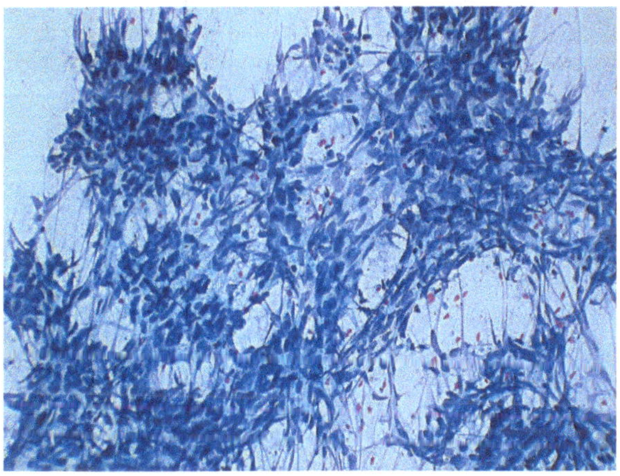

Fig. 6.23 In spindle cell carcinoma of the pancreas, the cells are large, elongated, and pleomorphic in shape, and are characterized by coarsely granular chromatin. P stain, ×400

with a definite spindle cell shape. The chromatin pattern is coarsely granular and prominent nucleoli are rarely seen (Fig. 6.23).

6.3 Renal Tumors

6.3.1 Clear-Cell Carcinoma

6.3.1.1 Clinicopathological Correlates

Clear-cell carcinoma is the most frequent malignancy of the kidney. It occurs only in adults, with the highest incidence in the sixth decade. Clinical manifestations appear late in the course of the disease and generally consist of pain in the flank and hematuria, a palpable mass is rarely detected. Indeed, the tumor is most frequently discovered incidentally in a patient undergoing imaging evaluation for other reasons. The onset with metastatic disease from an occult primary is the least frequent modality of clinical presentation. Tumors arising in the upper pole of the organ can grow into the suprarenal space to simulate an adrenal primary. On imaging, the tumor can appear solid, or partly or completely cystic. Histologically, there is a solid trabecular or syncytial proliferation of clear cells with a conspicuous component of capillaries. The tumor cells have a clear cytoplasm and may coexist with a minor component of cells having a granular cytoplasm (granular cells). Stromal blood extravasation and hemorrhagic necrosis of the tumor are frequently detected. The histopathological grade of the tumor, determined by evaluation of nuclear shape and size, has a great impact on prognosis [49].

6.3.1.2 Cytomorphology

The cytological picture on FNB is prototypical of those tumors with a clear-cell morphology (see Chapter 5) (Fig. 6.24). However, the samples are generally contaminated by blood and necrotic debris, and cellularity may be sparse [50]. The neoplastic cells tend to lose their characteristic features in tumors of high grade and may instead be highly variable in shape, with enlarged or bizarre nuclei and a sparse amphophilic cytoplasm (Fig. 6.25). In the sarcomatoid variants of the tumor, highly pleomorphic spindle and epithelioid cells with bizarre and giant elements may predominate (Fig. 6.26) [50]. CNB sampling is generally not required for a definitive diagnosis provided that the cytological picture is properly correlated with the imaging data. Clear-cell carcinoma shows some preferential sites of metastatic involvement, namely, the adrenal and thyroid glands, lung, ovary, and liver [49].

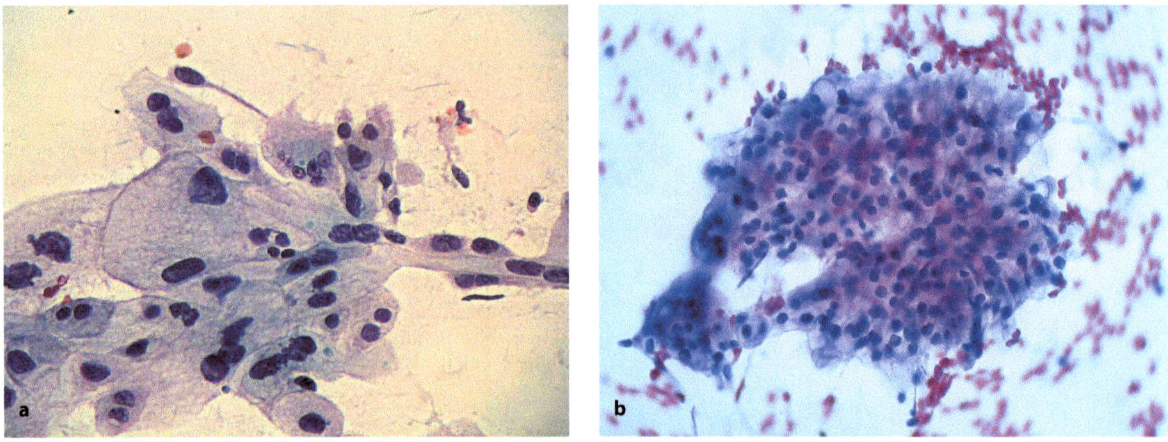

Fig. 6.24 a High-power view of medium to large cells displaying an abundant and clear cytoplasm. P stain, ×1000. b A large three-dimensional aggregate of clear cells. Note that in thicker areas the cytoplasm no longer looks clear but instead appears eosinophilic. P stain, ×400

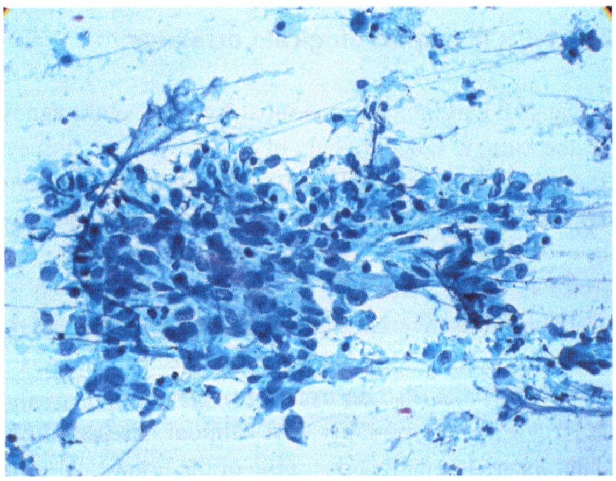

Fig. 6.25 In poorly differentiated tumors, the cells are large and their cytoplasm is amphophilic. Note the marked nuclear pleomorphism. P stain, ×400

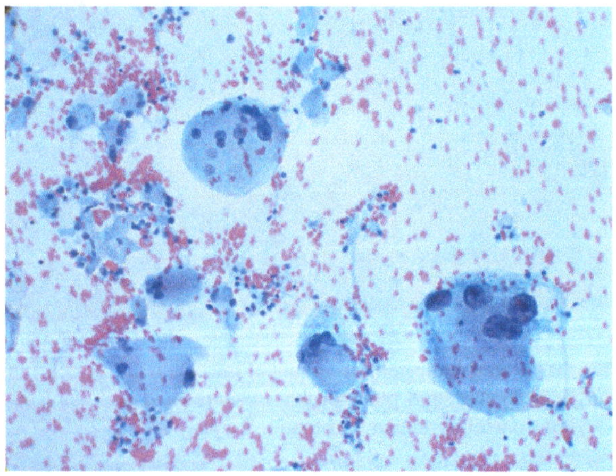

Fig. 6.26 In high-grade sarcomatoid variants of renal cell carcinoma, the picture may be dominated by giant multinucleated cells

In these sites, the tumor should be differentiated from primary clear-cell malignancies in the above-mentioned organs. An immunohistochemical evaluation is of help in the differential diagnosis; it must be performed on cell-block paraffin sections from core-biopsy or needle-rinse samples. Clear-cell carcinoma is typically CK±/EMA+/VIM+/CD10+; adrenal cortical carcinoma, CK-/EMA-/VIM+/CD10-; and hepatocellular carcinoma, CK-/EMA-/VIM±/CD10+ [51]. Additional markers that are not expressed in renal cell carcinoma help differentiate this tumor from other malignancies possibly sharing the same clear-cell morphology: TTF-1 (bronchogenic and thyroid carcinomas), calretinin (mesothelioma), placental alkaline phosphatase (yolk-sac tumor and seminoma), the melanoma markers S100P, HMB-45, and Melan-A (clear-cell and balloon-cell malignant melanoma), neuroendocrine markers (large-cell and clear-cell neuroendocrine carcinoma), and specific hormone products such as thyroglobulin (clear-cell carcinoma of the thyroid of follicular derivation), calcitonin (medullary thyroid carcinoma), and parathyroid hormone (parathyroid carcinoma).

6.3.2 Papillary Carcinoma

6.3.2.1 Clinicopathological Correlates

Papillary carcinoma can occur in individuals of any age, with the highest incidence in the fifth and sixth decades of life. It represents 10–15% of renal malignancies and is less aggressive than classical clear-cell carcinoma [49]. The tumor mass is typically cortical in location or may appear to grow outside the organ. Histologically, the tumor consists of a tubulo-papillary growth often containing dispersed psammoma bodies. Epithelial cells covering the papillary structures and tubules are of intermediate size, cuboid to cylindrical in shape, with a small nucleus and pale to clear or finely granular cytoplasm. A specific variant of the tumor is composed of oncocytic/oncocytoid cells. Papillary structures have a connective-tissue stalk containing numerous histiocytes with a foamy cytoplasm. Tumor cells show the characteristic CK7+/CD10+ immunohistochemical profile [51].

6.3.2.2 Cytomorphology

The FNB yield of papillary carcinoma generally shows an abundant cellularity, with a prevalence of aggregates having a two- or three-dimensional configuration [50]. The cells are small to intermediate in size and their shape is oval or spindly elongated. They have an amphophilic or basophilic fragile cytoplasm and their nuclei are oval to elongated, with finely granular or vesicular chromatin. Focally within the aggregates, the elongated cells tend to form peripheral palisades, tufts, or pseudorosettes, which are the only hints of a papillary or micropapillary pattern of growth (Fig. 6.27a). Non-cohesive cells are also observed in

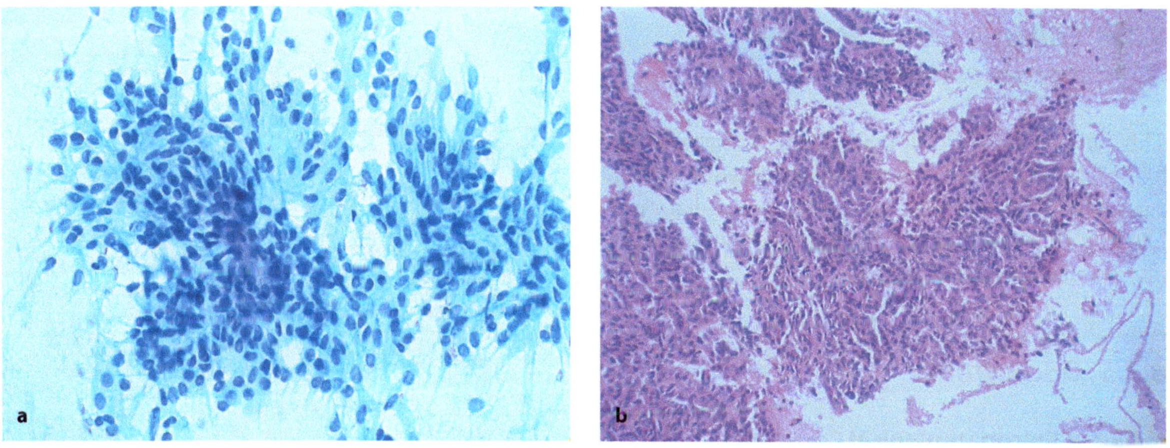

Fig. 6.27 **a** Three- and two dimensional clusters of elongated cells that tend to form palisades or pseudorosettes. P stain, ×400. **b** Cell-block paraffin section, from the same case as in **a**, allows for better identification of the characteristic micropapillary pattern of tumor growth. H&E stain, ×400

the background, as are foamy histiocytes. The examination of cell-block paraffin sections, when available, is of help in confirming the diagnosis (Fig. 6.27b).

6.3.3 Chromophobe-Cell Carcinoma

Chromophobe-cell carcinoma is a rare malignancy, accounting for no more than 5% of renal tumors [49]. Its clinical presentation is similar to that of clear-cell carcinoma. Its salient feature is a peculiar proliferating cell type of intermediate size with a small nucleus and an abundant cytoplasm that is microvacuolar, reticulated, or floccular in appearance. These tumor cells grow in laminar structures.

The cytological features upon FNB of this tumor have been reported only rarely in the literature [50,52]. The cellularity is moderate to high, with the cells arranged in small clusters and as single cells. The cytoplasm of the tumor cells is abundant, and the cell membrane is thickened. The nuclei are hyperchromatic, with occasional intranuclear inclusions.. The cytoplasm is positively stained by colloidal iron and shows strong immunohistochemical expression of CK7. Additional immunohistochemical properties are a positive reaction for c-kit and negative expression of PAX-2 [53]. A variant of chromophobe-cell carcinoma is characterized by cytoplasmic eosinophilia and the tumor has an oncocytic/oncocytoid appearance. Like oncocytoma cells, chromophobe-cell carcinoma cells show immunoreactivity for progesterone receptor and CD117 [54].

6.3.4 Collecting-Duct (Bellini's) Adenocarcinoma

This rare variant of renal malignancy is characterized by a biphasic growth of adenocarcinoma and urothelial carcinoma. It is a highly aggressive tumor that originates within the renal medulla and shows early involvement of hilar structures.

6.3.5 Oncocytoma

6.3.5.1 Clinicopathological Correlates

Renal oncocytoma in the pure form is a benign tumor [49]. It is typically located in the renal cortex and is generally discovered incidentally by imaging techniques. By definition, tumor growth is locally aggressive but does not produce distant metastases. Histologically, it consists of a solid proliferation of oncocytic cells organized in laminar, trabecular, or syncytial patterns. The stroma is sparsely vascularized and edematous. Tumor cells are intermediate to large in size, round to polygonal in shape, and contain an abundant granular cytoplasm. The nuclei are regular and occasionally contain prominent nucleoli.

6.3.5.2 Cytomorphology

The cytological picture on FNB is prototypical of tumors with an oncocytic/oncocytoid cell morphology (see Chapter 5) (Fig. 6.28). However, a definitive diagnosis of oncocytoma cannot be made with certainty based upon partial sampling of the tumor, such as in the setting of FNB, since other primary malignant tumors of the kidney, namely, clear-cell carcinoma, papillary carcinoma, and chromophobe-cell carcinoma, may contain an oncocytic/oncocytoid cellular component indistinguishable from that of conventional oncocytoma. Therefore, pathological evaluation of the entirely excised tumor is generally required for a conclusive diagnosis.

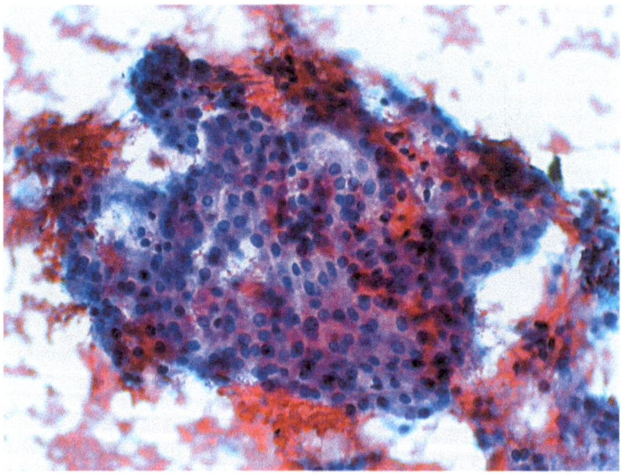

Fig. 6.28 Three-dimensional cluster of cells with monotonous round nuclei and an abundant granular and eosinophilic cytoplasm. P stain, ×400

6.3.6 Angiomyolipoma

Angiomyolipoma is a rare pseudotumor of variable size (1–20 cm in its largest diameter) that is usually asymptomatic and in about half the cases occurs in the setting of the tuberous sclerosis complex. Histologically, it consists of a hamartomatous proliferation of spindle and epithelioid cells admixed with adipocytes and lipoblasts, as well as malformed vessels [55,56]. Angiomyolipoma should be considered in aspirates of renal and extrarenal masses when an admixture of blood vessels, fat, and smooth muscle cells is encountered. Nonetheless, the FNB procedure is rarely diagnostic and no more than about 20 cases have been reported in the literature [57]. The cytological picture can be classified within the category of samples with spindle cell and epithelioid cell morphologies. The cells are arranged in loosely cohesive clusters. Nuclear atypia is occasionally identified, as well as naked nuclei and intranuclear inclusions. The cytoplasm of the spindle and epithelioid elements is delicate and sometimes vacuolated [56,57]. The differential diagnosis includes other tumors composed of similar spindle and epithelioid cells (leiomyoma and leiomyosarcoma), or lipoma and liposarcomas. The constituting cells typically display cytoplasmic positivity for the melanoma-associated markers HMB-45 and Melan-A but are S100P-negative; in addition, they are positive for the expression of calponin and muscle-specific actin (HHF35) [55]. The epithelioid and spindle cells preferentially stain for melanoma-associated and smooth muscle antigens, respectively [55]. The detection of this particular immunohistochemical profile plays a decisive role in making the correct diagnosis.

6.3.7 Special Problems in the Differential Diagnosis of Renal Tumors

Primary renal tumors can show a range of cytohistological microscopic patterns: clear-cell, tubulo-papillary, oncocytic/oncocytoid, spindle cell, round cell, and poorly differentiated gland-forming adenocarcinomatous [50]. The first two patterns are most commonly encountered in daily practice and reflect the microscopic appearance of conventional clear-cell carcinoma and papillary carcinoma. Moreover, the oncocytic/oncocytoid cellular pattern can be seen in several tumor types other than oncocytoma (see above). In FNB material, immunohistochemical studies can be of help in the differential diagnosis of difficult cases, provided that cell-block preparations are available. Table 6.1 summarizes the immunohistochemical reactivity of the different renal tumors for vimentin, CD10, CK7, c-kit, and AMACR (α-methylacyl-CoA racemase), according to Allory et al. [58]. While CD10 is expressed in all tumor types, although with differing intensity, the other markers are preferentially or exclusively expressed in selected tumors. For example, AMACR positivity strongly favors a diagnosis of papillary carcinoma. In AMACR-negative tumors, one should consider conventional clear cell carcinoma if the cell profile is VIM+/CK7-/c-kit-, and chromophobe-cell carcinoma or oncocytoma if it is VIM-/CK7+/c-kit+. These latter two tumors share an unusual positivity for progesterone receptor [54] but, according to Memeo et al. [53], chromophobe-cell carcinoma is PAX2-negative and oncocytoma PAX2-positive. It should be noted that mesenchymal neoplasms, such as angiomyolipomas, as well as metastatic lesions, such as malignant melanoma, may display frankly epithelioid cellular features and cytoplasmic granularity, thus simulating a primary oncocytic/oncocytoid neoplasm of the kidney. In addition, adrenal cortical neoplasms are to be added to the list of oncocytic tumors and, in fact, are sometimes confused clinically, radiologically, and pathologically with a renal neoplasm arising at the upper pole of the kidney. The *spindle cell pattern* is rather commonly encountered in high-grade sarcomatoid variants of conventional clear-cell carcinoma, but also in metastatic malignant melanoma and pleomorphic sarcoma metastatic to or secondarily infiltrating the kidney. The

Table 6.1 Immunohistochemical reactivity of renal tumors [58]

	Vimentin	CD10	CK7	c-kit	AMACR
Clear-cell carcinoma	2	2	0	0	0
Papillary carcinoma	2	2	2	0	2
Chromophobe-cell carcinoma	0	1	2	2	0
Oncocytoma	0	1	1	2	0

Percent positivity: 0 ≤5% of cells; 1= 5–50%; 2 ≥50%

round-cell morphology is seen in neuroendocrine carcinoma and primitive neuroectodermal tumor/Ewing sarcoma (PNET/ES) [59]. The latter is a very rare renal malignancy. The correct diagnosis is based upon detection of the immunohistochemical profile Vimentin+/CD45-/S100P-/Melan-A-/CD99+/CK±/CD117+/CD99+ and demonstration of the t(11;22)(q24;q12) translocation by molecular characterization. The FNB cytological features of a histologically proven case of PNET/ES of the kidney are illustrated in the internet at the *Foro de Diagnostico por Imagen (Fotopat)* website [60].

6.4 Adrenal Gland Tumors

Primary tumors may originate from the cortex or the medulla of the adrenal gland [61]. The former are defined as adenoma and carcinoma and are easily investigated by FNB. The latter, i.e., pheochromocytoma, should not be punctured due to the potential risk of inducing a life-threatening hypertension crisis and fatal hemorrhage ("pheochromocytoma crisis"). Paraganglia are strictly correlated with the adrenal medulla but are located outside the gland in the retroperitoneum. Tumors derived from the paraganglia show the same features as pheochromocytoma. Most mass lesions of the adrenal gland are metastatic malignancies and are sampled at the time of tumor staging. Immunohistochemical studies can provide an important contribution to the distinction between primary and metastatic lesions and to the identification of the tumor's primary site. Thus, collecting material by FNB for cell-block and conventional smear preparations is of paramount importance.

6.4.1 Adenoma of the Adrenal Cortex

6.4.1.1 Clinicopathological Correlates

Adenoma of the adrenal cortex occurs in adults, with an equal male:female distribution. The tumor is frequently responsible for an endocrine syndrome (hyperaldosteronism, Cushing's syndrome, virilization, etc.). Adenoma of the adrenal cortex is usually detected by imaging techniques and typically measures no more than 4 cm in its largest diameter. The presence of such a mass, when correlated to endocrine symptoms, is highly suggestive for the tumor and should not prompt further evaluation by FNB, which is, instead, used to investigate an adrenal tumor mass in patients in whom endocrine symptoms are absent [62]. FNB sampling is also indicated to rule out a small adrenal cortical carcinoma, which is more typically unassociated with endocrine symptoms. Histologically, adenoma of the adrenal cortex consists of a solid proliferation of cells of intermediate size, polygonal in shape and containing an eosinophilic or clear cytoplasm [62].

6.4.1.2 Cytomorphology

Sampling by FNB can be performed percutaneously or under endoscopic ultrasound assistance [63] and generally yields a highly cellular smear. The cells are often non-cohesive or in loose sheets. Naked nuclei are evident in the background as are lipofuscin pigment deposits and lipid vacuoles. By definition, in the sample there is no evidence of tumor necrosis. According to Wu et al., 1998 [64], the combined cytological features of bare nuclei; foamy, vacuolated background; and large, cohesive tissue fragments with sinusoidal endothelial cells in a small (<3.5 cm) adrenal nodule are highly specific for a FNB diagnosis of benign adrenal cortical nodule. The nuclei are round and small with a finely granular chromatin, but the occasional presence of nuclei that are larger or of bizarre shape is not uncommon. This latter observation does not represent a criterion of possible malignancy; rather, adrenal cortical carcinoma should only be suspected when tumor necrosis is prominent and nuclear chromatin is definitely coarsely granular. A potential problem of confusing primary adrenocortical neoplasms with metastases from hepatocellular carcinoma and vice versa has been reported by Dusenberry and Dekker [62]. In addition, extraneous, benign cells of hepatic origin that contaminate the needle sample may be misinterpreted as adrenal cortical adenoma cells [65].

6.4.2 Carcinoma of the Adrenal Cortex

6.4.2.1 Clinicopathological Correlates

Carcinoma of the adrenal cortex is a rare and aggressive malignancy generally encountered in adults 50–60 years of age and older [61]. Only in a minority of cases is the tumor associated with a clinically significant secretion of glucocorticoids or androgens. At presentation, the tumor is commonly of large size (>5 cm) and contains extensive areas of necrosis that may induce a pseudocystic change [61]. Histologically, carcinoma of the adrenal cortex consists of a solid cellular proliferation of cells in a trabecular or alveolar pattern together with a huge vascular component. The cells are intermediate to large, their cytoplasm is optically clear, or it may be granular and eosinophilic or amphophilic. The nuclei are large and frequently pleomorphic. Multinucleated cells are commonly encountered. Intratumoral coagulative necrosis is prominent.

6.4.2.2 Cytomorphology

The cytological appearance of the tumor in FNB samples is best classified within the clear-cell or oncocytic/oncocytoid morphology [66,67]. In fact, the cytological picture in smears resembles that of renal cell carcinoma due to several overlapping features, including an abundant clear cytoplasm, large nuclei with prominent nucleoli, bare nuclei, and prominent vascularity. According to Sharma et al., 1997 [66], adrenal cortical carcinoma is typically characterized by: the presence of cells in sheets with a central, thin-walled vascular core (endocrine vascular pattern); a monomorphic cell population; eccentric nuclei; focal dramatic anisonucleosis; and focal spindling with crushing of the cell nuclei (Fig. 6.29a). By contrast, renal cell carcinoma is mainly characterized by an acinar pattern with only a focal endocrine pattern, well-defined cytoplasmic angles and projections, and cytoplasmic vacuolations. Pleomorphism, if present, is gradual and seen uniformly in all the cells. In other cases, the cytoplasm of adrenal gland carcinoma cells is not clear but rather granular and eosinophilic and oncocytoid (Fig. 6.29b). In this author's experience, adrenal cortical carcinoma is also often confused with a metastatic carcinoma originating in the lung, especially in patients presenting with concomitant masses in the lung and adrenal gland. Due to massive necrosis of the adrenal mass, any attempt to perform an immunohistochemical investigation on cell-block material may be unsuccessful, and the distinction is rarely obtained by sampling only the adrenal mass. Finally, in the presence of only slight atypia in the cellular sample and no necrotic changes, adrenal cortical carcinoma should be distinguished from adrenal cortical adenoma. In general, the latter is associated with an endocrine syndrome and the size of the mass, as determined by imaging techniques, is <4 cm. Tumors of larger size should be considered benign only with great caution [61].

6.4.3 Pheochromocytoma

FNB sampling of pheochromocytoma is potentially hazardous to the patient; consequently, there are very few reports in the literature describing the cytological

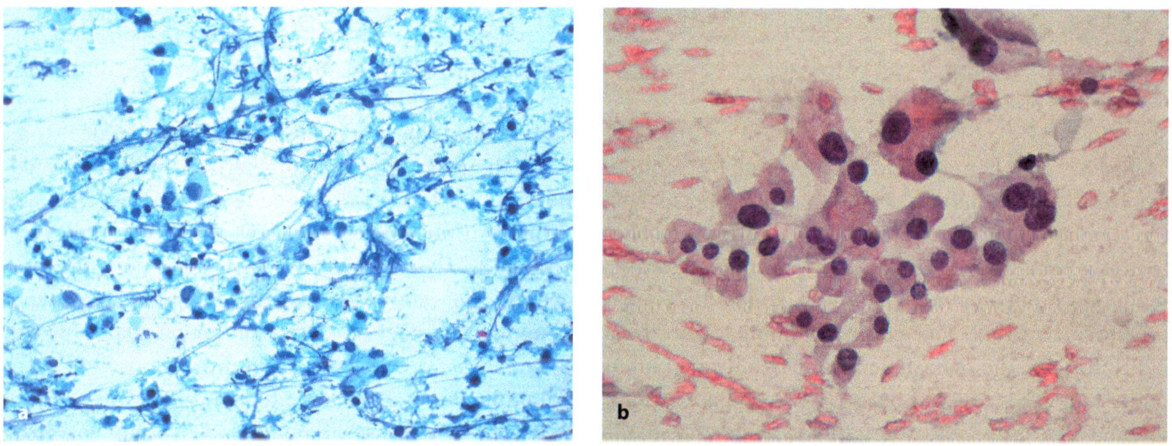

Fig. 6.29 a Large pleomorphic cells are seen in a highly necrotic background in a FNB sample of a typical case of adrenal cortical carcinoma. P stain, ×400. b Medium-sized and polygonal cells with a granular cytoplasm may be seen in some cases of adrenal cortical carcinoma. P stain, ×400

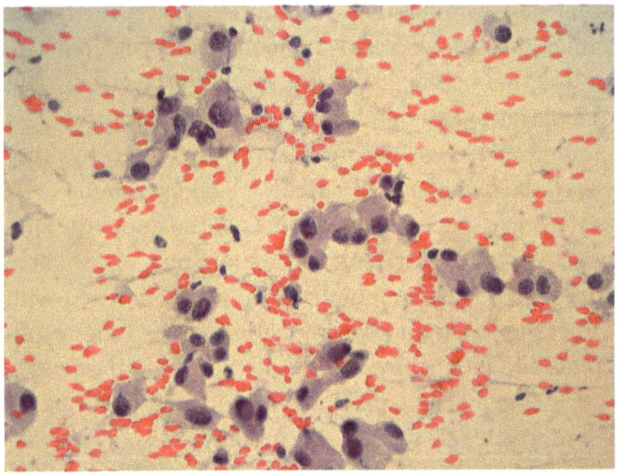

Fig. 6.30 Large oncocytoid cells with nuclear pleomorphism are seen in small clusters. FNB smear in a case of pheochromocytoma. P stain, ×400

features of this tumor [63,68]. Pheochromocytoma rarely appears as an incidental and asymptomatic mass and in most patients it is responsible for the typical endocrine syndrome induced by the hypersecretion of adrenaline. The cellular yield upon FNB is sparse and rich in blood. The cells are aggregated or non-cohesive and have an oncocytic/oncocytoid cytomorphology. Nuclear pleomorphism and intranuclear pseudoinclusions are common findings. The cytoplasm is granular and rather abundant (Fig. 6.30). The presence of synaptophysin and chromogranin in cytoplasmic granules, as demonstrated by immunohistochemistry of cell-block material, provides a conclusive diagnosis of the tumor.

6.4.4 Metastatic Malignancies

Metastatic tumors of the adrenal gland are by far more frequently encountered than primary tumors. In fact, the adrenal gland is a preferential site of metastatic seeding for a large number of primary tumors, including bronchogenic, mammary, pancreatic, hepatocellular, ovarian, and colon carcinomas. In about half the cases, the metastatic lesions are located bilaterally and are small (<2 cm). HCC or renal cell carcinoma can grow into the adrenal gland due to its contiguity, thus inducing a unilateral tumor mass that simulates an adrenal primary [69]. In FNB samples, adrenal cortical tumors can share the clear-cell and oncocytic/oncocytoid cell morphologies characteristic of these latter malignancies. Immunohistochemistry performed on cell-block material aids in differentiating primary vs. metastatic malignancies, as adrenal cortical carcinoma is typically non-reactive for cytokeratins, EMA, or CD10, and is strongly and diffusely positive for vimentin [70]. In addition, adrenal cortical tumor cells are positive for the expression of Melan-A, calretinin, inhibin, and bcl-2 [71]. Adrenal cortical carcinoma can be easily distinguished from renal cell carcinoma secondarily infiltrating the gland by investigating the immunohistochemical reactivity for EMA and CD10, as both are consistently absent in the former tumor [70]. Metastatic HCC can be diagnosed if oncocytoid cells show both CD10 and Hep-par positivity. Adrenal cortical carcinoma can also share the large-cell morphology of metastatic bronchogenic carcinoma; in this context, positive immunostaining for cytokeratin and EMA favors a bronchogenic primary, and TTF-1 positivity, when present, provides confirmatory evidence. Finally, the detection of a glandular cell, small cell, or epithelioid and spindle cell morphology completely supports the diagnosis of a metastatic malignancy and identification of the primary tumor site should be obtained based on the use of properly planned immunohistochemical panels (see Chapter 5).

6.5 Ovarian Tumors

Ovarian tumors commonly present as a cystic mass and are easily and properly evaluated preoperatively by imaging techniques. Fine-needle aspiration and partial evacuation of these tumors under ultrasound guidance for cytological investigation is often inconclusive due to the poor cellularity of the sample. Moreover, the procedure is characterized by a low sensitivity as well as a low negative predictive value, and actually often fails to identify the proliferating cell type [72,73]. However, in young women, the procedure can safely differentiate functional and other benign ovarian cysts from malignant ones [74–76]; nonetheless, fine-needle aspiration biopsy is not a common practice in the preoperative evaluation of ovarian cystic masses. Sampling of ovarian masses by FNB is instead indicated for investigating large tumors, or tumors that are totally or partially solid, at least partially necrotic, and unilateral. In these cases, the main diagnostic problems include benignancy vs. malignancy, the definition of histotype, whether tumor growth involves the ovary, and, if the tumor is frankly malignant, whether it is a primary or a metastatic malignancy. The diagnostic yield of FNB of solid areas is greatly amplified if sampling is adequate enough to provide both direct smears and a cell-block preparation from a needle rinse. The latter material is essential for the immunohistochemical categorization of tumor cells.

6.5.1 Serous Tumors

Solid variants of serous ovarian tumors are either well-differentiated or poorly differentiated carcinomas. They are frequently bilateral and associated with ascites. Cytological evaluation of ascitic fluid is often adequate for a proper diagnosis. Histologically, the tumor consists of a tubulo-papillary or microcystic proliferation of cylindrical cells with frequent psammoma bodies [77]. Cytologically, the FNB picture is that of tumors with a glandular-cell morphology, papillary pattern (see Chapter 5). The cytological features of poorly differentiated tumors include hypercellularity, abundant papillary fragments, and a necrotic background (Fig. 6.31a). The characteristics of the tumor cells are a high nuclear/cytoplasmic ratio, anisonucleosis, and prominent nucleoli (Fig. 6.31b).

6.5.2 Mucinous Tumors

Solid variants of mucinous tumors are generally mucinous carcinoma. At onset, this malignancy is often unilateral and large. Proliferating cells belong to two categories, the intestinal type and the mullerian (endocervical-like) type, with the former occurring more frequently [77]. Cytologically, the cells of either type are classified as having a glandular-cell morphology and a mucinous pattern (see Chapter 5). Mucin, cellular detritus, and foamy histiocytes are prominent in the background. Cells form tubular or papillary aggregates or, rarely, syncytial sheets (Fig. 6.32). The nuclei of cells of benign proliferations as well as those of tumors of low-grade malignancy are regular in size and shape, with small nucleoli. Any attempt to differentiate mucinous tumors of borderline malignancy from frankly malignant tumors upon FNB samples should be highly discouraged and the diagnosis should be limited to descriptive terms [74]. In addition, there should be a high index of suspicion that a mucinous tumor is actually a metastasis from another organ in order to prevent misdiagnosis of a metastatic neoplasm as a primary ovarian tumor. The most frequent sites for the primary tumor are the gastrointestinal tract and the pancreas. Immunohistochemically, the *intestinal-type* variant of ovarian mucinous tumor has a CK7+/CK20+ profile, with frequent concomitant CDX2 positivity and occasional positivity for chromogranin. The *endocervical-type* variant is CK7+/CK20-/CDX2- and

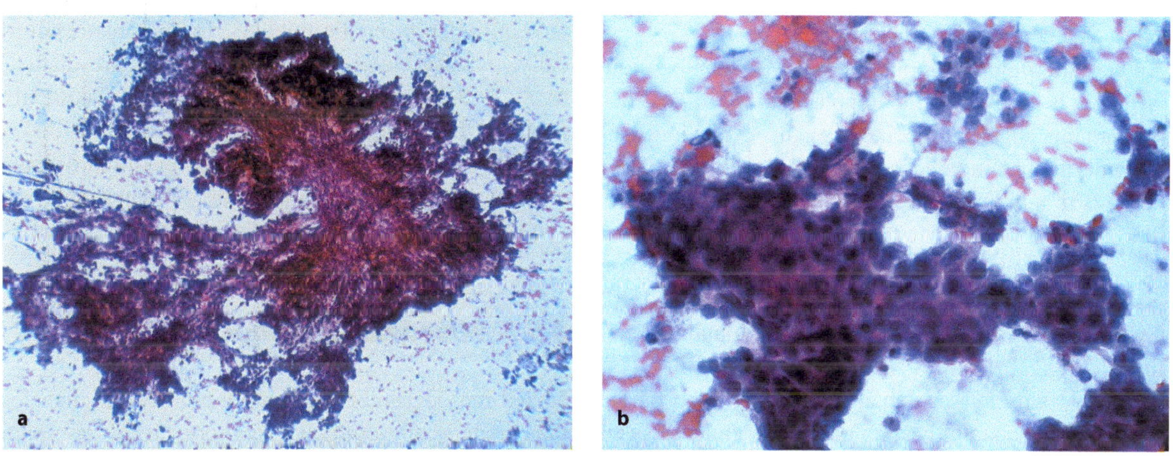

Fig. 6.31 **a** A large papillary cluster containing pleomorphic elongated cells; necrotic debris is seen in the background. P stain, ×200. **b** At higher-power view, tumor cells display a high nuclear/cytoplasmic ratio, with anisonucleosis and prominent nucleoli. P stain, ×400

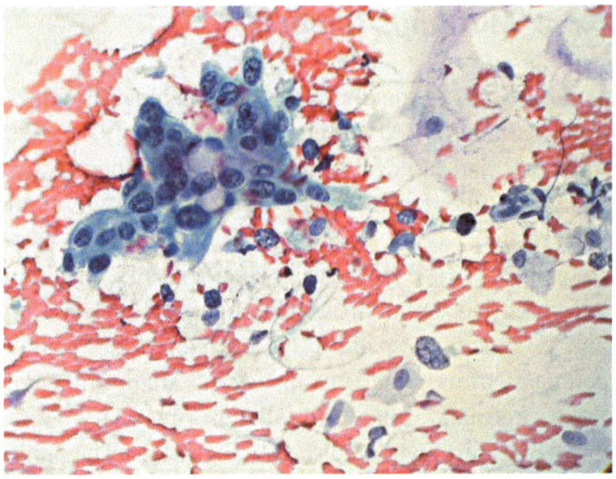

Fig. 6.32 A small aggregate of epithelial glandular cells showing intracytoplasmic mucin vacuoles. P stain, ×500

may show concomitant positivity for estrogen receptors [77]. The term “pseudomyxoma ovarii” refers to the induction of a tumor mass secondary to mucin extrusion into the ovarian stroma from mucinous glands of a mucinous tumor, with a subsequent sclerosing reaction. The term “pseudomyxoma peritonei” refers to the extrusion of mucin and epithelial cells into the peritoneal cavity, eliciting a fibroplastic reaction that simulates a solid tumor. The latter can develop in association with ovarian mucinous and appendiceal mucinous tumors or as a consequence of extraintestinal diffusion of a mucinous “colloid” adenocarcinoma of the large intestine.

6.5.3 Endometrioid Carcinoma

An endometrioid carcinoma of the ovary can be quite large but is rarely bilateral at presentation. In 10–20% of patients, it is associated with a concomitant endometrial carcinoma [78]. Histologically, the tumor consists of a tubular, glandular, papillary proliferation of cylindrical cells with a basally located nucleus and a sparse amphophilic or eosinophilic cytoplasm. There is often a squamoid or squamous cell component [78]. Cytologically, the FNB samples show glandular-cell morphological features and a tubulo-glandular or papillary pattern (see Chapter 5), with a possible concomitant squamoid cell or definitely squamous cell component [74–76]. The nuclear/cytoplasmic ratio and nuclear characteristics depend on the tumor grade. The tumor cells may contain large clear vacuoles and sometimes appear as clear cells. In addition, there is a variant characterized by oncocytic/oncocytoid cells. Immunohistochemically, tumor cells express CK7 and EMA and are non-reactive for CK20, inhibin, WT1, and calretinin [78].

6.5.4 Clear-Cell Carcinoma

Clear-cell carcinoma of the ovary occurs in middle aged and elderly women and is always associated with endometriosis [78]. It presents as a large solid and cystic tumor mass which in about one-third of patients is bilateral. Histologically, there is a heterogeneous population of clear cells, cells having an eosinophilic granular cytoplasm, and hobnail-type cells associated in a solid, tubular, papillary, or microcystic pattern of growth. The cytological picture of the FNB samples is typical of those belonging to the category with clear-cell morphology. The tumor cells have a well-defined external membrane surrounding an optically clear cytoplasm containing variable amounts of fine vacuoles, and round nuclei with distinct or prominent nucleoli (Fig. 6.33a). So-called raspberry bodies (globular, hyaline basement membrane stromal structures, either naked or surrounded by neoplastic epithelial cells) [79] and a tigroid background in Giemsa-stained samples [80] are characteristic cytological features. The combination of clear, atypical cells and a basement membrane stroma is highly specific to this neoplasm. In CNB samples, the clear cells are cuboid, cylindrical, or polygonal with nuclei of variable size and shape (Fig. 6.33b). Hobnail-like cells have a hyperchromatic nucleus. Immunohistochemically, ovarian clear-cell carcinoma cells are distinctively CK7+/EMA+/CD10- and are frequently positive for cytokeratin 34βE12. This profile is quite distinctive and of help in distinguishing ovarian clear-cell carcinoma from renal cell and yolk-sac carcinomas.

6.5.5 Mixed Mesodermal Tumors

Mixed mesodermal tumors are biphasic malignancies that include an epithelial component of common epithelial origin (serous, mucinous, endometrioid, or undifferentiated) and a mesenchymal component that can be homologous (fibrosarcoma, leiomyosarcoma)

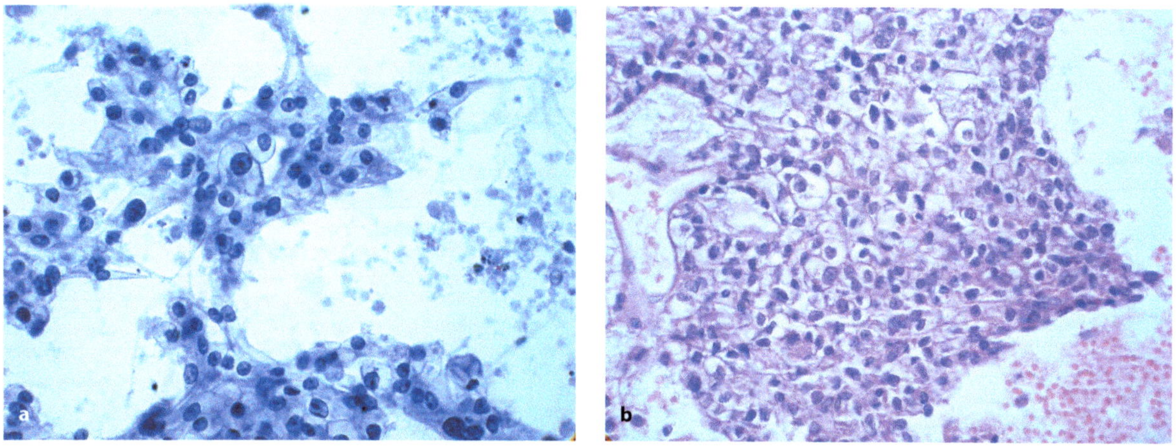

Fig. 6.33 a Cells appear polygonal in shape and have a clear cytoplasm; the nuclei are variable in size and contain single prominent nucleoli. P stain, ×400. b Cell-block paraffin section, from the same case as in a, allows better identification of the characteristic clear cell morphology of the tumor cells. H&E stain, ×400

or heterologous (chondrosarcoma, rhabdomyosarcoma). These rare tumors occur almost exclusively in the elderly [78]. Cytologically, there may be a composite morphological picture reflecting the peculiar intrinsic features of the tumor; alternatively, only one component may be represented in the FNB sample. Only a few cases of this tumor have been reported in the medical literature [81,82].

6.5.6 Transitional Cell Tumors

Transitional cell tumors of the ovary fall into two distinct clinicopathological categories: Brenner tumors and transitional cell carcinomas. The latter is variably associated with a squamous cell component or an undifferentiated carcinoma. Residual areas of typical Brenner tumor must be demonstrated in order to define the tumor as primary in the ovary [78]. For this reason, incomplete sampling, such as by FNB, is unable to properly identify the tumor. Although the cytological sample is morphologically interpretable as a transitional cell tumor, a possible secondary involvement by a urothelial carcinoma cannot be ruled out. Immunohistochemical investigation of p63 expression may be of help in this respect because it is a characteristic finding of urothelial carcinoma but not of transitional cell carcinoma of the ovary [83].

6.5.7 Granulosa Cell Tumor

6.5.7.1 Clinicopathological Correlates

There are two distinct variants of granulosa cell tumor, namely, the *juvenile* variant, which occurs in younger women, in the second and third decades of life, and the *adult* variant, occurring in women beginning at about age 40 [84]. The former is associated with hyperandrogenism and virilization, the latter with hyperestrogenism accompanied by metrorrhagia in postmenopausal or amenorrhea in premenopausal women. In the adult variant, there is a prevailing monolateral ovarian involvement and a large tumor is detected at clinical onset. The tumor is of low-grade malignancy and is poorly aggressive. Histologically, the proliferating cells are small to intermediate in size and round, spindled, or polygonal and epithelioid in shape. Their nuclei show a characteristic "coffee bean" outline due to the presence of deep clefts. The tumor proliferation is organized in microfollicular or macrofollicular structures in which Call-Exner bodies can be seen. Growth occurs in a solid trabecular pattern or may be totally cystic [84]. Immunohistochemically, the tumor cells are inconsistently positive for CK8,18 but show positive cytoplasmic expression of actin and inhibin, membrane positivity for CD99, and nuclear staining for calretinin [84].

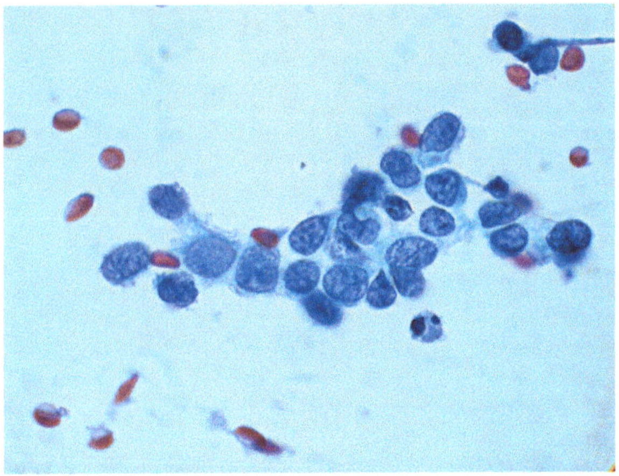

Fig. 6.34 A cluster of small cells with scant cytoplasm and characteristic nuclear grooves. FNB sample from a granulosa cell tumor of the ovary. P stain, ×1000

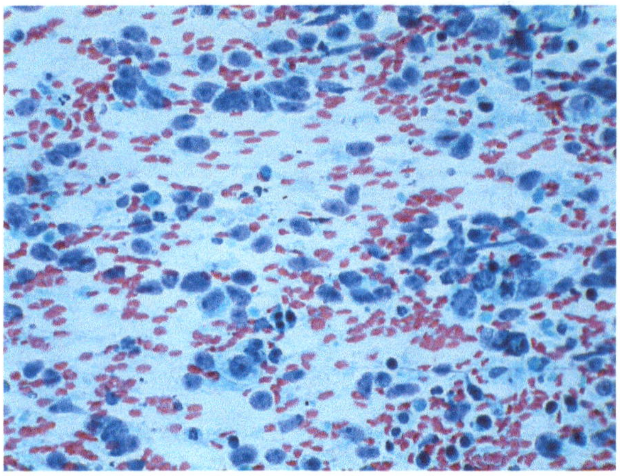

Fig. 6.35 Tumor cells are non cohesive and intermediate in size; they display a fragile cytoplasm which can appear vacuolated; nuclei are characteristically round in shape and are centered by a single well evident nucleolus. FNB sample from ovarian disgerminoma, P stain, ×400.

6.5.7.2 Cytomorphology

The cytological appearance in FNB suggests a tumor having a small-cell morphology (Fig. 6.34). A correct diagnosis cannot be made unless definite Call-Exner bodies and nuclear grooves are detected. The cytopathological features of granulosa cell tumors in primary or metastatic sites have been described in a limited number of previous reports [85–88].

6.5.8 Undifferentiated Small-Cell Carcinoma

Undifferentiated small-cell carcinoma is a rare and highly aggressive ovarian malignancy occurring most frequently in the young adult age group. Clinically, these patients typically present with hypercalcemia, with normal parathyroid function and a large unilateral ovarian mass [78]. Cytological evaluation of the FNB sample shows a tumor with a small-cell morphology and a pattern of marked cellular dissociation as well as marked nuclear atypia. The tumor cells are small and round to oval or spindle-shaped. The cytoplasm is sparse and the nuclei are highly pleomorphic, with small nucleoli; the chromatin is dense or coarsely granular. Necrotic debris is seen in the background. Immunohistochemically, the tumor cells poorly express CK8, 18 but are positive for WT1, EMA, and calretinin (with both nuclear and cytoplasmic positivity). Neither inhibin, nor CD99, nor TTF-1 is expressed [89].

6.5.9 Dysgerminoma

Dysgerminoma is the most common ovarian tumor of germ cell origin. It presents as a rapidly growing, unilateral, and solid mass that is characteristically associated with an increased serum lactate dehydrogenase titer. The tumor is prone to early involvement of the reproperitoneal lymph nodes and liver. Histologically and cytologically, it recapitulates the morphology of testicular seminoma, classical variant. The FNB sample shows tumor cells that are totally non-cohesive, of intermediate size, with a round nucleus and a well-evident and centrally located nucleolus (Fig. 6.35). The cytoplasm is fragile and can appear vacuolated. A concomitant granulomatous inflammation and necrotic detritus are frequently detected within the tumor. Immunohistochemically, the tumor cells show slight and inconsistent expression of CK8, 18 whereas placental alkaline phosphatase and c-kit expression are constant features [89].

6.5.10 Squamous Cell Carcinoma Arising in a Mature Teratoma

Mature cystic teratomas are benign tumors accounting for about 25–30% of ovarian masses. They are easily identified preoperatively and are almost never sampled by FNB. The secondary development of malignancy of a somatic component within the teratoma is a rare but well-known occurrence, and up to 80% of secondary carcinomas are of the squamous-cell type [90]. These tumors typically occur in women over 50 years of age. The chance in this age group of a secondary malignancy developing in a mature teratoma should always be taken into consideration.

6.5.11 *Metastatic Malignancies*

The ovary is a preferential site of metastatic involvement by tumors originating both within and outside the abdominal cavity. The most common primary sites are the breast, the colon and rectum, the stomach, and the endometrium. Less frequently, ovarian metastases are induced by tumors of the vermiform appendix, the pancreatic and biliary tracts, and the kidney. The clinical onset is typically characterized by the development of a bilateral ovarian mass of moderate size (<10 cm) in a patient previously treated (usually within 2 years) for a carcinoma in the above-mentioned sites. Less frequently, a metastatic ovarian tumor originates from an occult primary and represents the first manifestation of the disease. This is typical of the so-called Krukenberg tumor, which occurs in young women and is prevalent in the right ovary [91]. The stomach is the most common site of the primary tumor, which may be totally asymptomatic. Histologically, the tumor is composed of a diffuse proliferation of signet-ring cells that elicit an intensely desmoplastic reaction in the ovarian stroma. FNB sampling usually fails to document the epithelial component of the tumor due to massive sclerosis within the ovarian mass; instead, core-biopsy sampling is essential for a correct diagnosis. Colonic carcinoma infiltrating the ovary contiguously is practically indistinguishable from a primary mucinous tumor, with the only difference being a more pronounced necrosis and a conspicuous intralesional inflammation. Immunohistochemically, an ovarian mucinous carcinoma frequently, but not always, has a CK7+/CK20- profile whereas colorectal carcinomas have the reverse pattern, i.e., CK7-/CK20+. CDX2 is expressed in both tumor types [77]. A carcinoma of the breast that metastasizes into the ovary is practically indistinguishable from a primary endometrioid carcinoma and both are positive for the expression of estrogen receptor. In these cases, positive expression of GCDFP15 provides conclusive evidence of the tumor's mammary origin [91].

6.6 Tumors Growing into the Peritoneal Cavity

6.6.1 *Gastrointestinal Stromal Tumors*

6.6.1.1 Clinicopathological Correlates

Tumors of the gastrointestinal stroma occur most frequently in the stomach and small intestine (respectively, in 60–70% and 20–30% of patients) and in no more than 10% of patients in the remaining segments of the digestive tract (esophagus, colon, and rectum) [92]. By definition, these tumors originate from mesenchymal components of the gastrointestinal tract and thus show no sign of neural or smooth-muscle differentiation. They consist of a proliferation of epithelioid and spindle cells that grow in a solid, fascicular, storiform, alveolar, or hemangiopericytoma-like pattern. A pseudocystic transformation of the tumor mass is rather common in tumors arising from the stomach. A malignant course, initially characterized by multiple relapses within the abdominal cavity (with tumors arising intramurally in the intestinal wall or on the peritoneal surface) and, later on, by metastatic involvement of the liver and lung, is seen in 30–40% of these patients [92]. This malignant behavior occurs more frequently in elderly patients and in those with tumors >5 cm in diameter, located distally in the intestinal tract, and characterized by necrotic changes and/or high mitotic activity.

6.6.1.2 Cytomorphology and Immunohistiochemistry

FNB, performed percutaneously or via endoscopic ultrasound guidance, is a well-established and widely accepted procedure for the diagnosis of these tumors [93,94]. The cytological picture in FNB samples is prototypical of tumors with an epithelioid and spindle cell morphology (see Chapter 5). The tumor cells tend to cluster in small aggregates, are rather monomorphous in appearance (Fig. 6.36a), and have a small and elongated nucleus lacking prominent nucleoli. In

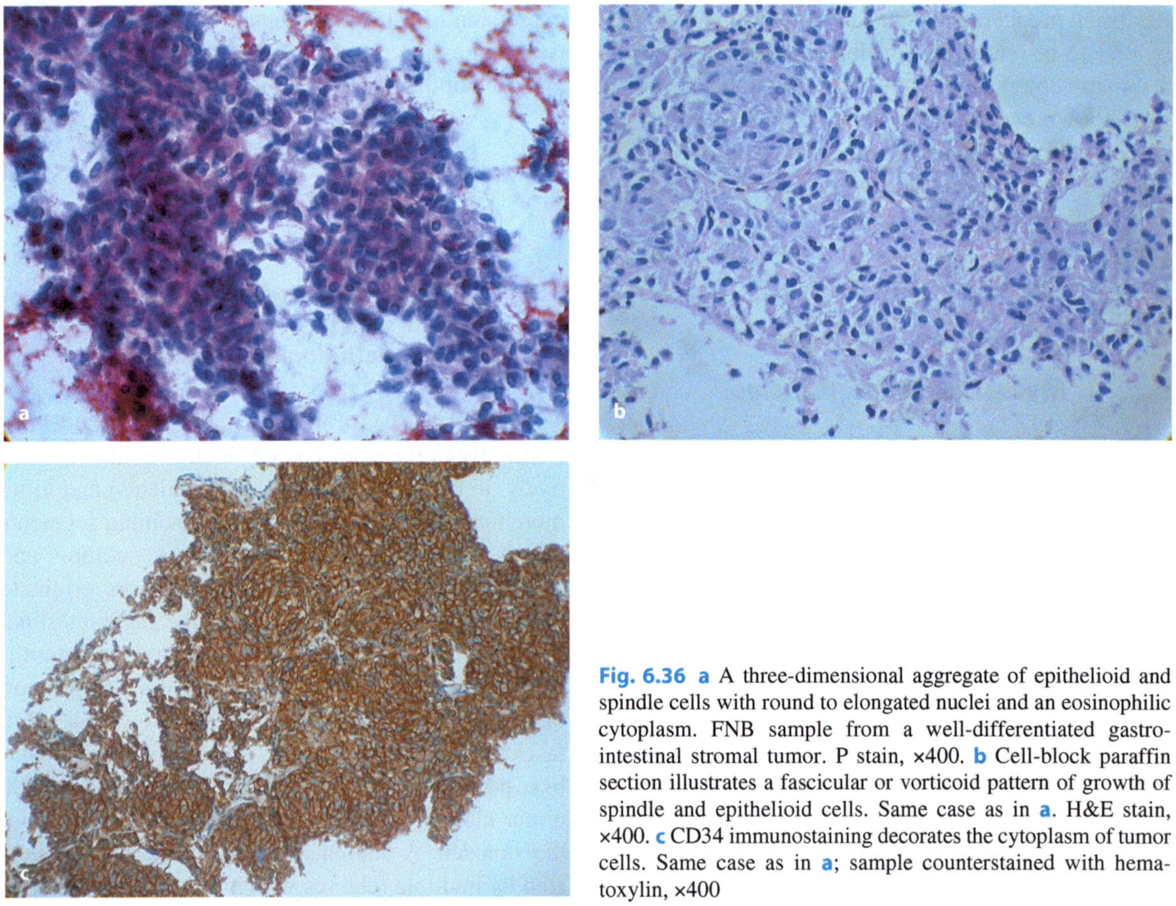

Fig. 6.36 **a** A three-dimensional aggregate of epithelioid and spindle cells with round to elongated nuclei and an eosinophilic cytoplasm. FNB sample from a well-differentiated gastrointestinal stromal tumor. P stain, ×400. **b** Cell-block paraffin section illustrates a fascicular or vorticoid pattern of growth of spindle and epithelioid cells. Same case as in **a**. H&E stain, ×400. **c** CD34 immunostaining decorates the cytoplasm of tumor cells. Same case as in **a**; sample counterstained with hematoxylin, ×400

cell-block material, they exhibit a fascicular and vorticoid pattern of growth (Fig. 6.36b). Gastrointestinal stromal tumors are characterized by the overexpression and mutations of c-kit. FNB samples are amenable to mutational analysis, as shown by Schmitt et al., 2007 [95]. The immunohistochemical profile is marked by the expression of vimentin and the frequent coexpression of CD34 (Fig. 6.36c) and CD117 (c-kit). Smooth-muscle actin and desmin are expressed in 40–50% of the tumors while S100P is not expressed. This profile aids in the differentiation of gastrointestinal stroma tumors from smooth-muscle tumors (leiomyoma and leiomyosarcoma) [96], as the latter express muscle markers but not CD34 and CD117, and from peripheral nerve sheath tumors, which are characterized by a S100P+/GFAP+/CD34- immunohistochemical profile. According to Meara et al., 2007 [97], p53 immunostaining may be useful in predicting the outcome of gastrointestinal stroma tumors diagnosed by FNB.

6.6.2 Intra-Abdominal (Mesenteric) Fibromatosis

Intra-abdominal fibromatosis is a benign expanding tumor mass typically originating from the mesentery. These tumors also may arise sporadically in individuals who have previously undergone abdominal surgery and in the setting of Gardner's syndrome. The tumor is usually classified preoperatively by imaging techniques as a gastrointestinal stromal tumor [98,99]. FNB samples are characterized by sparse cellularity, with rare fragments of regular wavy fibrocyte-like spindle cells without atypia. CNB is required to acquire a sufficient tissue amount for diagnostic evaluation. The tumor consists of a solid proliferation of spindle cells immersed in an enormous amount of collagen stroma. The immunohistochemical profile of intra-abdominal fibromatosis is similar to that of gastrointestinal stromal tumor (including c-kit expression) but the tumor cells do not express CD34.

6.6.3 *Peritoneal Lesions*

6.6.3.1 Multicystic Mesothelioma

This is a quite rare psedotumoral lesion that almost exclusively occurs in women of reproductive age, many of whom have a history of endometriosis and/or previous surgery involving the gastrointestinal tract [100]. The tumor consists of a multicystic mass growing on the pelvic peritoneum. The cysts are delimited by flat or cuboid mesothelial cells having a typical CK7+/calretinin+ immunohistochemical profile and positivity for estrogen receptors. To this author's knowledge, the FNB cytology of this lesion has been reported just once [101]. The differential diagnosis includes cystic lymphangioma, developmental cysts, and infectious cysts.

6.6.3.2 Malignant Mesothelioma

Malignant mesothelioma can develop in the peritoneum as either a primary malignancy or a secondary involvement by a pleural tumor or mesothelioma of the tunica vaginalis testis. The cytological diagnosis is obtained by examining the cellular content of the ascitic fluid. The tumor quite rarely presents as a solid mass without associated ascites and is therefore not a target for percutaneous FNB.

6.6.3.3 Desmoplastic Small Round-Cell Tumor

This is a quite rare malignancy mainly occurring in male teenagers or young adults. It is a highly aggressive tumor that originates in the pelvic region and secondarily involves the entire peritoneal cavity and retroperitoneum [102]. Visceral metastatic involvement of the liver, pancreas, or ovary occurs as a late event. The tumor consists of a proliferation of cells of intermediate to small size, with round and hyperchromatic nuclei and sparse cytoplasm. These cells grow in cords that are separated by a desmoplastic stroma. Immunohistochemically, they coexpress epithelial markers and desmin (in globular cytoplasmic deposits) and WT1 [102]. Detection of the EWS-WT1 gene fusion transcript is required for the diagnosis [102]. The sample collected by FNB shows a small round-cell morphology, with a pleomorphic pattern and marked cellular non-cohesion [103]. The tumor cells are sometimes clustered, with a rosette-like feature. The diagnostic yield of FNB can also be used to detect the EWS/WT1 chimeric transcript in tumor cells by molecular analysis [104].

6.7 Tumors of the Abdominal Wall

Relapse of adenocarcinoma of the gastrointestinal tract, pancreas, and ovary following excisional surgical procedures is a frequent occurrence involving the scar of a previous laparotomy. These tumors commonly produce an expanding mass that originates from the anterior abdominal wall and grows into the abdominal cavity. A concomitant ascites may be observed. FNB is a simple and convenient procedure to correctly diagnose these tumors, thereby expediting decision-making regarding additional adjuvant therapy. The so-called *Sister Mary Joseph's nodule* represents a peculiar presentation of many types of relapsing gynecological and gastrointestinal malignancies as well as those of the pancreatic and biliary tracts. The lesion consists of a palpable mass that bulges into the umbilicus as a result of metastatic involvement of the subcutaneous fat and muscular wall in the umbilical area. The lesion can even represent the primary manifestation of an occult malignancy and is commonly associated with multiple nodular involvement of the parietal peritoneum. FNB is the procedure of choice to obtain a correct diagnosis [105–107] (Fig. 6.37).

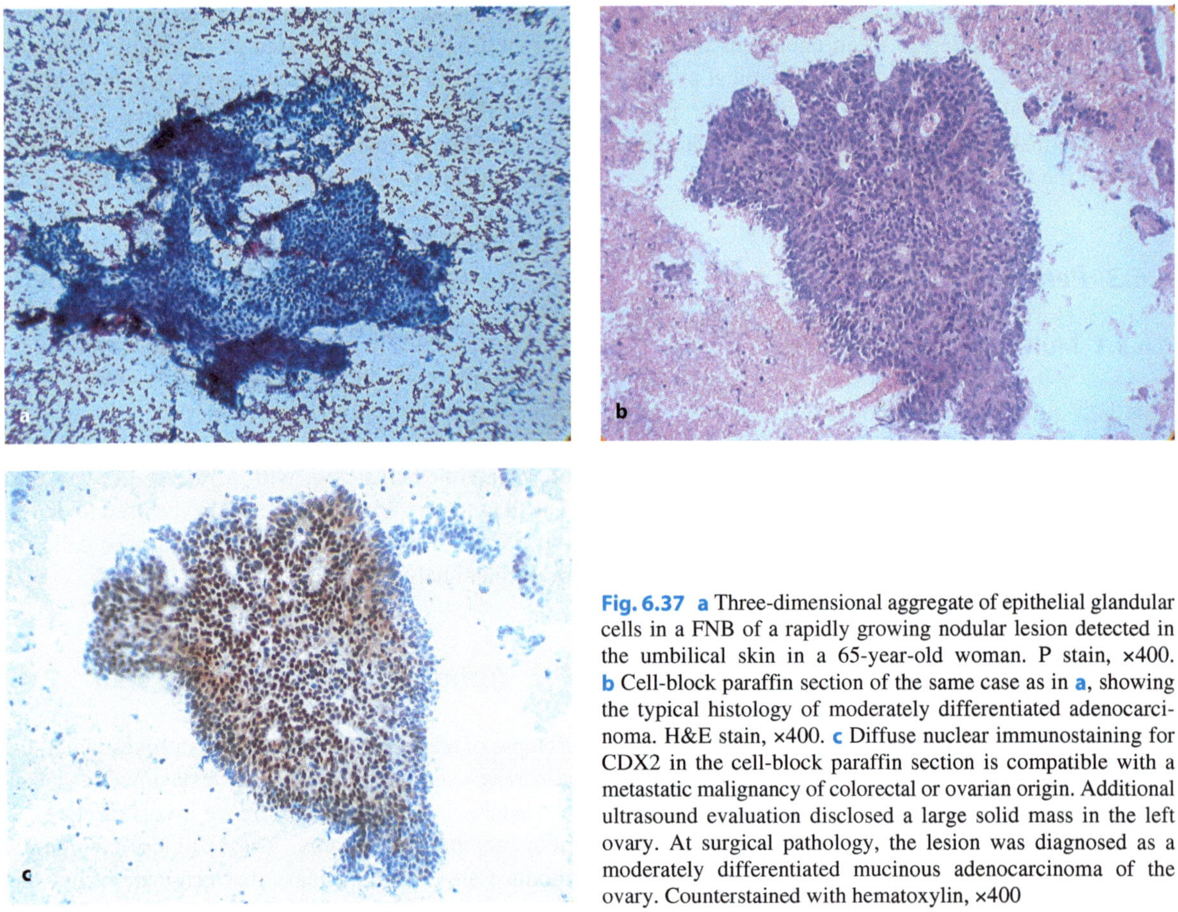

Fig. 6.37 **a** Three-dimensional aggregate of epithelial glandular cells in a FNB of a rapidly growing nodular lesion detected in the umbilical skin in a 65-year-old woman. P stain, ×400. **b** Cell-block paraffin section of the same case as in **a**, showing the typical histology of moderately differentiated adenocarcinoma. H&E stain, ×400. **c** Diffuse nuclear immunostaining for CDX2 in the cell-block paraffin section is compatible with a metastatic malignancy of colorectal or ovarian origin. Additional ultrasound evaluation disclosed a large solid mass in the left ovary. At surgical pathology, the lesion was diagnosed as a moderately differentiated mucinous adenocarcinoma of the ovary. Counterstained with hematoxylin, ×400

6.8 Tumors of the Retroperitoneal Space

6.8.1 Malignant Lymphomas

The retroperitoneum is a frequent site of origin for non-Hodgkin's lymphoma of B-cell lineage, especially follicular lymphoma. In this site, the latter can elicit a florid desmoplastic reaction, which is responsible for a pathological picture resembling that of idiopathic retroperitoneal fibrosis.

6.8.2 Soft-Tissue Tumors

The most common soft-tissue tumors occurring within the retroperitoneal space are lipomatous tumors, leiomyosarcoma, solitary fibrous tumor, and tumors of the peripheral nerve sheath, all of which can be sampled by FNB, both percutaneously and by endoscopic ultrasound. The latter approach is used especially for tumors occurring in the perigastric and periduodenal compartments. Well-differentiated *liposarcoma* in the retroperitoneum is almost exclusively of the lipoma-like variant and grows as a space-occupying tumor mass that has already become quite large at the time of diagnosis. Lipomatous tumors can be diagnosed readily by FNB but the role of this procedure in the identification of variants of liposarcomas and in the distinction of benign vs. malignant tumors is not sufficiently reliable [108]. Liposarcoma undergoes dedifferentiation; this is especially true of long-standing tumors and/or tumors at sites of previous surgical tumor excision. Dedifferentiation is evidenced by a pleomorphic cellular component composed of spindle cells and giant cells with a tendency to tumor necrosis. The malignant fibrous-histiocytoma-like variant of liposarcoma is characterized by the proliferation of large pleomorphic cells with a foamy cytoplasm; these cells are admixed with a substantial component of lymphocytes and granulocytes. Pseudocystic transformation of the tumor is not unusual such that tumor cells are unexpectedly found in cytological samples prepared by centrifugation of the evacuated fluid (Fig. 6.38). Dedifferentiated liposarcoma is practically indistinguishable from other high-grade sarcomas of the retroperitoneal space, such as leiomyosarcoma and malignant peripheral nerve tumors. The sample collected by FNB shows a spindle cell morphology with a pleomorphic pattern and includes large and bizarre cells. FNB is an accurate and useful diagnostic procedure for these tumors [109]. Primary *leiomyosarcoma* of the retroperitoneum is a highly aggressive malignancy. The cytological picture in FNB samples is prototypical of tumors with a spindle cell morphology (see Chapter 5) (Fig. 6.39) [110] but sometimes an epithelioid cellular component may predominate. In the latter case, leiomyosarcoma should be differentiated from a gastrointestinal stromal tumor secondarily infiltrating the retroperitoneal space. Benign *schwannoma* or neurilemmoma is not uncommonly found in the retroperitoneum. The FNB sample shows a spindle cell morphology with a monophasic pattern lacking cellular atypia [111]. In the event of partial or complete pseudocystic change, a proper diagnosis cannot be obtained based on FNB. In addition, nuclear atypias can be detected especially in the "ancient" variant and they pose challenging problems of interpretation, especially in FNB material [112]. *Adult rhabdomyosarcoma* can be added to the list of soft-tissue sarcomas arising primarily in the retroperitoneal space. This quite rare malignancy is easily diagnosed on FNB provided that cell-block material is made available for immunostaining. The cytological picture in FNB samples is prototypical of tumors with a small-cell morphology, i.e., a pleomorphic pattern with marked cellular dissociation (Fig. 6.40a). Immunohistochemistry shows tumor cells with cytoplasmic positivity for CD99 (Fig. 6.40b) and desmin (Fig. 6.40c) but the diagnosis should be supported by positivity for at least one of the following skeletal-muscle-specific markers: myoglobin, MyoD1, fast skeletal muscle myosin, or muscle-specific myogenin [113].

6.8.3 Germ Cell Tumors

Germ cell tumors commonly occur in the retroperitoneum in adult men as a consequence of metastatic spread from a testicular tumor [114]. The latter may be clinically unapparent due to its small size or to necrotic and/or sclerotic transformation ("burned out" testicular primary) [115]; thus, the extragonadal tumor is interpreted as a primary lesion. Extragonadal germ cell tumors characteristically present as a midline mass in the retroperitoneal compartment and sometimes appear

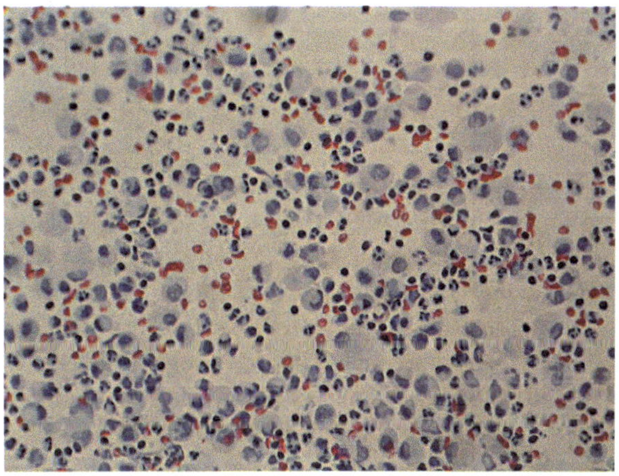

Fig. 6.38 Large and pleomorphic cells with a vacuolated cytoplasm were unexpectedly found in the smears obtained after centrifugation of a clear fluid evacuated from a pseudocystic mass detected in the retroperitoneum in a 52-year-old woman. The tumor was subsequently diagnosed as a dedifferentiated liposarcoma with diffuse pseudocystic change. P stain, ×400

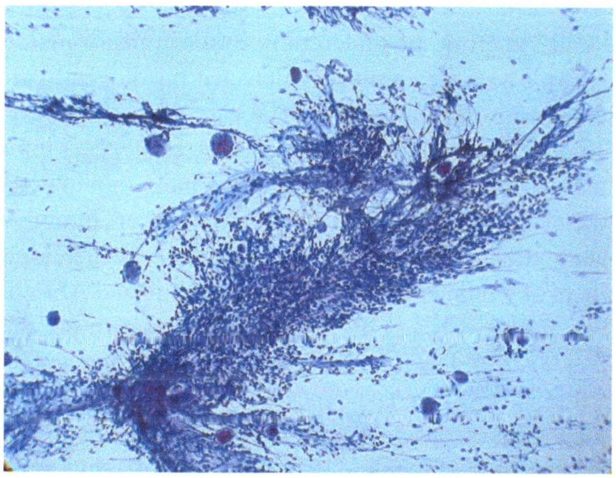

Fig. 6.39 FNB sample of a large retroperitoneal tumor infiltrating the posterior muscular wall of the abdomen. A large aggregate of pleomorphic spindle cells is seen; several round normal striated muscle cells are present in the background. P stain, ×400

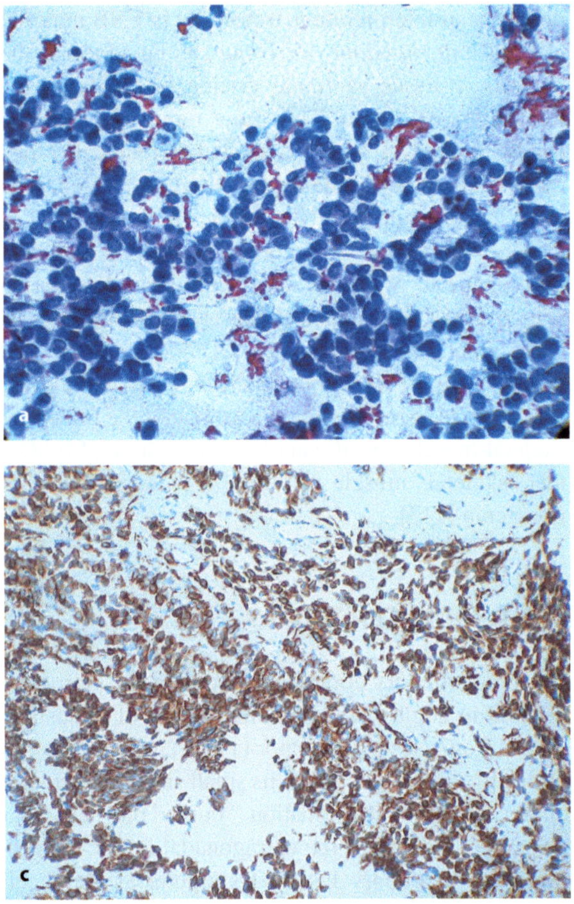

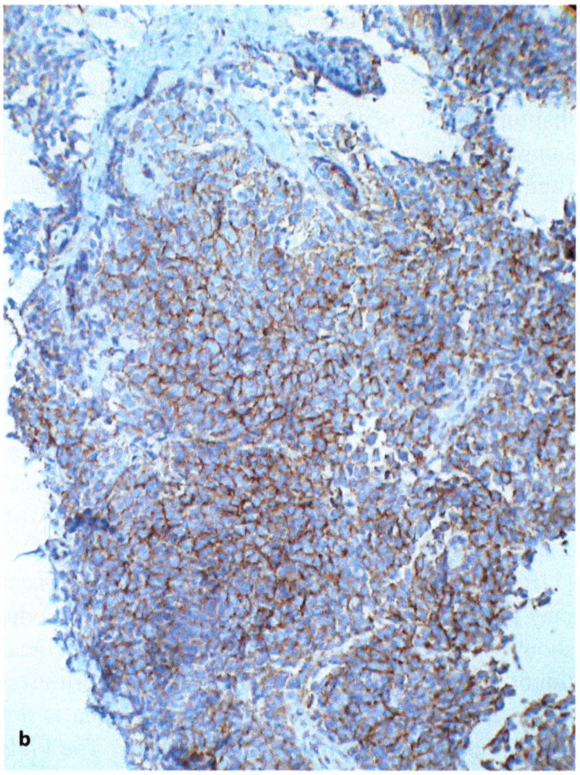

Fig. 6.40 **a** FNB sample collected from a large retroperitoneal tumor in a 25-year-old man, showing round to elongated pleomorphic small cells characterized by marked dissociation. **b** Same case as in **a**. Immunostaining reactivity for CD99 in tumor cells in a cell-block paraffin section. Counterstained with hematoxylin, ×400. **c** Same sample as in **a** and **b**. Immunostaining reactivity for desmin. Counterstained with hematoxylin, ×400

totally necrotic or undergoing cystic transformation [114]. The most commonly detected histological varieties are seminoma, embryonal carcinoma, teratocarcinoma, and yolk-sac tumor. The detection of a tumor mass in the midline in a young adult male should raise the suspicion of an extragonadal germ cell tumor, a contention supported by the detection of increased titers of β human chorionic gonadotrophin and AFP. In this setting, FNB is highly reliable in confirming the diagnosis; in fact, several reports have documented its value [116–118]. The procedure allows for the easy identification of seminoma, embryonal carcinoma, and choriocarcinoma while the diagnosis of immature teratoma and mixed germ cell tumors can pose a significant problem because of sampling error on needle aspiration [118]. FNB of metastatic seminoma generally yields a highly cellular smear. The background is typically rich in cellular detritus (Fig. 6.41a), which is particularly evident in air-dried smears stained by the May Grünwald Giemsa method (Fig. 6.41b). The tumor cells are non-cohesive and appear to be mixed with lymphocytes. They are small to intermediate in size and contain large and round nuclei generally centered by a prominent nucleolus (Fig. 6.41a,b). Positive immunostaining for placental alkaline phosphatase aids in confirming the diagnosis (Fig. 6.41c). The cellular sample obtained by FNB sampling of embryonal carcinoma consists of aggregates with a glandular cell morphology. The tumor cells have a large nucleus with an irregular profile and display a well-evident nucleolus. The cytoplasm is fragile and sparse and may contain clear vacuoles or hyaline globules (Fig. 6.42). The diagnosis of metastatic yolk-sac tumor is particularly difficult in FNB smears but it can be supported by the detection of typical microcystic, glandular-alveolar (Fig. 6.43), or

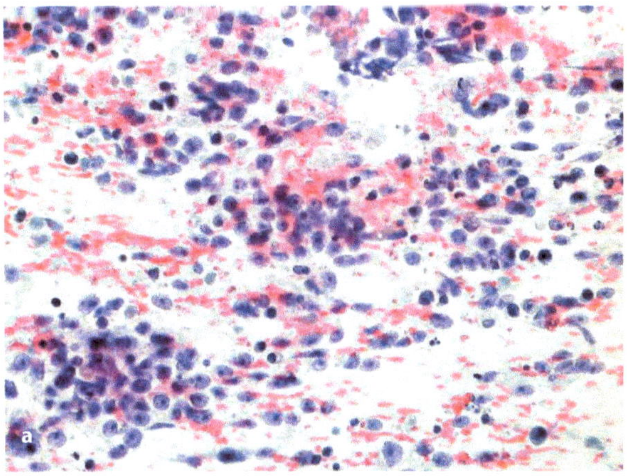

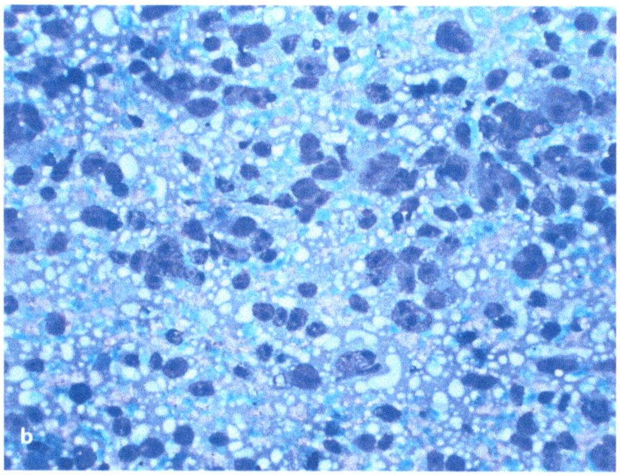

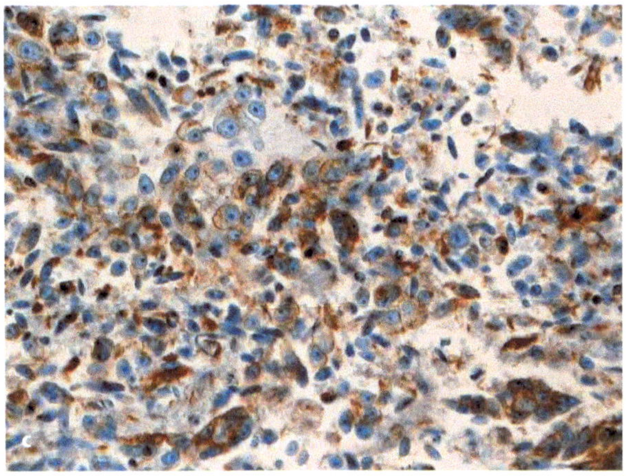

Fig. 6.41 **a** FNB sample of metastatic seminoma into a retroperitoneal lymph node. The harvest consists of medium-sized cells with a small amount of cytoplasm, a round nucleus, and a central prominent nucleolus. P stain, ×400. **b** The background of smears of FNB seminoma samples has a typical tigroid appearance in air-dried slides stained with the May Grünwald Giemsa method. **c** Immunostaining for placental alkaline phosphatase of a cell-block paraffin section demonstrates a positive cytoplasmic reaction in seminoma cells. Counterstained with hematoxylin, ×400

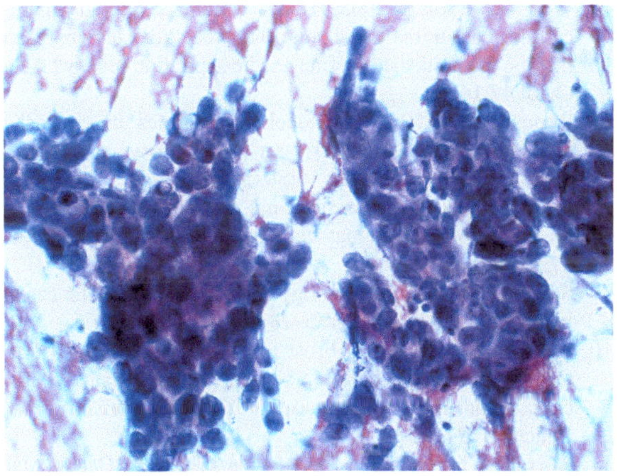

Fig. 6.42 FNB sample of an embryonal carcinoma that has metastasized into a retroperitoneal lymph node. The cells have a large nucleus with an irregular profile and display a well-evident nucleolus. The cytoplasm is fragile and sparse and may contain clear vacuoles or hyaline globules

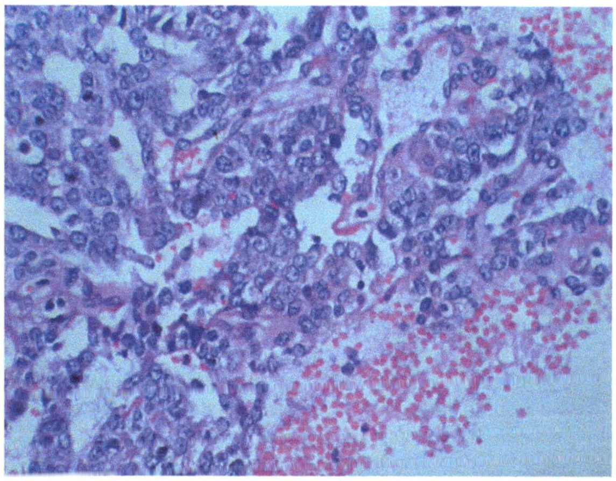

Fig. 6.43 Cell-block paraffin section of a FNB sample of a yolk-sac tumor that has metastasized into a retroperitoneal lymph node, displaying a glandular-alveolar pattern

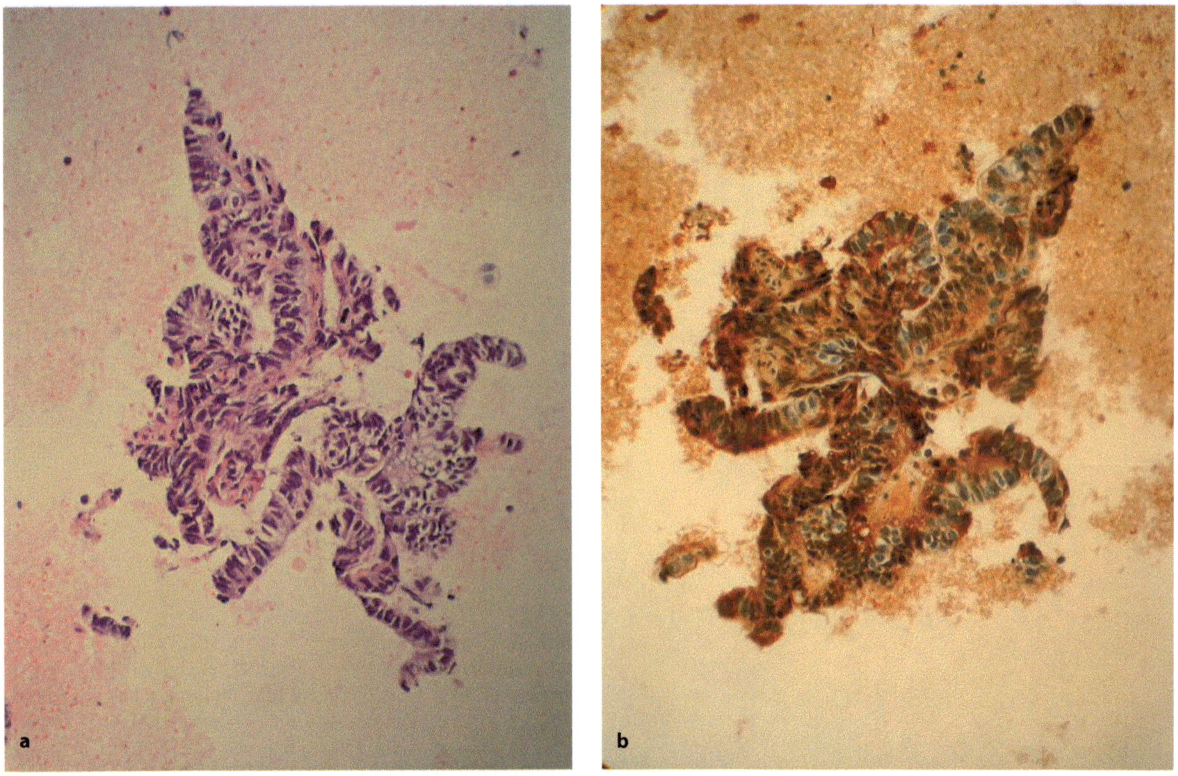

Fig. 6.44 a Cell-block paraffin section of a FNB sample of a yolk-sac tumor that has metastasized into a retroperitoneal lymph node, displaying a papillary pattern. b Same case as in a. Immunostaining for AFP shows a positive cytoplasmic reaction of the tumor cells

papillary (Fig. 6.44a) patterns if core-biopsy specimens of the tumor are obtained. Positive immunostaining for AFP (Fig. 6.44b) provides supportive evidence for the diagnosis.

References

1. Kakar S, Ferrell LD (2007) Tumors of the liver, gallbladder and biliary tree. In: Fletcher CDM (ed) Diagnostic Histopathology of Tumors. Churchill Livingstone Elsevier, pp 417–462.
2. Wang P, Meng ZQ, Chen Z et al (2008) Diagnostic value and complications of fine needle aspiration for primary liver cancer and its influence on the treatment outcome–a study based on 3011 patients in China. Eur J Surg Oncol 34:541–546.
3. Caturelli E, Ghittoni G, Roselli P et al (2004) Fine needle biopsy of focal liver lesions: the hepatologist's point of view. Liver Transpl 10:S26–29.
4. Kuo FY, Chen WJ, Lu SN et al (2004) Fine needle aspiration cytodiagnosis of liver tumors. Acta Cytol 48:142–148.
5. de Boer WB, Segal A, Frost FA, Sterrett GF (1999) Cytodiagnosis of well differentiated hepatocellular carcinoma: can indeterminate diagnoses be reduced? Cancer 87:270–277.
6. Wee A, Nilsson B (2003) Highly well differentiated hepatocellular carcinoma and benign hepatocellular lesions. Can they be distinguished on fine needle aspiration biopsy? Acta Cytol 47:16–26.
7. Roncalli M (2004) Hepatocellular nodules in cirrhosis: focus on diagnostic criteria on liver biopsy. A Western experience. Liver Transpl 10:S9–S15.
8. Wanless IR (2007) International consensus on histologic diagnosis of early hepatocellular neoplasia. Hepatol Res 37:S139–141.
9. Sakamoto M (2007) Pathology of early hepatocellular carcinoma. Hepatol Res 37:S135–138.
10. de Boer WB, Segal A, Frost FA, Sterrett GF (2000) Can CD34 discriminate between benign and malignant hepatocytic lesions in fine-needle aspirates and thin core biopsies? Cancer 90:273–278.
11. Borscheri N, Roessner A, Röcken C (2001) Canalicular immunostaining of neprilysin (CD10) as a diagnostic marker for hepatocellular carcinomas. Am J Surg Pathol 25:1297–1303.
12. Chu PG, Ishizawa S, Wu E, Weiss LM (2002) Hepatocyte antigen as a marker of hepatocellular carcinoma: an immunohistochemical comparison to carcinoembryonic antigen, CD10, and alpha-fetoprotein. Am J Surg Pathol 26:978–988.

13. Lau SK, Prakash S, Geller SA, Alsabeh R (2002) Comparative immunohistochemical profile of hepatocellular carcinoma, cholangiocarcinoma, and metastatic adenocarcinoma. Hum Pathol 33:1175–1181.
14. Anatelli F, Chuang ST, Yang XJ, Wang HL (2008) Value of glypican 3 immunostaining in the diagnosis of hepatocellular carcinoma on needle biopsy. Am J Clin Pathol 130:219–223.
15. Ligato S, Mandich D, Cartun RW (2008) Utility of glypican-3 in differentiating hepatocellular carcinoma from other primary and metastatic lesions in FNA of the liver: an immunocytochemical study. Mod Pathol 21:626–631.
16. Kandil D, Leiman G, Allegretta M et al (2007) Glypican-3 immunocytochemistry in liver fine-needle aspirates: a novel stain to assist in the differentiation of benign and malignant liver lesions. Cancer 111:316–322.
17. Roncalli M, Borzio M, Di Tommaso L (2007) Hepatocellular dysplastic nodules. Hepatol Res 37:S125–134.
18. Tot T (2002) Cytokeratins 20 and 7 as biomarkers: usefulness in discriminating primary from metastatic adenocarcinoma. Eur J Cancer 38:758–763.
19. Lei JY, Bourne PA, diSant'Agnese PA, Huang J (2006) Cytoplasmic staining of TTF-1 in the differential diagnosis of hepatocellular carcinoma vs cholangiocarcinoma and metastatic carcinoma of the liver. Am J Clin Pathol 125:519–525.
20. Wieczorek TJ, Pinkus JL, Glickman JN, Pinkus GS (2002) Comparison of thyroid transcription factor-1 and hepatocyte antigen immunohistochemical analysis in the differential diagnosis of hepatocellular carcinoma, metastatic adenocarcinoma, renal cell carcinoma, and adrenal cortical carcinoma. Am J Clin Pathol 118:911–921.
21. Durnez A, Verslype C, Nevens F et al (2006) The clinicopathological and prognostic relevance of cytokeratin 7 and 19 expression in hepatocellular carcinoma. A possible progenitor cell origin. Histopathology 49:138–151.
22. Piscaglia F, Bolondi L (2007) Recent advances in the diagnosis of hepatocellular carcinoma. Hepatol Res 37:S178–192.
23. Okuda H, Obata H (1982) Hepatocellular carcinoma arising in noncirrhotic and highly cirrhotic livers: a comparative study of histopathology and frequency of hepatitis B markers. Cancer 49:450–455.
24. Tanaka H, Tsukuma H, Teshima H et al (1997) Second primary cancers following non-Hodgkin's lymphoma in Japan: increased risk of hepatocellular carcinoma. Jpn J Cancer Res 88:537–542.
25. Bruno G, Andreozzi P, Graf U, Santangelo G (1999) Hepatitis C virus: a high risk factor for a second primary malignancy besides hepatocellular carcinoma. Fact or fiction? Clin Ter 150:413–418.
26. Kloppel G, Klimstra DS (2007) Tumors of the exocrine pancreas. In: Fletcher CDM (ed) Diagnostic Histopathology of Tumors. Churchill Livingstone Elsevier, pp 463–484.
27. Brits CJ, Franz RC (1976) Pale nodular nuclei-diagnostic of adenocarcinoma of the pancreas? Acta Cytol 20:462–468.
28. Mitchell ML, Bittner CA, Wills JS, Parker FP (1988) Fine needle aspiration cytology of the pancreas. A retrospective study of 73 cases. Acta Cytol 32:447–451.
29. Robins DB, Katz RL, Evans DB et al (1995) Fine needle aspiration of the pancreas. In quest of accuracy. Acta Cytol 39:1–10.
30. Paksoy N, Lilleng R, Hagmar B, Wetteland J (1993) Diagnostic accuracy of fine needle aspiration cytology in pancreatic lesions. A review of 77 cases. Acta Cytol 37:889–893.
31. Ylagan LR, Edmundowicz S, Kasal K et al (2002) Endoscopic ultrasound guided fine-needle aspiration cytology of pancreatic carcinoma: a 3-year experience and review of the literature. Cancer 96:362–369.
32. Fisher L, Segarajasingam DS, Stewart C et al (2009) Endoscopic ultrasound guided fine needle aspiration of solid pancreatic lesions: Performance and outcomes. J Gastroenterol Hepatol 24:90–96
33. Lin F, Staerkel G (2003) Cytologic criteria for well differentiated adenocarcinoma of the pancreas in fine-needle aspiration biopsy specimens. Cancer 99:44–50.
34. Yun SS, Remotti H, Vazquez MF et al (2007) Endoscopic ultrasound-guided biopsies of pancreatic masses: comparison between fine needle aspirations and needle core biopsies. Diagn Cytopathol 35:276–282.
35. Seth AK, Argani P, Campbell KA (2008) Acinar cell carcinoma of the pancreas: an institutional series of resected patients and review of the current literature. J Gastrointest Surg 12:1061–1067.
36. Stelow EB, Bardales RH, Shami VM et al (2006) Cytology of pancreatic acinar cell carcinoma. Diagn Cytopathol 34:367–372.
37. Labate AM, Klimstra DL, Zakowski MF (1997) Comparative cytologic features of pancreatic acinar cell carcinoma and islet cell tumor. Diagn Cytopathol 16:112–116.
38. Salla C, Chatzipantelis P, Konstantinou P et al (2007) Endoscopic ultrasound-guided fine-needle aspiration cytology in the diagnosis of intraductal papillary mucinous neoplasms of the pancreas. A study of 8 cases. JOP 8:715–724.
39. Garcea G, Ong SL, Rajesh A et al (2008) Cystic lesions of the pancreas. A diagnostic and management dilemma. Pancreatology 8:236–251.
40. Belsley NA, Pitman MB, Lauwers GY et al (2008) Serous cystadenoma of the pancreas: limitations and pitfalls of endoscopic ultrasound-guided fine-needle aspiration biopsy. Cancer 114:102–110.
41. Yasuhara Y, Sakaida N, Uemura Y et al (2002) Serous microcystic adenoma (glycogen-rich cystadenoma) of the pancreas: study of 11 cases showing clinicopathological and immunohistochemical correlations. Pathol Int 52:307–312.
42. Gherardi G (2005) Retroperitoneal tumor mass in 63-years old man. http://pat.uninet.edu/zope/pat/casos/C158/index.html
43. Chen F, Frankel WL, Wen P (2004). Pathologic quiz case: a multicystic mass of the pancreatic body in a 70-year-old man. Serous microcystic adenoma of the pancreas. Arch Pathol Lab Med 128:83–85
44. Eble JN, Bonsib SM (1998) Extensively cystic renal neoplasms: cystic nephroma, cystic partially differentiated nephroblastoma, multilocular cystic renal cell carcinoma, and cystic hamartoma of renal pelvis. Semin Diagn Pathol 15:2–20.
45. Kloppel G, Heitz PU (2007) Tumors of the endocrine pancreas. In: Fletcher CDM (ed) Diagnostic Histopathology of Tumors. Churchill Livingstone Elsevier, pp 1123–1138
46. Chang F, Chandra A, Culora G et al (2006) Cytologic diagnosis of pancreatic endocrine tumors by endoscopic ultra-

sound-guided fine-needle aspiration: a review. Diagn Cytopathol 34:649–58.
47. Stelow EB, Bardales RH, Stanley MW (2005) Pitfalls in endoscopic ultrasound-guided fine-needle aspiration and how to avoid them. Adv Anat Pathol 12:62–73.
48. Schmitt AM, Anlauf M, Rousson V et al (2007) WHO 2004 criteria and CK19 are reliable prognostic markers in pancreatic endocrine tumors. Am J Surg Pathol 31:1677–1682.
49. Eble JN, Young RH (2007) Tumors of the urinary tract. In: Fletcher CDM (ed) Diagnostic Histopathology of Tumors. Churchill Livingstone Elsevier, pp 1123–1138.
50. Masoom S, Venkataraman G, Jensen J et al (2009) Renal FNA-based typing of renal masses remains a useful adjunctive modality: evaluation of 31 renal masses with correlative histology. Cytopathology 20:50–55.
51. Kim MK, Kim S (2002) Immunohistochemical profile of common epithelial neoplasms arising in the kidney. Appl Immunohistochem Mol Morphol 10:332–338.
52. Salamanca J, Alberti N, López-Ríos F et al (2007) Fine needle aspiration of chromophobe renal cell carcinoma. Acta Cytol 51:9–15.
53. Memeo L, Jhang J, Assaad AM et al (2007) Immunohistochemical analysis for cytokeratin 7, KIT, and PAX2: value in the differential diagnosis of chromophobe cell carcinoma. Am J Clin Pathol 127:225–229.
54. Mai KT, Teo I, Belanger EC, Robertson SJ et al (2008) Progesterone receptor reactivity in renal oncocytoma and chromophobe renal cell carcinoma. Histopathology 52:277–282.
55. Stone CH, Lee MW, Amin MB et al (2001) Renal angiomyolipoma: further immunophenotypic characterization of an expanding morphologic spectrum. Arch Pathol Lab Med 125:751–758.
56. Crapanzano JP (2005) Fine-needle aspiration of renal angiomyolipoma: cytological findings and diagnostic pitfalls in a series of five cases. Diagn Cytopathol 32:53–57.
57. Wadih GE, Raab SS, Silverman JF (1995) Fine needle aspiration cytology of renal and retroperitoneal angiomyolipoma. Report of two cases with cytologic findings and clinicopathologic pitfalls in diagnosis. Acta Cytol 39:945–950.
58. Allory Y, Bazille C, Vieillefond A et al (2008) Profiling and classification tree applied to renal epithelial tumours. Histopathology 52:158–166.
59. Dehner LP (2004) Primitive neuroectodermal tumour (Ewing sarcoma). In: Eble et al (eds) Tumours of the urinary System and Male Genital Organ. WHO Classification of Tumours. IARC Press, Lyon, pp 83–84.
60. Gherardi G (2005) Fine–needle aspiration cytology of a tumor in the left kidney http://pat.uninet.edu/zope/pat/casos/C210/index.html
61. Lack LE (2007) Tumors of the Adrenal Gland. In: Fletcher CDM (ed) Diagnostic Histopathology of Tumors. Churchill Livingstone Elsevier, pp 1099–1122.
62. Dusenbery D, Dekker A (1996) Needle biopsy of the adrenal gland: retrospective review of 54 cases. Diagn Cytopathol 14:126–134.
63. Stelow EB, Debol SM, Stanley MW (2005) Sampling of the adrenal glands by endoscopic ultrasound-guided fine-needle aspiration. Diagn Cytopathol 33:26–30.
64. Wu HH, Cramer HM, Kho J, Elsheikh TM (1998) Fine needle aspiration cytology of benign adrenal cortical nodules. A comparison of cytologic findings with those of primary and metastatic adrenal malignancies. Acta Cytol 42:1352–1358.
65. Chen KT (2005) Extraneous cells of hepatic origin in adrenal fine needle aspiration as a diagnostic pitfall: a case report. Acta Cytol 49:449–451.
66. Sharma S, Singh R, Verma K (1997) Cytomorphology of adrenocortical carcinoma and comparison with renal cell carcinoma. Acta Cytol 41:385–392.
67. Saboorian MH, Katz RL, Charnsangavej C (1995) Fine needle aspiration cytology of primary and metastatic lesions of the adrenal gland. A series of 188 biopsies with radiologic correlation. Acta Cytol 39:843–51.
68. Jiménez-Heffernan JA, Vicandi B, López-Ferrer P et al (2006) Cytologic features of pheochromocytoma and retroperitoneal paraganglioma: a morphologic and immunohistochemical study of 13 cases. Acta Cytol 50:372–378.
69. Mai KT, Landry DC, Robertson SJ et al (2001) A comparative study of metastatic renal cell carcinoma with correlation to subtype and primary tumor. Pathol Res Pract 197:671–675.
70. Yang B, Ali SZ, Rosenthal DL (2002) CD10 facilitates the diagnosis of metastatic renal cell carcinoma from primary adrenal cortical neoplasm in adrenal fine-needle aspiration. Diagn Cytopathol 27:149–152.
71. Zhang PJ, Genega EM, Tomaszewski JE et al (2003) The role of calretinin, inhibin, melan-A, bcl-2, and c-kit in differentiating adrenal cortical and medullary tumors: an immunohistochemical study. Mod Pathol 16:591–597.
72. Ganjei P, Dickinson B, Harrison T et al (1996) Aspiration cytology of neoplastic and non–neoplastic ovarian cysts: is it accurate? Int J Gynecol Pathol 15:94–101.
73. Papathanasiou K, Giannoulis C, Dovas D et al (2004) Fine needle aspiration cytology of the ovary: is it reliable? Clin Exp Obstet Gynecol 31:191–193.
74. Wojcik EM, Selvaggi SM (1994) Fine-needle aspiration cytology of cystic ovarian lesions. Diagn Cytopathol 11:9–14.
75. Ganjei P (1995) Fine-needle aspiration cytology of the ovary. Clin Lab Med 15:705–726.
76. Martínez-Onsurbe P, Ruiz Villaespesa A, Sanz Anquela JM et al (2001) Aspiration cytology of 147 adnexal cysts with histologic correlation. Acta Cytol 45:941–947.
77. Clement PB, Young RH (2008) Surface epithelial-stromal tumors: general features, serous tumors, and mucinous tumors. In: Atlas of Gynecologic surgical pathology, Elsevier, Philadelphia, pp 322–332.
78. Clement PB, Young RH (2008) Surface epithelial-stromal tumors: endometrioid, clear cell transitional, squamous, rare, undifferentiated, and mixed cell types. In: Atlas of Gynecologic Surgical Pathology, Elsevier, Philadelphia, pp 333–357.
79. Jiménez-Heffernan JA, Vicandi B, González-Peramato P et al (2004) Cytologic features of clear cell carcinoma of the female genital tract. Diagnostic value of the "raspberry body" in nonexfoliative cytologic specimens. Acta Cytol 48:47–51.
80. Khunamornpong S, Thorner PS, Suprasert P, Siriaunkgul S (2005) Clear-cell adenocarcinoma of the female genital tract: presence of hyaline stroma and tigroid background in

various types of cytologic specimens. Diagn Cytopathol 32:336–340.
81. Mourad WA, Sneige N, Katz RL et al (1994) Fine-needle aspiration cytology of recurrent and metastatic mixed mesodermal tumors. Diagn Cytopathol 11:328–332.
82. Silva RG, Dahmoush L, Gerke H (2006) Pancreatic metastasis of an ovarian malignant mixed Mullerian tumor identified by EUS-guided fine needle aspiration and Trucut needle biopsy. JOP 7:66–69.
83. Liao XY, Xue WC, Shen DH et al (2007) p63 expression in ovarian tumours: a marker for Brenner tumours but not transitional cell carcinomas. Histopathology 51:477–483.
84. Clement PB, Young RH (2008) Sex cord-stromal and steroid tumors. In: Atlas of Gynecologic Surgical Pathology, Elsevier, Philadelphia, pp 386–412.
85. Ozkara SK, Turan G (2008) Cystic fluid and fine needle aspiration cytopathology of cystic adult granulosa cell tumor of the ovary: a case report. Acta Cytol 52:247–250.
86. Ali S, Gattuso P, Howard A et al (2008) Adult granulosa cell tumor of the ovary: fine-needle-aspiration cytology of 10 cases and review of literature. Diagn Cytopathol 36:297–302.
87. Ylagan LR, Middleton WD, Dehner LP (2002) Fine-needle aspiration cytology of recurrent granulosa cell tumor: case report with differential diagnosis and immunocytochemistry. Diagn Cytopathol 27:38–41.
88. Shimizu K, Yamada T, Ueda Y et al (1999) Cytologic features of ovarian granulosa cell tumor metastatic to the lung. A case report. Acta Cytol 43:1137–1141.
89. McCluggage WG, Young RH (2005). Immunohistochemistry as a diagnostic aid in the evaluation of ovarian tumors. Semin Diagn Pathol 22:3–32.
90. Hackethal A, Brueggmann D, Bohlmann MK et al (2008) Squamous-cell carcinoma in mature cystic teratoma of the ovary: systematic review and analysis of published data. Lancet Oncol 9:1173–1180.
91. Clement PB, Young RH (2008) Metastatic tumors to the ovary (including pseudomyxoma peritonei, hematolymphoid neoplasms, and tumors with functioning stroma). In: Atlas of Gynecologic Surgical Pathology, Elsevier, Philadelphia, pp 425–452.
92. Fenoglio-Preiser CM, Noffsinger AE, Stemmermann GN et al (2008) Mesenchymal Tumors. In: Gastrointestinal Pathology, an Atlas and Text. Wolters Kluwer Lippincott Williams & Wilkins, Chicago, pp 1203–1219.
93. Chatzipantelis P, Salla C, Karoumpalis I et al (2008) Endoscopic ultrasound-guided fine needle aspiration biopsy in the diagnosis of gastrointestinal stromal tumors of the stomach. A study of 17 cases. J Gastrointestin Liver Dis 17:15–20.
94. Akahoshi K, Sumida Y, Matsui N et al (2007) Preoperative diagnosis of gastrointestinal stromal tumor by endoscopic ultrasound-guided fine needle aspiration. World J Gastroenterol 13:2077–2082.
95. Schmitt FC, Gomes AL, Milanezi F et al (2007) Mutations in gastrointestinal stromal tumors diagnosed by endoscopic ultrasound-guided fine needle aspiration. Minerva Med 98:385–388.
96. Stelow EB, Murad FM, Debol SM et al (2008) A limited immunocytochemical panel for the distinction of subepithelial gastrointestinal mesenchymal neoplasms sampled by endoscopic ultrasound-guided fine-needle aspiration. Am J Clin Pathol 129:219–225.
97. Meara RS, Cangiarella J, Simsir A et al (2007) Prediction of aggressiveness of gastrointestinal stromal tumours based on immunostaining with bcl-2, Ki-67 and p53. Cytopathology 18:283–289.
98. Rodriguez JA, Guarda LA, Rosai J (2004) Mesenteric fibromatosis with involvement of the gastrointestinal tract. A GIST simulator: a study of 25 cases. Am J Clin Pathol 121:93–98.
99. Yantiss RK, Spiro IJ, Compton CC, Rosenberg AE (2000) Gastrointestinal stromal tumor versus intra-abdominal fibromatosis of the bowel wall: a clinically important differential diagnosis. Am J Surg Pathol 24:947–957.
100. Clement PB, Young RH (2008) Tumor-like lesions and tumors of the peritoneum (excluding mullerian lesions). In: Atlas of Gynecologic Surgical Pathology. Elsevier, Philadelphia, pp 474–490.
101. Devaney K, Kragel PJ, Devaney EJ (1992) Fine-needle aspiration cytology of multicystic mesothelioma. Diagn Cytopathol 8:68–72.
102. Lae ME, Roche PC, Jin L et al (2002) Desmoplastic small round cell tumor: a clinicopathologic, immunohistochemical, and molecular study of 32 tumors. Am J Surg Pathol 26:823–835.
103. Granja NM, Begnami MD, Bortolan J (2005). Desmoplastic small round cell tumour: Cytological and immunocytochemical features. Cytojournal 2:6.
104. Ferlicot S, Coué O, Gilbert E et al (2001) Intraabdominal desmoplastic small round cell tumor: report of a case with fine needle aspiration, cytologic diagnosis and molecular confirmation. Acta Cytol 45:617–621.
105. Schneider V, Smyczek B (1990) Sister Mary Joseph's nodule. Diagnosis of umbilical metastases by fine needle aspiration. Acta Cytol 34:555–558.
106. Scudeler D, Wakely PE Jr (2006) Fine needle aspiration biopsy of gastrointestinal stromal tumor presenting as an umbilical mass (Sister Mary Joseph's Nodule). Ann Diagn Pathol 10:100–103.
107. Gupta RK, Lallu S, McHutchison AG, Prasad J (1991) Fine needle aspiration of Sister Mary Joseph's nodule. Cytopathology 2:311–314.
108. Kapila K, Ghosal N, Gill SS, Verma K (2003) Cytomorphology of lipomatous tumors of soft tissue. Acta Cytol 47:555–562.
109. Fleshman R, Mayerson J, Wakely PE Jr (2007) Fine-needle aspiration biopsy of high-grade sarcoma: a report of 107 cases. Cancer 111:491–498.
110. Domanski HA, Akerman M, Rissler P, Gustafson P (2006) Fine-needle aspiration of soft tissue leiomyosarcoma: an analysis of the most common cytologic findings and the value of ancillary techniques. Diagn Cytopathol 34:597–604.
111. Li S, Ai SZ, Owens C, Kulesza P (2009) Intrapancreatic schwannoma diagnosed by endoscopic ultrasound-guided fine-needle aspiration cytology. Diagn Cytopathol 37:132–135.
112. Dodd LG, Marom EM, Dash RC et al (1999) Fine-needle aspiration cytology of "ancient" schwannoma. Diagn Cytopathol 20:307–11.
113. Furlong MA, Mentzel T, Fanburg-Smith JC (2001) Pleomorphic rhabdomyosarcoma in adults: a clinicopathologic

study of 38 cases with emphasis on morphologic variants and recent skeletal muscle-specific markers. Mod Pathol 14:595–603.
114. Rosai J (2004) Peritoneum, retroperitoneum, and related structures. In: Rosai and Ackerman's Surgical Pathology, Chapter 26. Mosby, Edinburgh, New York, pp 2399–2400.
115. Fabre E, Jira H, Izard V et al (2004) 'Burned-out' primary testicular cancer. BJU Int 94:74–78.
116. Chao TY, Nieh S, Huang SH, Lee WH (1997) Cytology of fine needle aspirates of primary extragonadal germ cell tumors. Acta Cytol 41:497–503.
117. Collins KA, Geisinger KR, Wakely PE Jr (1995) Extragonadal germ cell tumors: a fine-needle aspiration biopsy study. Diagn Cytopathol 12:223–239.
118. Gupta R, Mathur SR, Arora VK, Sharma SG (2008) Cytologic features of extragonadal germ cell tumors: a study of 88 cases with aspiration cytology. Cancer 114:504–511.

Lung, Mediastinum, and Pleura

7

7.1 Introduction

Fine-needle biopsy (FNB) of thoracic lesions became commonplace in the USA in the 1980s due to the economic restraints imposed by the escalating financial burden of health care. The procedure was widely adopted due to its ability to yield expedient, minimally invasive, cost-conservative and tissue-specific diagnostic information, comparable to that obtained by histopathological evaluation, and to rationally and reliably direct the most appropriate form of patient management [1–31].

The main pulmonary targets for percutaneous FNB are lesions at any depth, most mediastinal masses, pleural-based solid nodular lesions, and any soft-tissue or bone lesion of the chest wall. In experienced hands, the procedure allows for a reliable identification of the cellular composition of primary pulmonary malignancies in a tissue-equivalent manner [1–4,7,11,12,15,16,18,23,24,27,29]. Preoperative knowledge of cell type and the extent of disease may assist the surgeon in planning the most appropriate intervention. If the patient is considered inoperable, the cellular sample collected by FNB is potentially sufficient to provide further identification of additional biological factors that may predict the therapeutic response. The chance of identifying the malignant cells as metastatic in nature is an additional advantage of pulmonary FNB, and the use of ancillary techniques may provide a reliable basis for identifying the tumor's primary site. Finally, an adequate FNB cellular sample can unexpectedly disclose the benign nature of the lesion, allowing the clinician to follow the patient conservatively.

The rationale for using FNB is to differentiate benign from malignant disease reliably and with minimal invasion, since the procedure can be performed on an outpatient basis. This advantage revolutionized the previous conventional diagnostic approach of radiologically detected pulmonary masses, which included exfoliative cytology combined with bronchoscopic investigation. This older approach was of very low sensitivity, ranging between 0.49 and 0.58 depending on the site of the lesion and its size [32]. FNB dramatically increased the accuracy of preoperative diagnosis, as its sensitivity ranges between 0.62 and 0.99, with an average of about 0.90, and its specificity values are very close to 100% [32]. The factors influencing diagnostic accuracy are the needle caliber, the site and the size of the lesion, and the number of passes [7,8,16,19,23–26,32]. Proper diagnostic triage can vary according to many factors, but the patient's compliance is crucial. In general, exophytic tumors located in the main bronchi and their major ramifications are best investigated by bronchoscopy while lesions located more peripherally in the bronchial tree represent the most appropriate targets for transthoracic FNB [33]. A computed tomography (CT) scan of the chest provides radio-graphic image enhancement to facilitate guidance of the needle to the target. As an alternative, ultrasound (US) guidance can assist FNB sampling of lung lesions that are adherent to the parietal pleura and chest wall [2,7].

7.1.1 Indications for FNB

The main indications for FNB sampling are the diagnostic evaluation of the following [33]:

- A solitary nodular lesion of the pulmonary parenchyma, pleura, or mediastinum that was recently detected, has grown rapidly, and raises suspicion of a primary malignancy.

- A solitary lesion or multiple solid nodular lesions that appeared in the above-mentioned sites in a patient who was previously treated for a pulmonary primary malignancy or another primary tumor in other anatomic districts and which is/are likely to represent disease relapse, without excluding, however, a new primary tumor or a pseudotumor.
- Centrally located perihilar tumor masses that raise suspicion of a primary malignancy for which alternative diagnostic procedures failed to provide a conclusive diagnosis.

Another indication for FNB sampling that is becoming increasingly important is the recruitment of a representative cellular sample in patients with inoperable non-small-cell bronchogenic carcinoma, to predict a possible response to targeted cancer therapies by molecular testing (EGFR and k-ras mutational analyses). This is performed using cutting needles.

Identification of the lesion's cellular composition will dictate assignment of the patient to thoracotomy, radiation, chemotherapy, surveillance, or continued diagnostic intervention. A general consensus is lacking on the use of FNB in the diagnostic evaluation of tumor masses of relatively small size, because in this context the patient would in any case be a candidate for lobectomy, which is performed for both diagnostic and therapeutic reasons [34]. This type of surgery, however, bears an estimated mortality risk of 2–3% and significant morbidity due to possible cardiovascular and respiratory complications. Thus, there is no reason why FNB should not be used in this context as a primary diagnostic modality, provided that the clinician is well aware of its possible low predictive value for some lesions [35]. In fact, the procedure may help in reliably identifying inflammatory conditions, pseudotumors, or even malignant lymphoma, thus warding off the risks intrinsic to the surgical procedure, which may not be justified.

7.1.2 Contraindications and Complications

The contraindications to performing aspiration biopsy of the thorax refer primarily to the lung [36]. At the top of the list are hemorrhagic diathesis, anticoagulant therapy, and pulmonary hypertension, which predispose the patient to intraparenchymal hemorrhage or hemoptysis following insertion and re-adjustment of the needle. Uncontrolled cough may deflect the needle from the target, thereby inflicting trauma to the pulmonary parenchyma. Arteriovenous malformations may threaten blood extravasation from the puncture wound, while advanced emphysema complicated by bullae may inflict pneumothorax.

7.1.3 Diagnostic Accuracy

The accuracy of transthoracic aspiration biopsy varies with the expertise of the radiologist in puncturing the lesion and acquiring a reliable sample, and with the competence and experience of the pathologist in the cytomorphological interpretation of the sample. The reader is referred to the exhaustive study published by Schreiber et al., 2003, on the subject [32]. Table 7.1 provides a summary of the reported data.

7.1.4 Technical Considerations

The patient is selected as a candidate for the procedure based on his/her clinical history, the size and location of the lesion, and exclusion of the above-discussed contraindications. The procedure is scheduled with the cytopathologist. The patient is positioned horizontally; the skin is prepared with betadine cleansing and anesthetized with 1% xylocaine, which is often directed into deeper tissues. The radiologist carefully selects the trajectory of the approach. The patient is continuously asked to cooperate. The needle traverses its selected trajectory to a predetermined depth under image-intensified guidance and is re-adjusted until there is unison of motion between the needle tip and the lesion during respiratory excursions. When the needle tip satisfactory resides within its destination, the stylet is removed and the syringe is attached. The plunger is withdrawn to create a vacuum and the needle is oscillated gently. The evacuation process is terminated the moment material enters the hub. The vacuum is allowed to re-equilibrate before the needle is removed. Following removal of the needle and the syringe, the needle is disconnected from the syringe to re-introduce air into the syringe. The harvest is then deposited onto the slide and a smear prepared. Immediate and 2-h post-biopsy chest films are taken to detect possible complications.

Table 7.1 Sensitivity and Specificity of Transthoracic Needle Aspiration and/or Biopsy for Diagnosis of Peripheral Bronchogenic Carcinoma adapted from Schreiber et al., 2003 [32], and including only studies with more than 100 cases reported

Reference no.	Patients, No.	Type of Needle	Sensitivity	Specificity
1	440	A	0.97	0.97
2	120	A	0.62	1.00
3	147	B	0.89	1.00
4	130	A	0.92	0.93
5	367	A	0.97	0.96
6	197	A	0.87	1.00
7	128	A	0.95	0.95
8	219	A, B, C	0.89	1.00
9	176	A	0.84	1.00
10	129	B, C	0.94	1.00
11	390	A, B	0.94	0.99
12	100	A	0.84	1.00
13	103	A	0.69	1.00
14	589	A, C	0.93	0.99
15	371	A, C	0.99	0.94
16	227	B	0.82	1.00
17	129	A, C	0.95	1.00
18	114	A	0.94	1.00
19	400	B	0.98	0.94
20	220	A	0.93	0.99
21	119	A	0.93	1.00
22	284	C	0.78	1.00
23	133	C	0.78	1.00
24	612	C	0.96	0.99
25	165	A	0.77	1.00
26	202	C	0.94	1.00
27	120	B	0.98	0.94
28	185	C	0.93	1.00
29	150	B	0.97	1.00
30	200	A, B	0.95	0.98

A = aspiration needle; *B* = aspiration biopsy needle; *C* = cutting biopsy needle

7.2 Lung

7.2.1 Classification and Clinical Presentation of Pulmonary Epithelial Malignancies

Among the myriad of diverse primary epithelial malignancies, the only clinically significant distinction is small-cell vs. non-small-cell carcinoma [37]. The former accounts for 15–20% of cases, and the latter for the remaining 70–80%. The distinction is based purely on therapeutic criteria because of the favorable chemotherapeutic implications for small-cell carcinoma and the reprieve from surgery. Conversely, non-small-cell malignancies are potentially resectable and treated by subsequent chemotherapy and radiotherapy. Moreover, patients with inoperable non-small-cell carcinomas may be candidates for new and promising "targeted therapy" regimens while those with small-cell carcinoma are not.

The main categories of lung carcinoma are listed in the WHO classification scheme, 2004 (Table 7.2) [37]. In the early stages of tumor development, all types of carcinoma may appear as a solitary mass that is centrally or peripherally located and variably demarcated from the surrounding parenchyma. Centrally located tumors originate from major bronchi and are typically responsible for partial or complete bronchial obstruction, which is the cause of obstructive symptoms, bronchopneumonia, and/or atelectasis rather early in the course of the disease. Peripherally located tumors are characterized by few or negligible obstructive phenomena and are generally asymptomatic in their early stages. With further evolution of the disease, new tumor lesions appear within the same

Table 7.2 WHO histological classification of tumors of the lung: malignant epithelial tumors [37]

- Squamous cell carcinoma
  - Papillary
  - Clear cell
  - Small-cell
  - Basaloid
- Small-cell carcinoma
  - Combined small-cell carcinoma
- Adenocarcinoma
  - Adenocarcinoma, mixed subtype
  - Acinar adenocarcinoma
  - Papillary adenocarcinoma
  - Bronchioloalveolar carcinoma
    - Non-mucinous
    - Mucinous
    - Mixed or indeterminate
  - Solid adenocarcinoma with mucin production
    - Fetal adenocarcinoma
    - Mucinous ("colloid") carcinoma
    - Mucinous cystoadenocarcinoma
    - Signet-ring adenocarcinoma
    - Clear cell adenocarcinoma
- Large-cell carcinoma
  - Large-cell neuroendocrine carcinoma
    - Combined large-cell neuroendocrine carcinoma
  - Basaloid carcinoma
  - Lymphoepithelioma-like carcinoma
  - Clear cell carcinoma
  - Large-cell carcinoma with rhabdoid features
- Adenosquamous carcinoma
- Sarcomatoid carcinoma
  - Pleomorphic carcinoma
  - Spindle cell carcinoma
  - Giant cell carcinoma
  - Carcinosarcoma
  - Pulmonary blastoma
- Carcinoid tumor
  - Typical carcinoid
  - Atypical carcinoid
- Salivary gland tumors
  - Mucoepidermoid carcinoma
  - Adenoid cystic carcinoma
  - Epithelial-myoepithelial carcinoma
- Preinvasive lesions
  - Squamous cell carcinoma in situ
  - Atypical adenomatous hyperplasia
  - Diffuse idiopathic pulmonary neuroendocrine hyperplasia

pulmonary lobe, in different lobes of the same lung, or in the contralateral lung. This parallels the development of lymph node involvement within the mediastinum and, finally, in distant organs, including the liver, the adrenals, and the brain.

Generally, the detection of a solitary nodule in the lung suggests a primary tumor while multiple nodular lesions are indicative of a metastatic malignancy, but there are several exceptions to this rule [38]. In fact, the early development of a lung primary may be characterized by the appearance of multiple nodular lesions; conversely, metastatic involvement of the lung from extrapulmonary malignancies may present as a solitary and slowly expanding tumor mass. Consequently, one should by no means rule out a priori the chance of metastasis following the detection of a solitary lesion or, vice versa, of a lung primary if the tumor consists of multiple nodules. In a minor proportion of cases, lung primary tumors may have an unusual appearance that can bewilder the clinical investigation and delay the diagnosis. Peripherally located tumors can involve the pleura very early in the course of the disease and grow along the serosal surface, closely simulating a mesothelioma (so-called mesothelioid adenocarcinoma) [39]. In the early stages of disease, tumors originating in the apex of the upper lobes may invade the pleura as well as the nerve and vascular structures of the base of the neck, causing symptoms that are apparently unrelated to a lung primary (Pancoast tumor and Horner's syndrome). Finally, early-stage adenocarcinoma of the lung may elicit an intense desmoplastic reaction thus simulating an intraparenchymal scar [37].

7.2.2 Adenocarcinoma

Bronchogenic adenocarcinoma can occur in a wide range of age groups and is preferentially located at the periphery of the lung. Histologically, this tumor generally corresponds to an otherwise typical adenocarcinoma composed of tubular and papillary structures of variable shape and size that are lined by cylindrical cells with intracellular mucin production [37,40]. A variably intense desmoplastic reaction is always present. In well-differentiated tumors, the cells are columnar to cuboidal in appearance, with a basal nucleus and a basophilic to clear cytoplasm possibly containing mucin droplets. In poorly differentiated tumors, the glandular pattern of growth is less evident and the tumors mainly consist of solid cords and trabeculae. Moreover, the cells have a reduced amount of cytoplasm and more pleomorphic nuclei.

The cytological picture on FNB is prototypical of

tumors having a glandular cell morphology, and there is a tendency to assume a tubulo-acinar (Fig. 7.1a–c), tubulo-papillary, mucinous, or solid structureless pattern. It is important to stress that the cytomorphology of a primary adenocarcinoma in the lung may overlap with the cytological appearance of a metastatic deposit of adenocarcinoma from various primary sites, including the breast, stomach, pancreas and biliary tract, small intestine, ovary, fallopian tube, and endocervix. The distinction between primary and metastatic malignancy generally requires proper clinical correlation and immunohistochemical studies (Fig. 7.1d,e).

Some variants of primary adenocarcinoma merit particular attention as they show distinct cytological

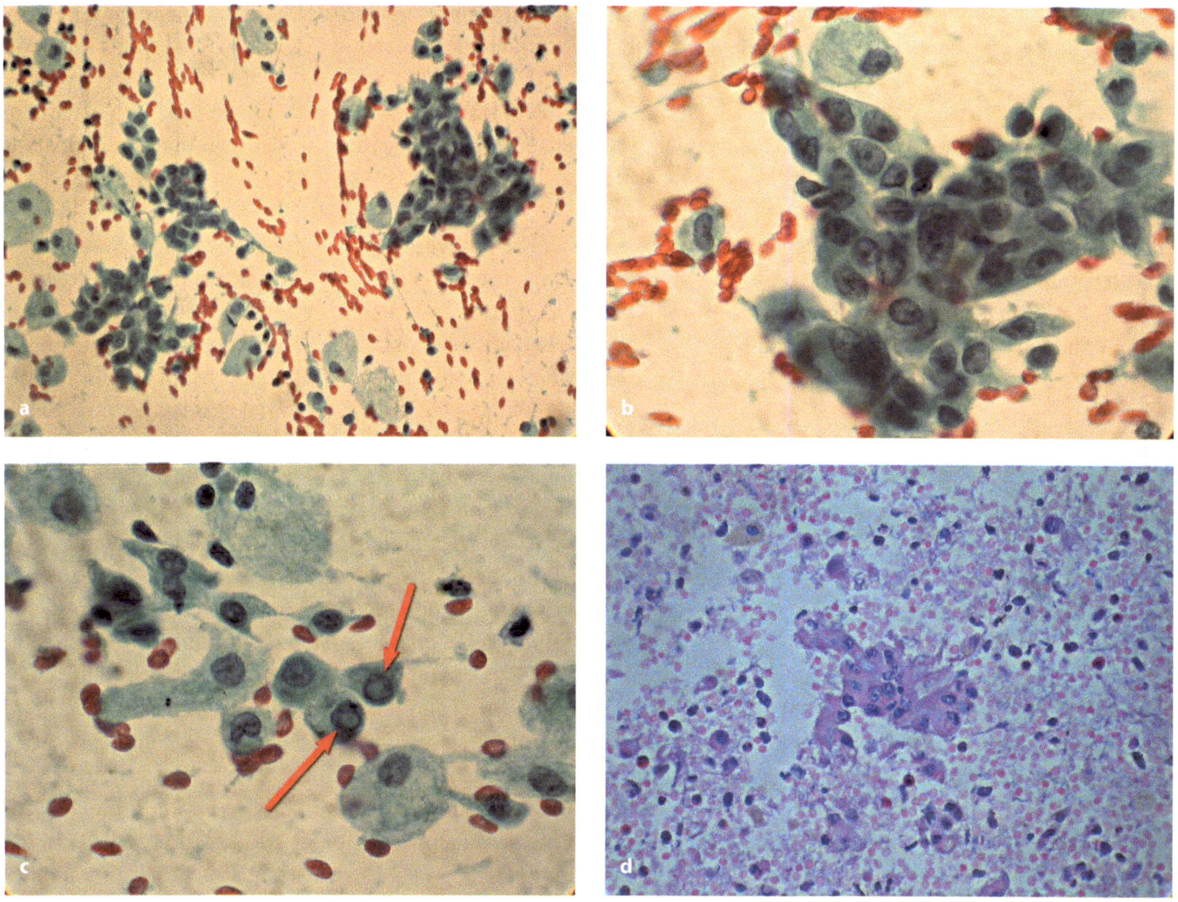

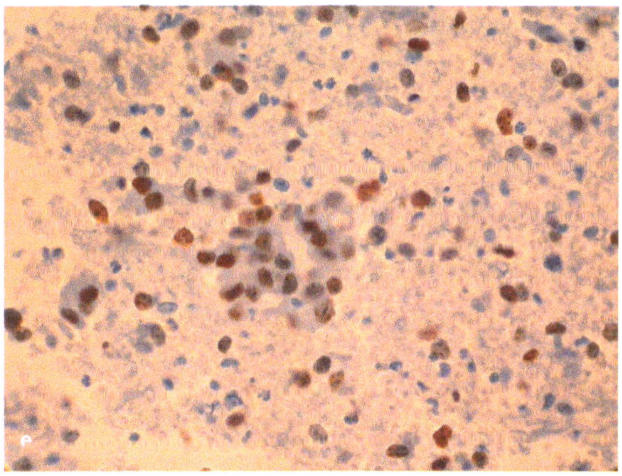

Fig. 7.1 a Tubulo-acinar aggregates of epithelial glandular cells are admixed with mononuclear histiocytes, which display a clear or microvacuolated cytoplasm. Smear, Papanicolaou (P) stain, ×400. **b** Glandular cells in acinar aggregates have round to oval nuclei with distinct nucleoli and a moderate amount of cytoplasm. Smear, P stain, ×400. **c** Occasionally, neoplastic epithelial cells are characterized by round intranuclear cytoplasmic inclusions (*arrows*); their cytoplasm is dense or microvacuolated, in contrast to the microvacuolated and clear cytoplasm of histiocytes. Smear, P stain, ×1000. **d** An acinar cellular aggregate is dispersed with necrotic debris. Paraffin section from a cell-block sample, hematoxylin & eosin (H&E) stain, ×400. **c** Tumor cells in aggregates and within the necrotic background show nuclear positivity for TTF1. Same sample as in **d**, counterstained with hematoxylin, ×400

features whose recognition is important in order to anticipate proper decision-making regarding treatment. These are discussed below.

7.2.2.1 Bronchioloalveolar Carcinoma

Clinicopathological Correlates

Bronchioloalveolar carcinoma represents a somewhat heterogeneous group of adenocarcinoma variants characterized by a high degree of cellular differentiation, the peculiar tendency to aerogenous spread, and evidence of advancement along the alveolar wall without destruction or effacement of the parenchymal architecture. There is a clear-cut female prevalence of the tumor, which is frequently asymptomatic at presentation. Radiologically, it can present as a single mass or as multiple lesions and may be unilateral or bilateral [37].

Cytomorphology

Mucinous Bronchioloalveolar Carcinoma

- Mucoid background (Fig. 7.2a) with histiocytes, possible inflammatory cells.
- Abundant cellularity.
- Cells almost equally distributed in aggregates (Fig. 7.2b) and as isolated elements (Fig. 7.2c).
- Cellular aggregates almost exclusively of two-dimensional type with a tendency to partial cellular non-cohesion at the periphery (Fig. 7.2b).
- Medium-sized and monomorphous cells with an abundant homogeneous or microvacuolated cytoplasm and a round to oval nucleus ("histiocytoid" appearance) (Fig. 7.2b–d).
- Nuclear size >2×RBC, with finely granular chromatin (Fig. 7.2d).
- Occasional intranuclear cytoplasmic inclusions (the cytoplasmic matrix within the inclusion often being eosinophilic) (Fig. 7.2e).

Non-mucinous Bronchioloalveolar Carcinoma

- Background rich in blood, with frequently detected pigment macrophages.
- Moderate to abundant cellularity.
- Cellular aggregation prevalent, with a tendency to three-dimensionality (pseudopapillae, morulae, tubules) and peripheral palisading (Fig. 7.3a).
- Two-dimensional aggregates of small size with a tendency to form "Indian files".
- Small to medium-sized monomorphous cells with scant cytoplasm (Fig. 7.3b).
- Medium-sized nuclei (>2×RBC), occasionally large and bizarre, oval to elongated in shape with a finely granular chromatin and possible small nucleoli (Fig. 7.3b,c).
- Nuclear membrane accentuation with frequent clefts (Fig. 7.3c) and nuclear cytoplasmic inclusions (Fig. 7.3d).

The above-described patterns can be seen as a component of lung adenocarcinoma or in a pure form. In addition, mucinous and non-mucinous tumor types frequently coexist in the same sample (Fig. 7.4). In the *mucinous variant*, there is often profuse cellularity; the tumor cells are organized in flat sheets and look highly monotonous. The internuclear distance within aggregates may be rather variable but nuclear molding is never seen. Nuclei vary only subtly in size and are consistently round or oval, with finely granular chromatin and slightly eccentric, punctate but intense nucleoli. When detected as isolated elements, the tumor cells characteristically assume a "histiocyte-like" or "histiocytoid" appearance due to their abundant cytoplasm and a relatively small and round and regularly shaped nucleus. These elements can easily be confused with atypical histiocytes; their proper recognition may need to be based upon immunocytochemical demonstration of cytokeratin products in the cytoplasm [41]. Mucous strands incorporating epithelial cells must be considered with caution in the separation of benign reactive bronchiolar cells (other than histiocytes) from malignant mucinous cells. In the *non-mucinous variant*, there is a great tendency for the cells to form three-dimensional aggregates; also, the cells look smaller due to a reduced amount of cytoplasm.

Nuclear inclusions occur in both variants although, in our experience, they seem to be more frequent in the non-mucinous variant. These inclusions are produced by invagination of the nuclear membrane. In the mucinous variant, the interiorized cytoplasmic matrix looks eosinophilic, thus contrasting with the clear staining features of the cytoplasm. The nuclear membrane is somewhat more accentuated in the non-mucinous

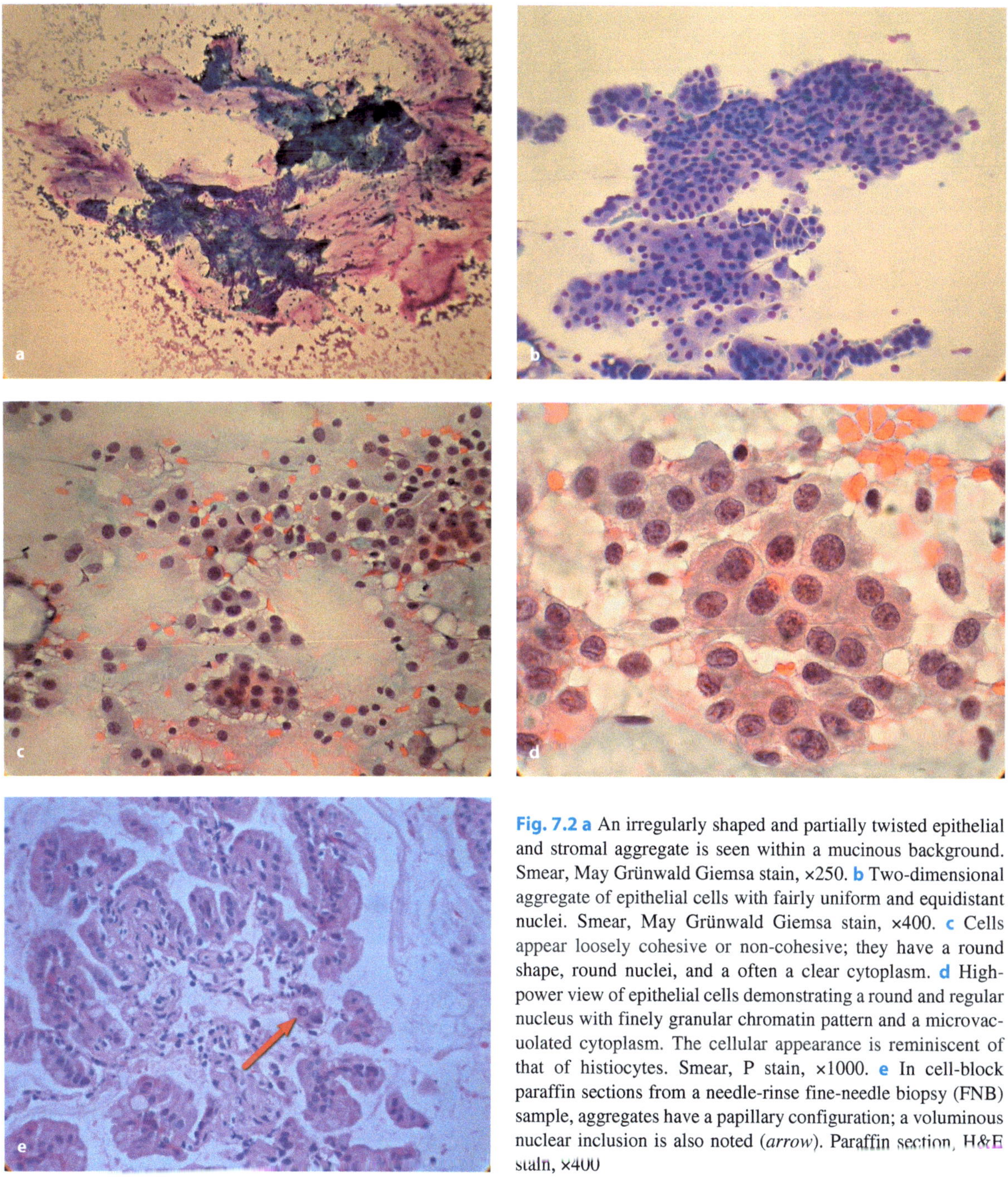

Fig. 7.2 a An irregularly shaped and partially twisted epithelial and stromal aggregate is seen within a mucinous background. Smear, May Grünwald Giemsa stain, ×250. **b** Two-dimensional aggregate of epithelial cells with fairly uniform and equidistant nuclei. Smear, May Grünwald Giemsa stain, ×400. **c** Cells appear loosely cohesive or non-cohesive; they have a round shape, round nuclei, and a often a clear cytoplasm. **d** High-power view of epithelial cells demonstrating a round and regular nucleus with finely granular chromatin pattern and a microvacuolated cytoplasm. The cellular appearance is reminiscent of that of histiocytes. Smear, P stain, ×1000. **e** In cell-block paraffin sections from a needle-rinse fine-needle biopsy (FNB) sample, aggregates have a papillary configuration; a voluminous nuclear inclusion is also noted (*arrow*). Paraffin section, H&E stain, ×400

variant and has an irregular outline due to multiple clefts. Similar intranuclear cytoplasmic inclusions occur in several non-bronchogenic neoplasms (papillary carcinoma of the thyroid, melanoma, etc.), in bronchogenic tumors (poorly differentiated adenocarcinoma, pleomorphic carcinoma), and in benign bronchiolar epithelium. Bronchioloalveolar carcinoma cells can be confused with reactive bronchiolar epithelium showing nuclear atypia [42,43]. To compound the issue, these benign cells frequently coexist in the same

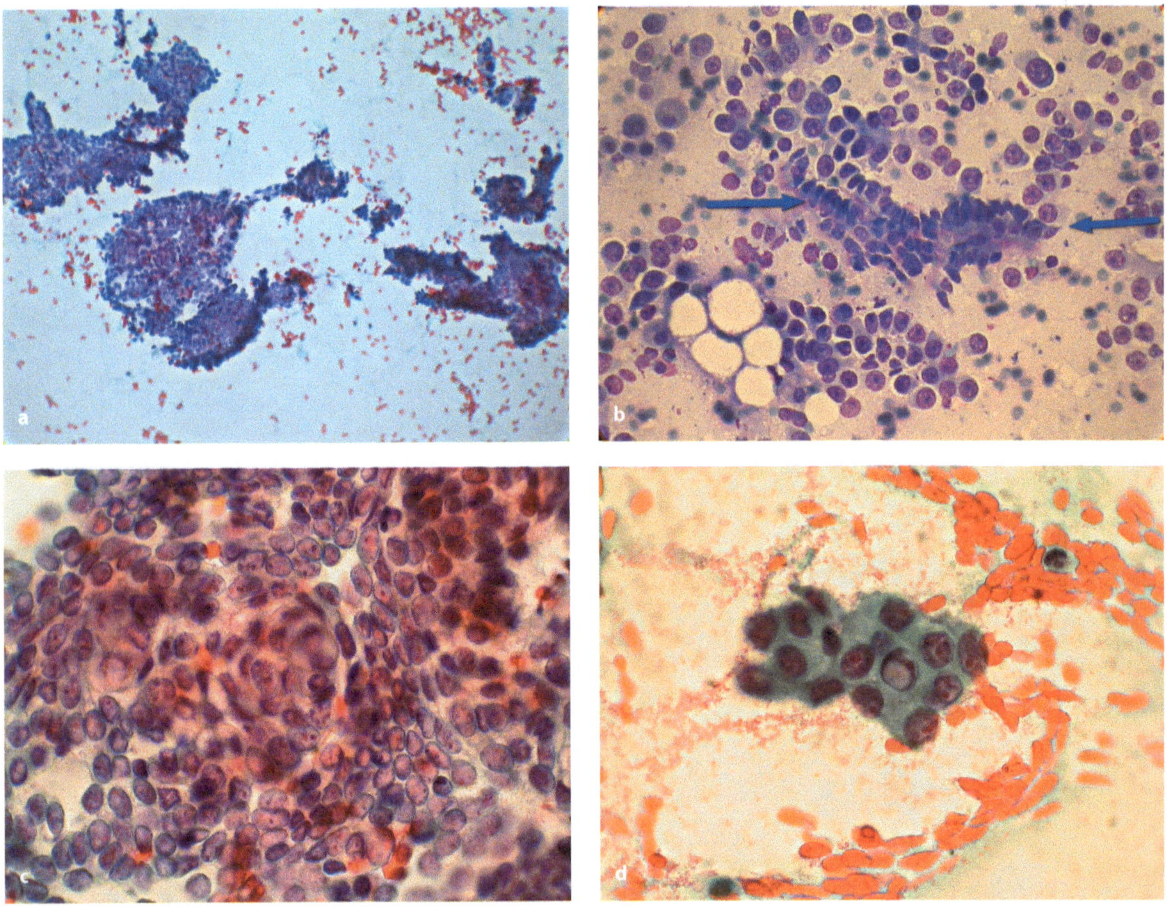

Fig. 7.3 **a** Irregularly shaped papillary, acinar, and two-dimensional aggregates are seen in this FNB sample collected from a non-mucinous brochioloalveolar carcinoma. Smear, P stain, ×400. **b** Higher magnification shows loosely cohesive medium-sized cells with large nuclei and scant cytoplasm. A strand of normal bronchiolar cells is also seen centrally in the image (*arrows*). Smear, May Grünwald Giemsa stain, ×1000. **c** Cells display round nuclei and have occasional small nucleoli. Smear, P stain, ×1000. **d** Acinar aggregate in a smear from a non-mucinous bronchioloalveolar carcinoma contains a cell with an evident nuclear inclusion. Smear, P stain, ×1000

FNB sample with malignant cells (Fig. 7.3b) and the distinction can be very difficult. In general, reactive bronchiolar cells cluster in small aggregates (while malignant cells form large clusters), contain a lesser amount of cytoplasm, and lack prominent nucleoli or a significant number of intranuclear cytoplasmic inclusions.

7.2.2.2 Poorly Differentiated Adenocarcinoma

- Background rich in blood, necrotic debris, or mucin.
- Variable extent of cellularity.
- Strong prevalence of three-dimensional aggregates (syncytia, trabeculae, papillae, large aggregates with arbitrary cellular arrangement) with nuclear overlapping and molding (Fig. 7.5a).
- Large, polyhedral to columnar cells with large nuclei (3–4×RBC) (Fig. 7.5a).
- Prominent anisokaryosis, anisonucleosis, abnormally disturbed nuclear cytoplasmic ratios (Fig. 7.5b,c).
- Coarsely granular chromatin with possible prominent basophilic nucleoli (Fig. 7.5b) and intranuclear cytoplasmic inclusions.
- Variable amount of cytoplasm that is amphophilic or basophilic in appearance or may contain mucin droplets displacing the nucleus.
- Variable amount of cells with a squamoid appearance.

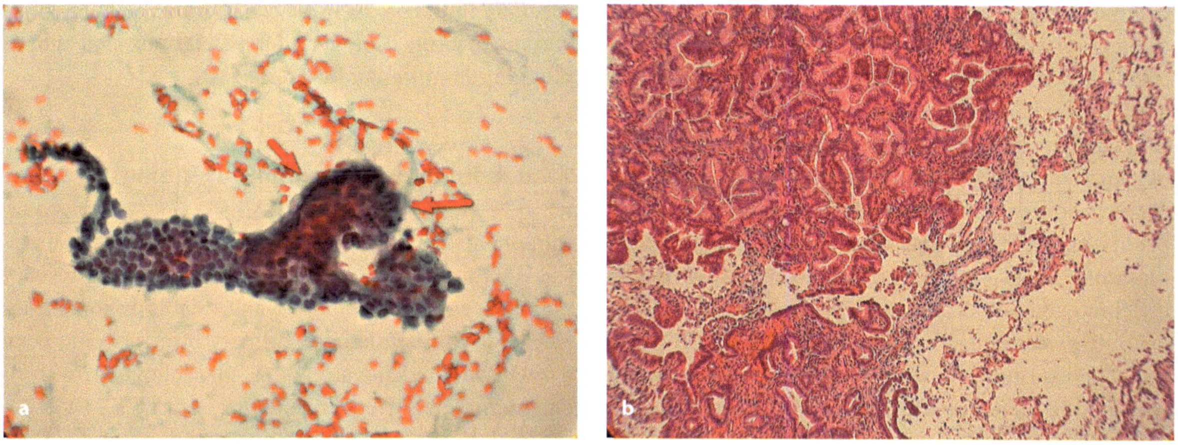

Fig. 7.4 a This single aggregate of tumor cells from a patient with mixed type bronchioloalveolar carcinoma shows a distinct component of non-mucinous cells (*left*) and of larger cells with more abundant cytoplasm, a clear mucinous content, and a pseudopapillary configuration (*arrows*). Smear, P stain, ×400. **b** Surgical specimen from the same patient as in **a**; the distinct mucinous component is seen in the upper half of the image and an obvious non-mucinous component in the lower half. Paraffin section, H&E stain, ×40

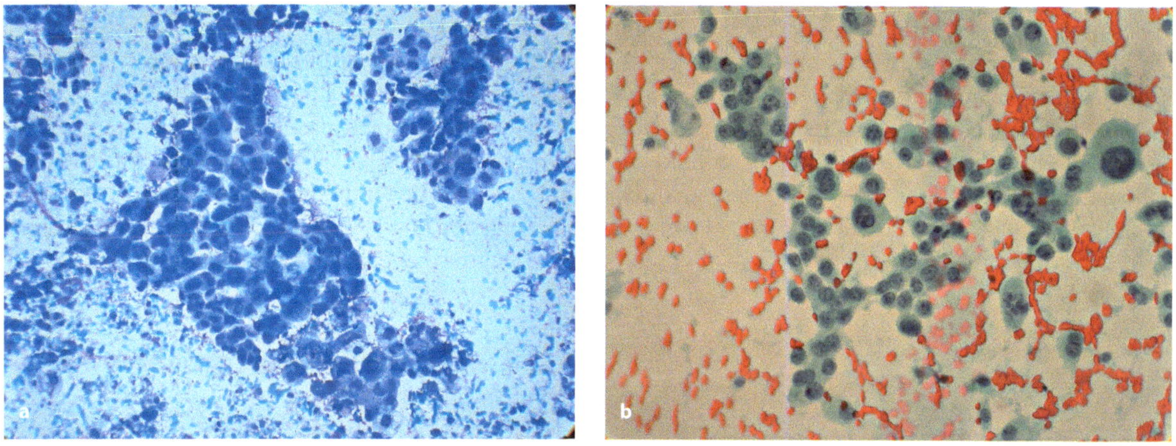

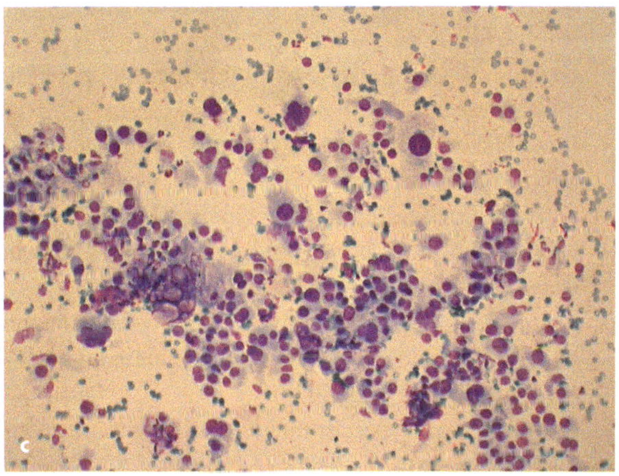

Fig. 7.5 a Aggregate of large epithelial glandular cells with focal nuclear overlap and pleomorphic cells with evident anisonucleosis. Smear, May Grünwald Giemsa stain, ×250. **b** The cells show a significant variation in nuclear size and shape, the chromatin pattern is coarsely granular and nucleoli are well evident. Smear, ×400, P stain. **c** Same case as in **b**; May Grünwald Giemsa stain outlines prominent variability in cellular configuration and nuclear size. Smear, ×400

Poorly differentiated adenocarcinoma is composed of medium to large cells forming cohesive and unstructured clusters without a definitive acinar configuration. The arrangement may be ambiguous, and the only clues to glandular differentiation may be the occasional evidence of intracytoplasmic mucin droplets, or focal abortive acinar formations with some resemblance to a central lumen. These tumor cells may contain intracytoplasmic inclusions. In FNB of moderately or poorly differentiated adenocarcinoma, particularly in the presence of extracellular mucin, the characteristic tumor cell harvest may be seen in conjunction with the appearance of multinucleated histiocytic giant cells. The latter may lead the observer to rule out a granulomatous inflammatory condition but, in fact, the multinucleated cells are a response to the extravasated mucin.

7.2.2.3 Mucinous (Colloid) Carcinoma

Mucinous carcinoma of the lung is a rare malignancy that generally grows as a solitary mass in the upper lobes of the lung [37,40]. The tumor can become quite large size before the appearance of symptoms. The FNB cytological picture, which is prototypical of tumors with a glandular cell morphology and a mucinous pattern, is highly reminiscent of colloid carcinoma of the breast (Fig. 7.6). The differential diagnosis thus includes a metastatic mucinous carcinoma (primary in the breast or large intestine), the mucinous variant of bronchioloalveolar carcinoma, and mucus plugging in inflammatory processes.

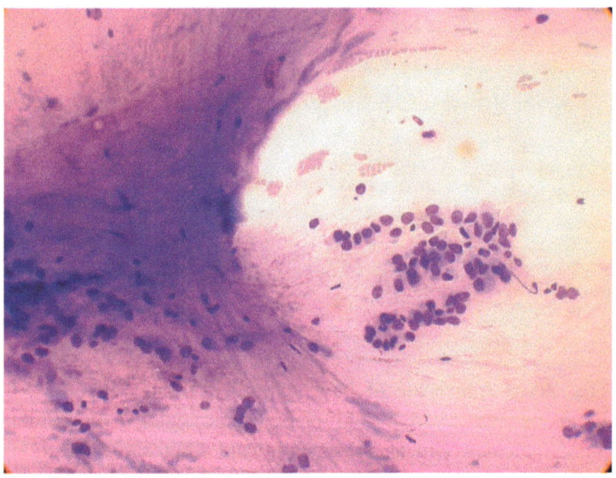

Fig. 7.6 Cohesive and non-cohesive medium-sized cells are seen in a mucoid (metachromatic) background in this FNB sample from a patient with primary bronchogenic colloid carcinoma. Smear, May Grünwald Giemsa stain, ×250

7.2.2.4 Immunohistochemical Findings

Immunohistochemistry performed on cell-block material is a greatly useful adjunct to the FNB diagnosis of pulmonary adenocarcinoma, and its role is sometimes pivotal in differentiating a primary bronchogenic from a metastatic adenocarcinoma. Bronchogenic adenocarcinoma cells frequently express the CK7+/CK20- profile but a significant proportion of tumors coexpress these two markers, while the CK7-/CK20+ profile is practically never seen [44,45]. Estrogen receptor positivity is seen in about 20% of cases [46]. TTF-1 positivity is detected in 70–85% of cases whereas some mucinous variants, namely, mucinous bronchoalveolar adenocarcinoma, are completely unreactive [47]. TTF-1 positivity can be used in the proper context to demonstrate a pulmonary origin of the adenocarcinoma cells but it should be kept in mind that TTF-1 is expressed in a minor proportion of ovarian carcinomas, of endometrioid and serous types [48,49]. The TTF-1+/CK5/6+/p63- profile is seen in about half the cases of bronchogenic adenocarcinoma and represents a specific profile for this tumor [50]. Finally, "aberrant" coexpression of TTF-1 and CDX2 is described in about 12% of bronchogenic adenocarcinomas [51].

7.2.3 Adenosquamous Carcinoma

- Background rich in blood, necrotic detritus, or pyknotic bare nuclei with inflammatory cells (Fig. 7.7a,b).
- Extent of cellularity variable, mainly poor to moderate.
- Prevalence of aggregated cells with a great tendency to form trabeculae, cords, or aggregates with arbitrary cellular arrangements (Fig. 7.7a).
- Medium to large cells, polygonal to elongated in shape.
- Round to oval, large, monotonous-looking nuclei with finely to coarsely granular chromatin and well-evident nucleoli (Fig. 7.7a).
- Possibility of hyperchromatic nuclei with an elongated shape (Fig. 7.7b).

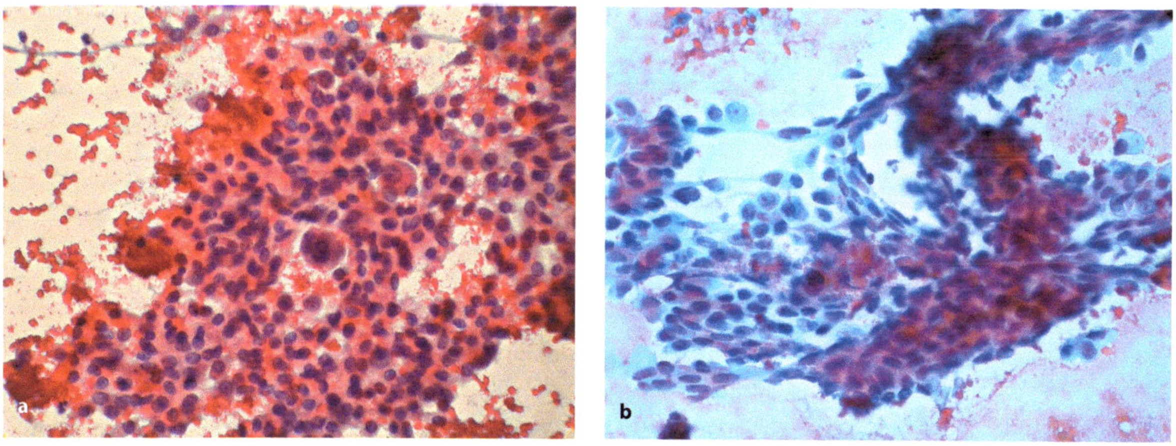

Fig. 7.7 a Large cluster showing a mixture of medium-sized polygonal cells with round nuclei containing prominent nucleoli and larger cells with more abundant and eosinophilic cytoplasm due to intracellular keratinization. Smear, P stain, ×400. **b** This large cluster is characterized by two components: round to oval cells in a two-dimensional aggregation pattern (*left*, adenocarcinoma component), and more elongated cells in multiple layers and with an eosinophilic cytoplasm (*right*, squamous cell carcinoma component). Smear, P stain, ×400

- Scant densely basophilic to amphophilic cytoplasm with a minor component of cells displaying cytoplasmic eosinophilia (Fig. 7.7b).

Adenosquamous carcinoma is defined as a carcinoma showing glandular and squamous cell differentiated components, with each comprising at least 10% of the tumor. The tumor is often peripheral in location and demonstrates a central scar.

7.2.4 Squamous Cell Carcinoma

Squamous cell carcinoma originates in the major bronchi in about two-thirds of cases and is peripherally located in the remaining one-third. Proximal airway masses often have an endobronchial component and are responsible for early obstructive symptoms. In a peripheral location, the tumor often undergoes central cavitation. Histologically, squamous cell carcinoma may show varying degrees of differentiation and extent of keratinization and it is completely similar to squamous cell malignancies arising in other anatomic sites [37,40].

The cytological picture on FNB is prototypical of tumors having a squamous cell morphology. Well-differentiated, poorly differentiated, keratinizing, and non-keratinizing variants are appropriately diagnosed cytologically. In keratinizing tumors, the cellular harvest is strikingly polymorphous and diverse. The background contains cytoplasmic fragments, inflammatory cells, and erythrocytes. Cells vary in shape from polygonal to stellate, with elongated forms exhibiting a tapering, eosinophilic, homogeneous cytoplasm. Large three-dimensional aggregates (Fig. 7.8a) or dissociated elements are observed. Angular, oval, sometimes lobulated nuclei vary considerably in size but are universally densely hyperchromatic and homogeneous (Fig. 7.8b). In tumors undergoing central cavitation and necrosis, sampling of the lesion interior may yield only necrotic tumor cells and the elements of diathesis. A characteristic features of bronchogenic squamous cell carcinoma is the more than occasional detection of round, medium to large elements with a densely hyperchromatic nucleus showing a smudged external profile and a clear cytoplasm closely resembling atypical koilocytes (Fig. 7.8b). In poorly differentiated tumors, the cells become smaller, the nuclei more fusiform and less hyperchromatic, and the tendency to dissociation more common, such that individually dispersed cells are seen among tenuous aggregates. Chromatin details may become more obvious, so that a coarsely granular texture and nucleoli are visible (Fig. 7.8c). Sometimes, the only clue to squamoid differentiation is the pattern of organization within loosely cohesive groups, with multiple stratifications and a tendency to a mosaic configuration.

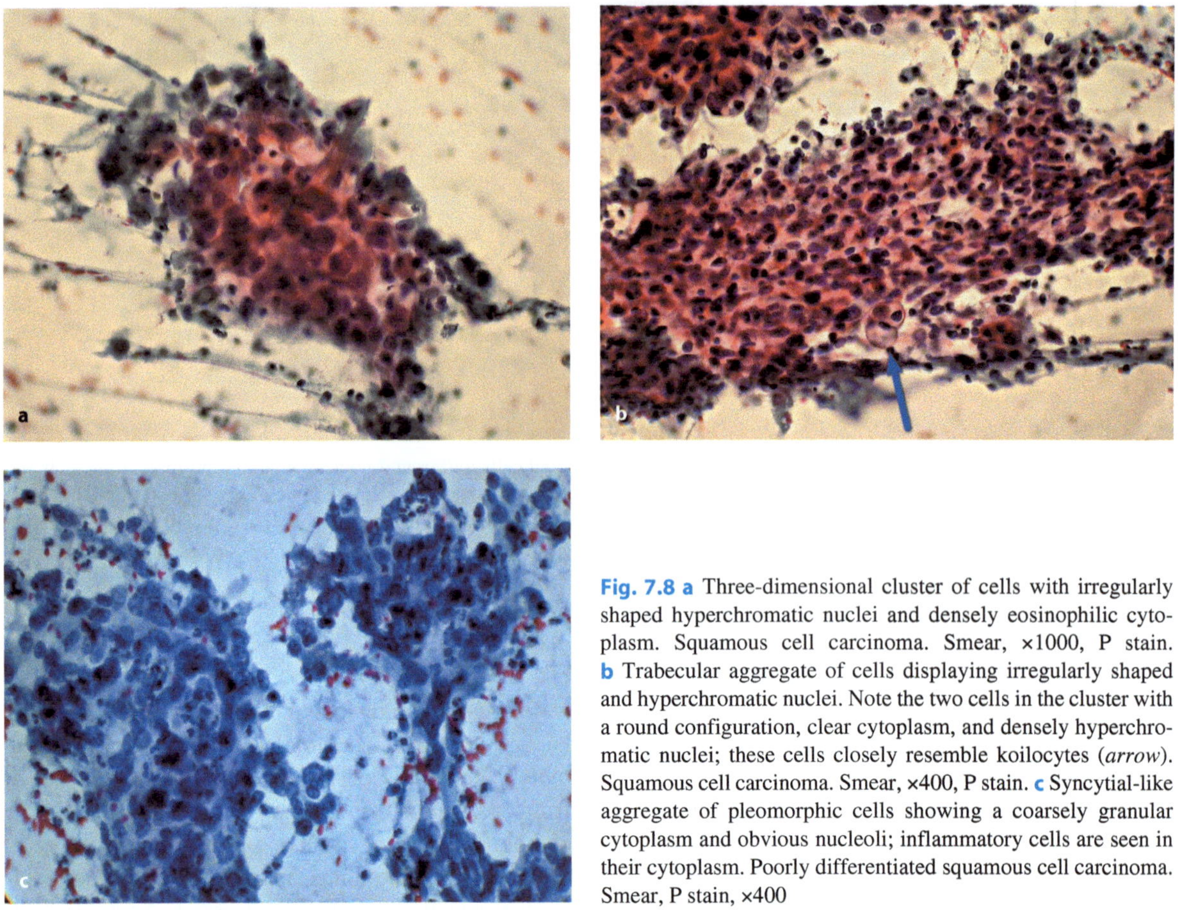

Fig. 7.8 a Three-dimensional cluster of cells with irregularly shaped hyperchromatic nuclei and densely eosinophilic cytoplasm. Squamous cell carcinoma. Smear, ×1000, P stain. **b** Trabecular aggregate of cells displaying irregularly shaped and hyperchromatic nuclei. Note the two cells in the cluster with a round configuration, clear cytoplasm, and densely hyperchromatic nuclei; these cells closely resemble koilocytes (*arrow*). Squamous cell carcinoma. Smear, ×400, P stain. **c** Syncytial-like aggregate of pleomorphic cells showing a coarsely granular cytoplasm and obvious nucleoli; inflammatory cells are seen in their cytoplasm. Poorly differentiated squamous cell carcinoma. Smear, P stain, ×400

The differential diagnosis of non-keratinizing squamous cell carcinoma includes poorly differentiated adenocarcinoma, small-cell carcinoma, and metastatic urothelial carcinoma. Immunohistochemistry performed on cell-block material is of help in properly identifying the tumor. In fact, bronchogenic squamous cell carcinoma cells are characteristically positive for CK5/6 and p63 [50] and practically never express TTF-1 nuclear positivity [47]. Testing for the presence of these three markers helps to distinguish squamous cell carcinoma from poorly differentiated adenocarcinoma and small-cell neuroendocrine carcinoma, whose profiles are, respectively, TTF-1+/CK5/6- /p63- and TTF-1+/CK5/6+ /p63- [50]. Finally, the distinction from metastatic urothelial carcinoma can be obtained by testing for CD10 and CK20, which are characteristically coexpressed in this tumor.

7.2.5 Large-Cell Carcinoma

- Background rich in blood or necrotic detritus with inflammatory cells.
- Prevalence of irregularly shaped two-dimensional aggregates with a tendency to loose cohesiveness at the periphery (Fig. 7.9a).
- Constituent cells large, pleomorphic, occasionally bizarre, with abundant cytoplasm (Fig. 7.9b).
- Large and pleomorphic nuclei with coarsely granular chromatin, prominent single or multiple nucleoli, with possibly numerous karryorhexis.
- Densely basophilic to amphophilic and/or microvacuolized cytoplasm with possible phagocytosis of granulocytes (emperipolesis) (Fig. 7.9b).

Large-cell carcinoma is an example of undifferentiated carcinoma completely or mainly consisting of

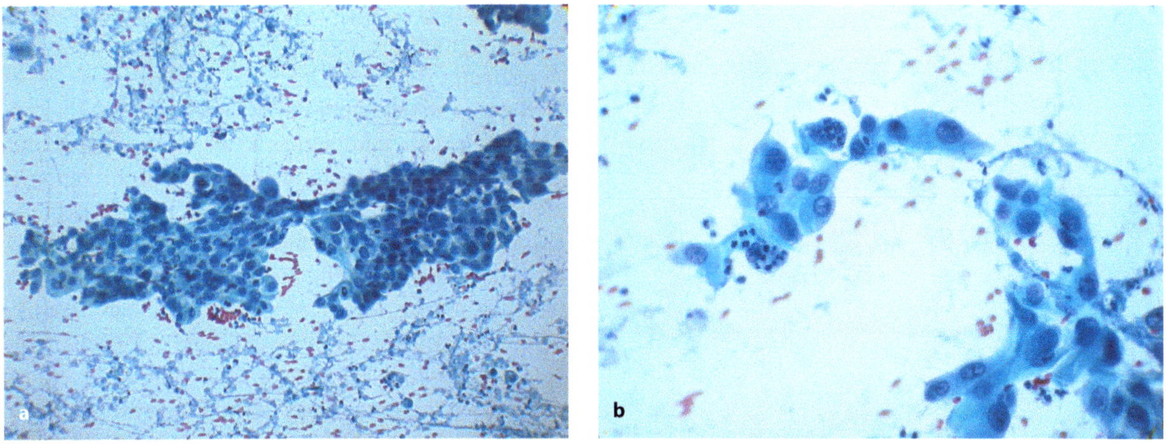

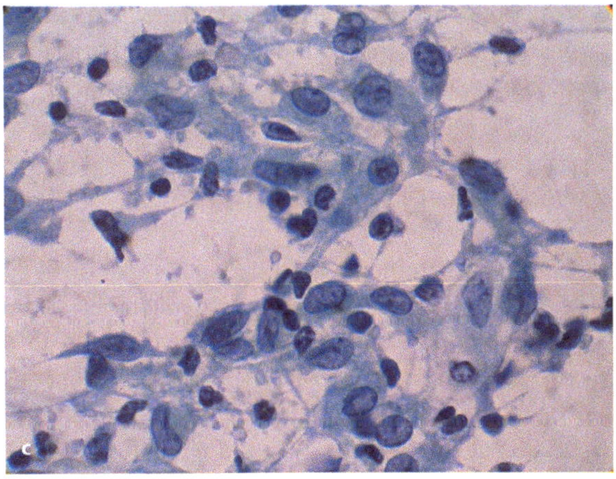

Fig. 7.9 a Two-dimensional aggregate of large cells with a pleomorphic and sometimes bizarre configuration and abundant basophilic cytoplasm. Large-cell carcinoma. Smear, P stain, ×400. **b** Occasionally, large cells may contain polymorphonuclear granulocytes in their cytoplasm ("emperipolesis"). Large-cell carcinoma. Smear, P stain, ×1000. **c** Large cells with vesicular nuclei containing occasional prominent nucleoli are admixed with small lymphocytes in a large-cell carcinoma displaying the lymphoepithelioma-like pattern. Smear, P stain, ×1000

large cells and lacking evidence of squamous or glandular cell differentiation. The tumor tends to appear in the periphery of the lung, where it grows rapidly. The main variants of the tumor are large-cell neuroendocrine carcinoma (see below), lymphoepithelioma-like carcinoma, and clear cell carcinoma. Lymphoepithelioma-like carcinoma is characterized by large cells displaying a large vesicular nucleus and prominent nucleoli, with a concomitant massive infiltration of small lymphocytes (Fig. 7.9c). Primary bronchogenic clear cell carcinomas are practically indistinguishable from clear cell carcinomas arising in other anatomic sites. Immunohistochemically, bronchogenic large-cell carcinoma cells express CK7 and TTF-1 [51, 52] but not CK5/6 or p63 [50].

7.2.6 Basaloid Cell Carcinoma

Most basaloid cell carcinomas arise in the proximal bronchi and display an endobronchial component. Histologically, they have a lobular, trabecular, or palisading pattern with foci of comedo-type necrosis. The tumor cells are small and monomorphic with a cuboid or somewhat fusiform shape [37,40]. Due to their proximal location, they are more often diagnosed by bronchoscopic biopsy but can represent an unexpected encounter in FNB practice, especially when the tumor is more peripherally located. The FNB picture (Fig. 7.10) is prototypical of tumors with a basaloid cell pattern. In the differential diagnosis, this tumor variant should be differentiated from primary or metastatic adenoid cystic carcinoma.

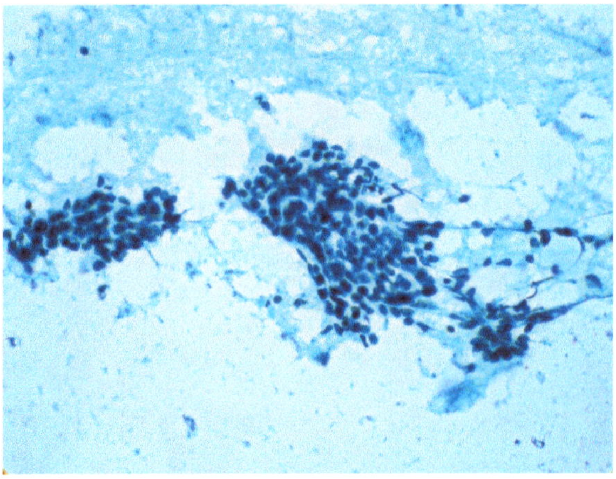

Fig. 7.10 Pleomorphic small-cell pattern with cohesive and non-cohesive cells is sometimes seen in poorly differentiated squamous cell carcinoma, thus simulating a small-cell neuroendocrine carcinoma. Smear, P stain, ×400

- Coarsely granular to densely hyperchromatic chromatin, multiple small nucleoli, frequent crushing artifacts.
- Barely visible amount of cytoplasm.

Spindle cell carcinoma is an unusual epithelial malignancy whose main feature is the proliferation of elongated cells resembling mesenchymal elements [37,40]. The tumor belongs to the category of sarcomatoid carcinomas of the lung, which includes a spectrum of morphologies of sarcoma or sarcoma-like neoplastic elements (spindle cells and giant cells). The spindle cells can take on a fascicular or storiform appearance that includes a fibrotic or myxoid stroma. The tumor is a peculiar variant of bronchogenic carcinoma but tumors with exactly the same features can originate in other visceral sites, such as the urinary tract, kidney, pancreas, and thyroid.

7.2.7 Spindle Cell Carcinoma

- Clean background with histiocytes and few inflammatory cells.
- Tendency to cellular cohesion, with large aggregates and three-dimensionality, or smaller aggregates with partial loss of cohesion (Fig. 7.11a).
- Large elongated cells with a definite spindle-like configuration (Fig. 7.11b).
- Elongated nuclei terminating with pointed ends.

7.2.8 Pleomorphic Carcinoma

Pleomorphic carcinoma is a variant of sarcomatoid carcinoma, with a significant component of large, giant, and bizarre cells (Fig. 7.12) in addition to a second component of an otherwise typical squamous cell carcinoma, adenocarcinoma, large-cell carcinoma, or spindle cell carcinoma [37]. In FNB samples, giant cells appear as non-cohesive elements with very large and polymorphous nuclei containing giant nucleoli. A huge inflammatory infiltrate accompanies the giant cells in some cases.

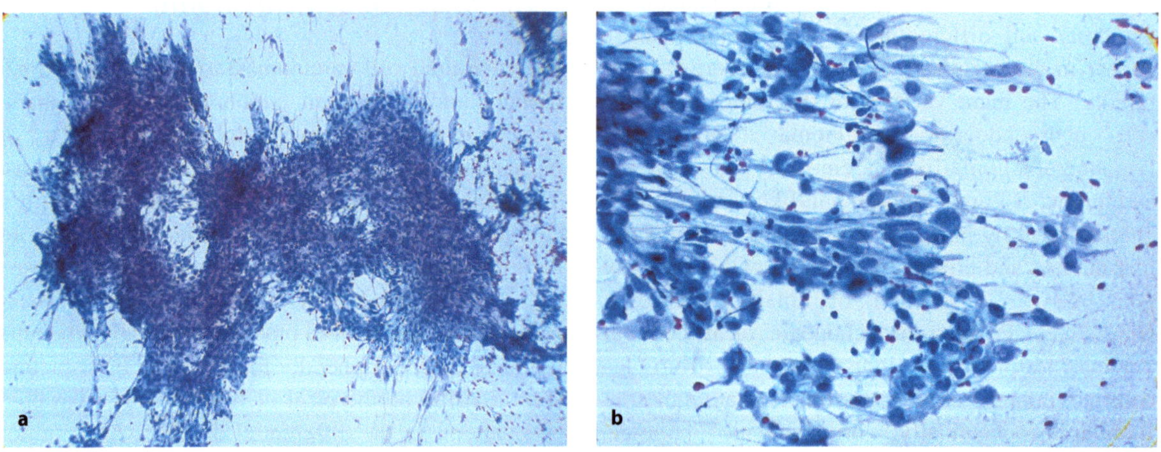

Fig. 7.11 a Large three-dimensional aggregate of cohesive and pleomorphic spindle cells in a sample obtained from a patient with spindle cell carcinoma. Smear, P stain, ×400. **b** High-power view of fairly elongated and large cells with a spindle-like morphology and containing similarly elongated and fusiform nuclei terminating with sharp ends. Spindle cell carcinoma. Smear, P stain, ×1000

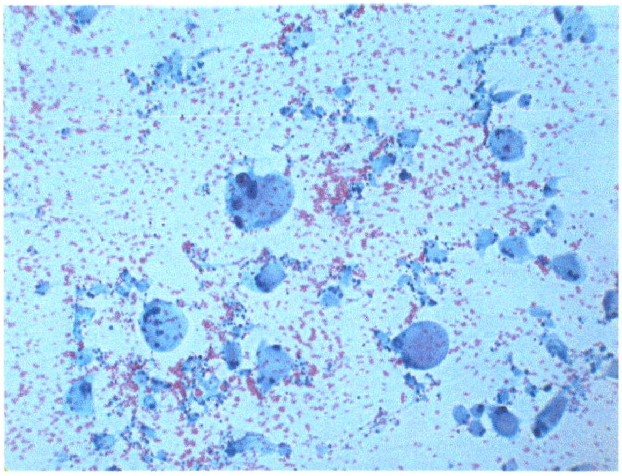

Fig. 7.12 Giant multinucleated cells often containing large and bizarre nuclei are characteristic of giant cell carcinoma. Smear, P stain, ×400

7.2.9 Neuroendocrine Tumors

Neuroendocrine tumors represent a spectrum of malignant neoplasms comprising poorly aggressive, low-grade malignancies (typical carcinoid tumor) and intermediate-grade (poorly differentiated neuro-endocrine carcinoma or "atypical" carcinoid tumors) to high-grade (small-cell and large-cell neuroendocrine carcinoma) malignancies [53]. With the exception of large-cell carcinoma, the cytological picture of these tumors on FNB is prototypical of tumors having a small-cell morphology. In particular, typical carcinoid tumors assume a monomorphous cell pattern with a tendency to cellular aggregation and mild nuclear atypia, while poorly differentiated and small-cell carcinomas assume a pleomorphic pattern with a tendency to cellular aggregation and marked nuclear atypia.

7.2.9.1 Typical Carcinoid

Typical carcinoid tumors mainly occur in major bronchi (central carcinoid) but are also often located peripherally in the lung (peripheral carcinoid). Central carcinoids are accessible to bronchoscopic biopsy and thus rather infrequently represent a target for transthoracic FNB. Peripheral carcinoid, by contrast, is commonly encountered in FNB practice. The diagnostic yield consists of a monotonous succession of uniform cells with minimal cytoplasm, resembling lymphocytes, but congregated in ribbons and amorphous clusters (Fig. 7.13a,b) [54–56]. Nuclei show delicate chromatin with well-evident nucleoli accentuated by paranucleolar and crisply delineated nuclear margins. Especially in peripherally located tumors, the harvest may consist of a population of uniform, short spindle cells sometimes congregated in abortive rosettes (Fig. 7.13c,d) [56]. The fusiform nuclei show definite margins and a coarsely granular chromatin with inconspicuous nucleoli. Metastatic involvement of mediastinal lymph nodes is detected at the time of diagnosis of carcinoid tumor in about 10–15% of patients [37,40]. These tumors are prone to produce distant metastases into the liver, bone, and brain even several years after surgical excision. Immunohistochemically, the tumor cells express low molecular weight cytokeratin and TTF-1 [47,50], in addition to common neuroendocrine markers. The differential diagnosis consists only of metastatic neuroendocrine tumors of carcinoid type. Testing for both TTF-1 and CDX-2 is of help in demonstrating a pulmonary (TTF-1+/CDX-2-) or intestinal (TTF-1-/CDX-2+) primary site of the tumor or in excluding both (TTF-1-/CDX-2-) [57].

7.2.9.2 Poorly Differentiated and Small-Cell Neuroendocrine Carcinoma

Poorly differentiated and small-cell neuroendocrine carcinomas commonly present in a central location, as they arise from major bronchi. They are highly aggressive tumors and metastases develop early in the course of the disease. For this reason, a majority of patients present with disease of advanced stage, i.e., with mediastinal lymph node involvement and visceral dissemination. In FNB samples, the tumor cells may be dispersed individually, randomly, and without architectural design but the tendency to cell aggregation prevails (Fig. 7.14a). The fragility of the cells results in the characteristic crushing artifact such that nuclear details are obliterated in most cellular elements (Azzopardi's phenomenon). Nuclear contours may vary from round to oval to fusiform, with elliptical and almond-shape configurations predominating. For those cells spared from degenerative hyperchromasia, the nuclear texture is generally delicate with evenly distributed chromatin. The diagnostic yield of these tumors fulfills the histopathological definition of

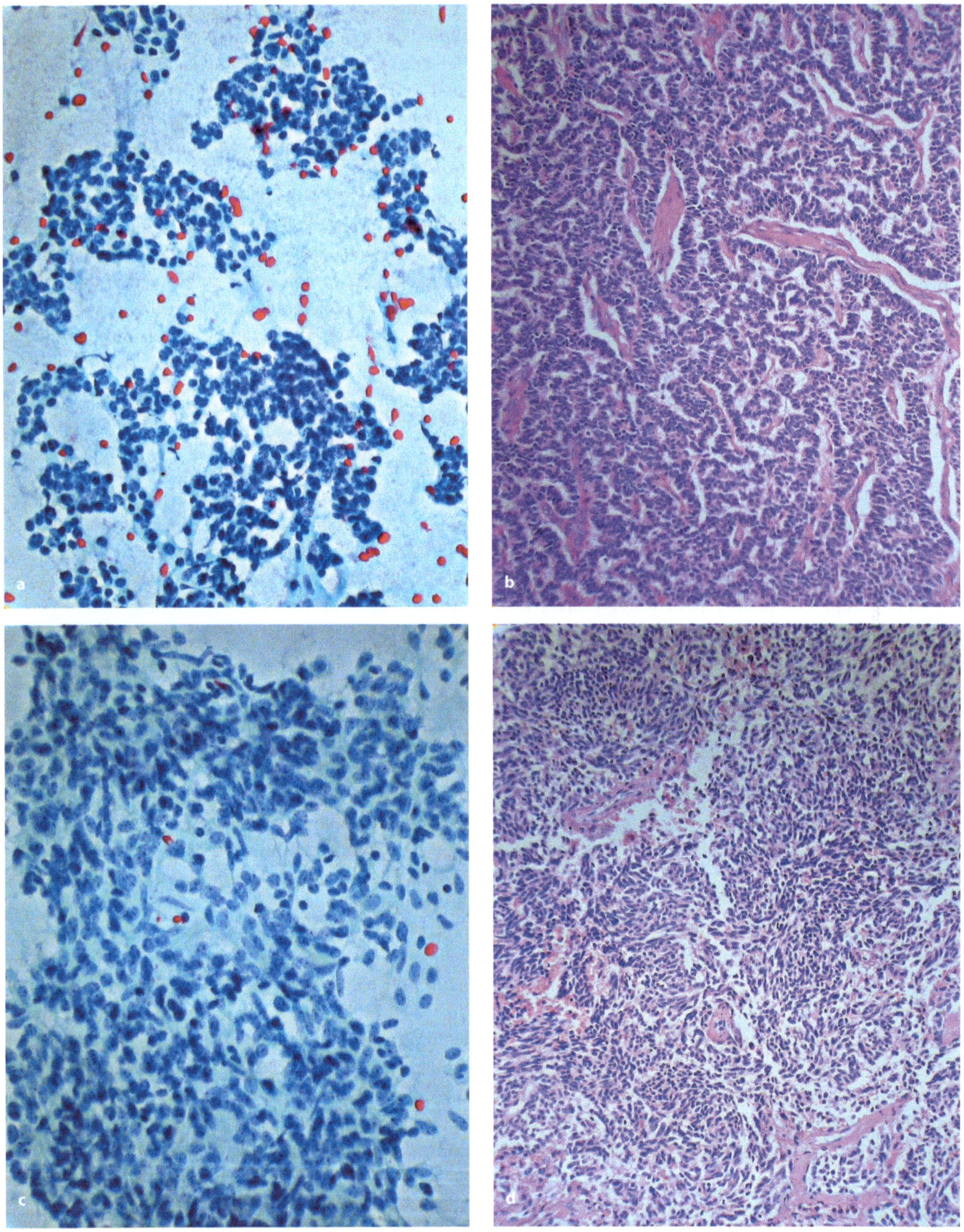

Fig. 7.13 a Monotonous-looking small and round cells displaying round nuclei with the characteristic "salt and pepper" chromatin texture and scant cytoplasm are characteristic of FNB samples from typical carcinoid tumor. Smear, P stain, ×400. **b** Histological features of typical carcinoid tumor: tumor cells grow in ribbons and files. Paraffin section, H&E stain, ×400. **c** A somewhat pleomorphic population of small cells with an elongated appearance and the characteristic granular chromatin texture is typical of FNB samples from spindle cell carcinoid tumor. Smear, P stain, ×400. **d** Histological features of spindle cell carcinoid tumor. Paraffin section, H&E stain, ×400

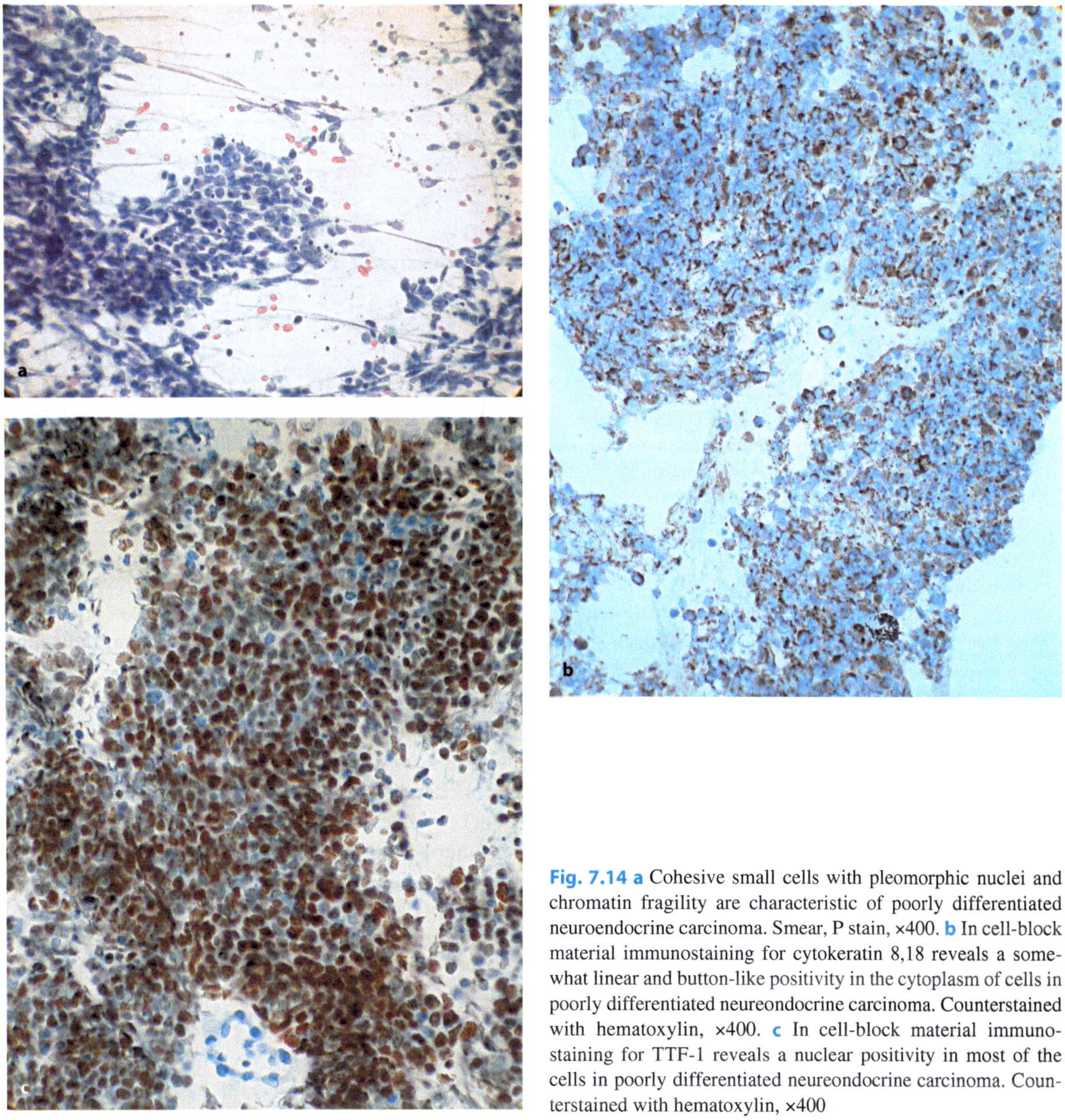

Fig. 7.14 a Cohesive small cells with pleomorphic nuclei and chromatin fragility are characteristic of poorly differentiated neuroendocrine carcinoma. Smear, P stain, ×400. **b** In cell-block material immunostaining for cytokeratin 8,18 reveals a somewhat linear and button-like positivity in the cytoplasm of cells in poorly differentiated neureondocrine carcinoma. Counterstained with hematoxylin, ×400. **c** In cell-block material immunostaining for TTF-1 reveals a nuclear positivity in most of the cells in poorly differentiated neureondocrine carcinoma. Counterstained with hematoxylin, ×400

poorly differentiated neuroendocrine carcinoma; the cells may appear larger and nuclei are more variable in size, contour, and configuration. Cellular non-cohesion is slightly more prevalent. Within the aggregates, nuclear molding is quite obvious [56,58]. Immunohistochemically, there is reduced expression of neuroendocrine markers and synaptophysin is more frequently detected than chromogranin. Among the commonly employed epithelial markers, only low molecular weight cytokeratins are expressed (CK8,18), and they tend to appear in a characteristic linear or punctate fashion (Fig. 7.14b). TTF-1 positivity is detected in most of the cells (Fig. 7.14c) [47,50]. The differential diagnosis encompasses poorly differentiated squamous cell carcinoma and other high-grade neuroendocrine malignancies, such as metastatic Merkel cell carcinoma. Testing for both TTF-1 and p63 is of help in differentiating these tumors from the former (small-cell neuroendocrine carcinoma is TTF-1+/p63- and squamous cell carcinoma is TTF-1-/p63+) [50], while

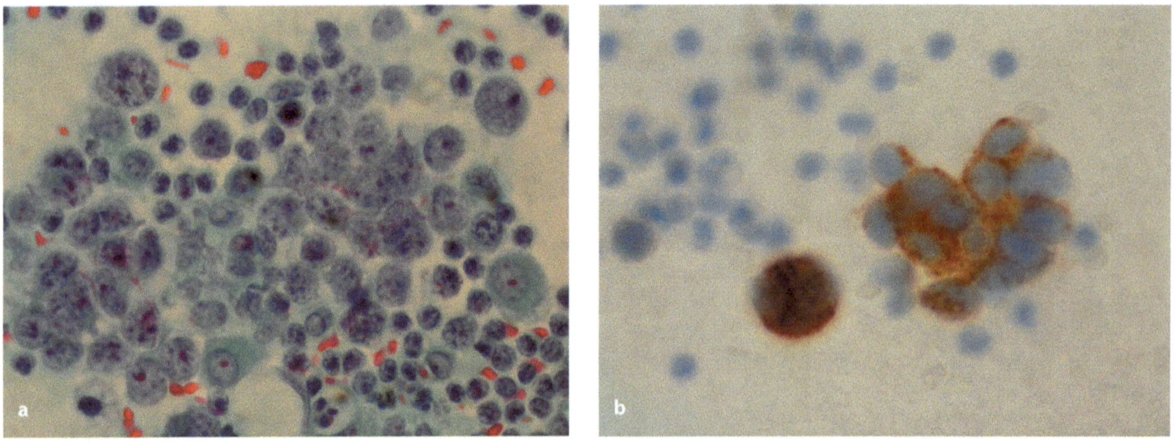

Fig. 7.15 a Effusion cytology in a patient with pleural involvement by large-cell neuroendocrine carcinoma of the lung; tumor cells show large nuclei with coarsely granular chromatin and prominent nucleoli. Smear, counterstained with hematoxylin, ×1000. **b** Same case as in **a**; immunostaining of the smear for chromogranin reveals a cytoplasmic granular positivity in the tumor cells. Smear, counterstained with hematoxylin, ×1000

the detection of a "button-like" positivity for cytokeratin [59], in particular CK20 [60], is a quite distinctive feature of Merkel cell carcinoma and excludes small-cell neuroendocrine carcinoma of the lung.

7.2.9.3 Large-Cell Neuroendocrine Carcinoma

Large-cell neuroendocrine carcinoma is a rare malignancy occurring almost exclusively in the elderly. Most of the tumors are localized peripherally in the lung and are clinically and radiologically indistinguishable from other types of non-small-cell carcinomas. They are responsible for an early dissemination into the pleural cavity. Histologically and cytologically [61], the tumors are characterized by a neuroendocrine morphology, high mitotic activity, and a neoplastic population of large polygonal cells with abundant cytoplasm and vesicular or finely granular chromatin. The cytological morphology and immunohistochemical findings in a pleural effusion obtained from a patient with this tumor are shown in Figure 7.15.

7.2.10 Pulmonary Metastatic Malignancies

Metastatic involvement of the lung by extrapulmonary neoplasms is commonly characterized by the appearance of multiple nodules and frequently associated with pleural effusion. Alternative and less common patterns of presentation take the form of a solitary nodule, cavitation, or cyst. The latter is an indication for FNB sampling to rule out a possible new primary tumor or a benign condition. Tumors most commonly inducing a solitary nodular metastasis are carcinoma of the colon, breast, and kidney, urothelial carcinoma, and melanoma. Cavitation is common in metastases from colorectal carcinoma, head and neck carcinomas, and uterine cervical carcinoma. Cystic nodules are reported as a common finding in metastases of endometrial stromal sarcoma and leiomyosarcoma and are complicated by pneumothorax [38].

In FNB samples, it is generally easy to diagnose metastatic disease and its differentiation from primary malignancy and infectious process can be accomplished readily and with confidence. Interpretative problems can arise, however, in the presence of a cytological picture of adenocarcinoma. As mentioned above, a reliable distinction between primary and metastatic adenocarcinoma is totally based upon the immunohistochemical survey. The adjunctive use of immunohistochemistry may also allow identification of the tissue of origin of the metastatic malignancy.

TTF-1 is currently the most reliable marker of the pulmonary origin of adenocarcinoma but it is essential to remember that, in FNB samples, follicular carcinoma of the thyroid metastatic to the lung may simulate a tumor of glandular cell morphology, tubulo-acinar pattern, and is strongly positive for this marker.

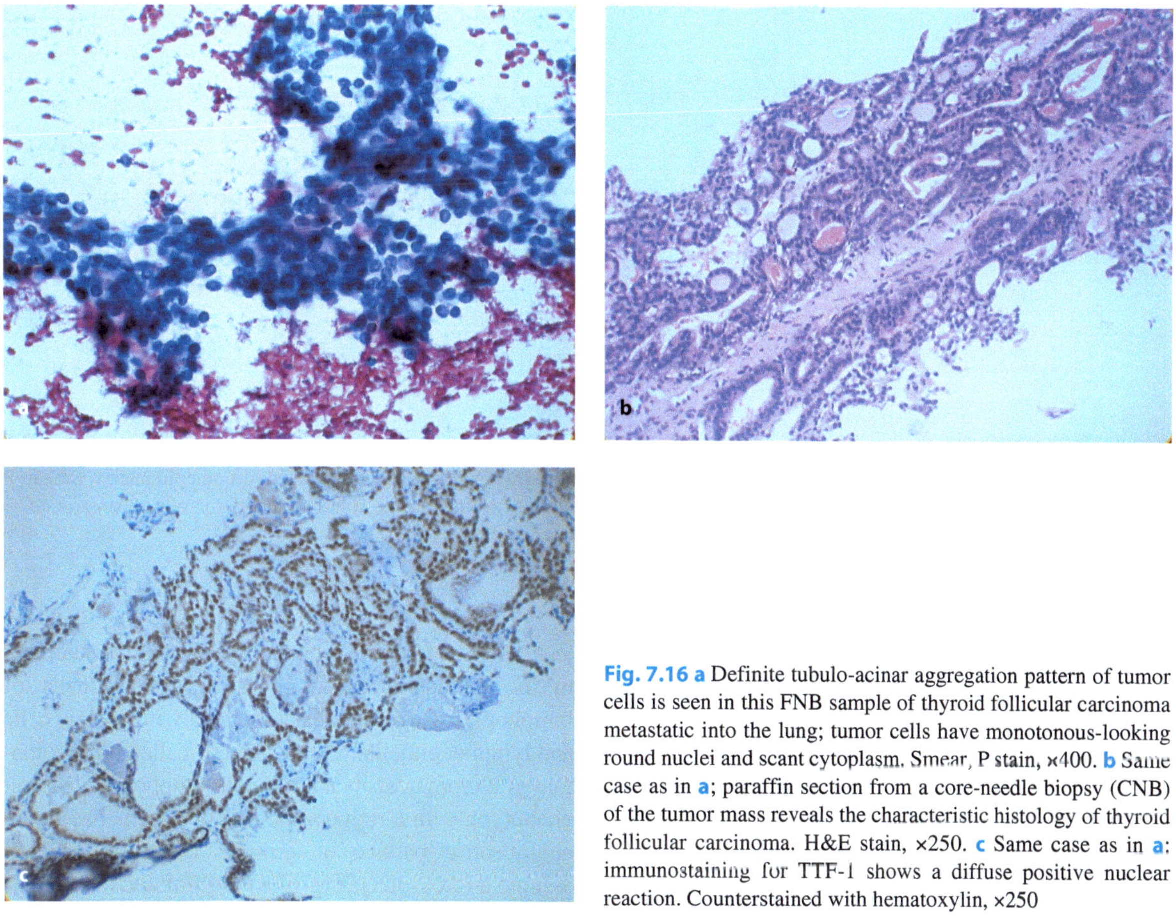

Fig. 7.16 a Definite tubulo-acinar aggregation pattern of tumor cells is seen in this FNB sample of thyroid follicular carcinoma metastatic into the lung; tumor cells have monotonous-looking round nuclei and scant cytoplasm. Smear, P stain, ×400. b Same case as in a; paraffin section from a core-needle biopsy (CNB) of the tumor mass reveals the characteristic histology of thyroid follicular carcinoma. H&E stain, ×250. c Same case as in a; immunostaining for TTF-1 shows a diffuse positive nuclear reaction. Counterstained with hematoxylin, ×250

Figure 7.16 illustrates a case featuring this peculiar cytomorphology and immunohistochemical reactivity, as demonstrated in a core-needle biopsy (CNB) sample.

7.2.11 Benign Lesions

7.2.11.1 Hamartoma

Pulmonary hamartomas are neoplastic mixtures of mature mesenchymal tissue elements normally found within the lung (cartilage, fibrovascular tissue, adipose tissue, smooth muscle, and bone). The lesion is most frequently localized peripherally. Due to its characteristic features (inert or indolently expansive homogeneous opacity), pulmonary hamartoma is readily diagnosed on X-rays and CT scan. However, when it is composed of an undifferentiated mesenchymal fibromyxoid component, the appearance may be interpreted as indeterminate for malignancy. FNB samples show fibromyxoid stromal fragments embedded in a mucoid matrix (Fig. 7.17) in addition to adipocytes and normal bronchial cells. Cartilage fragments are rarely detected. The cytological diagnosis is easily made in about 75% of the cases. In the remaining 25%, pulmonary hamartoma is a common source of false-positive diagnoses and it can be confused with carcinoid tumor and bronchioloalveolar carcinoma [62]. The latter enters the differential diagnosis when there is a concomitant proliferation of bronchiolar epithelium possibly containing nuclear vacuoles.

7.2.11.2 Inflammatory Conditions

These may present on imaging as a coin lesion and include nonspecific pulmonary abscess and granulomatous inflammation. Aspiration biopsy can

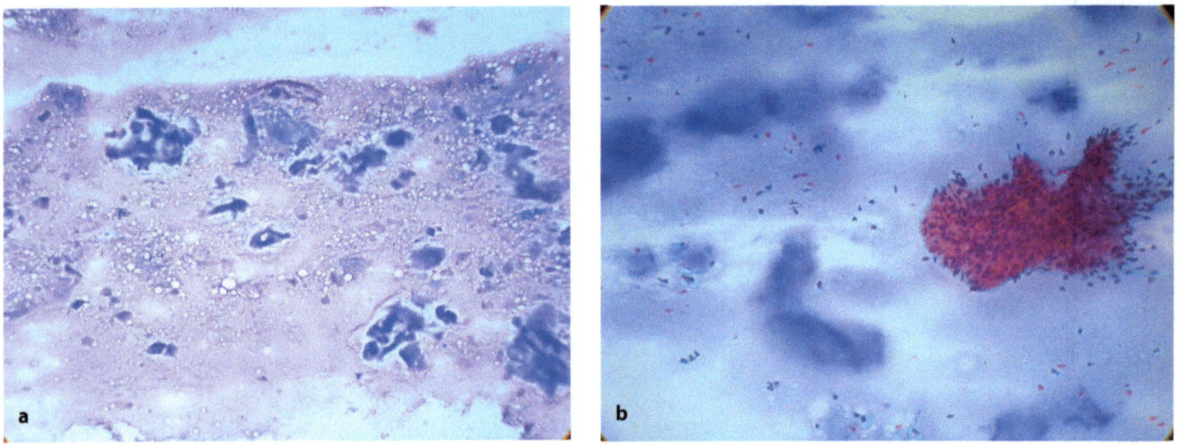

Fig. 7.17 a FNB sample from pulmonary hamartoma shows fibromyxoid stromal fragments dispersed in a mucoid matrix. Smear, P stain, ×250. **b** A cohesive aggregate of regularly shaped and monotonous fibrocyte-like spindle cells is seen in a background of mucoid matrix. FNB sample from pulmonary hamartoma; smear, P stain, ×250

successfully isolate specific etiological agents of infection for morphological and cultural identification, resulting in the selection of appropriate therapy, the avoidance of an incorrect diagnosis of cancer, and circumvention of surgery. Granulomatous inflammation is easily diagnosed by detecting epithelioid histiocytes in cohesive clusters, lymphocytes, a variable amount of granular, mucoid, or amorphous necrotic debris, and multinucleate giant cells. It is worth noting that squamous cell carcinoma can undergo massive cavitation with subsequent colonization by *Aspergillus* species and aspergilloma formation.

7.2.12 Rare Tumors

There is a relatively long list of unusual tumor entities occurring in the lung which thus far have been poorly investigated by FNB sampling; in fact, their cytological features are described in only few single case reports in the literature. This group includes epithelial tumors, such as acinic cell carcinoma and mucoepidermoid carcinoma, biphasic tumors (carcinosarcoma and pulmonary blastoma), tumors of uncertain histogenesis (sclerosing hemangioma, clear cell "sugar" tumor), some lymphoproliferative disorders, malignant melanoma, and unusual varieties of sarcoma.

Primary lymphoproliferative disorders of the lung are typically seen in the elderly, are mostly of the B-cell phenotype, and poorly aggressive. The pulmonary lesion is frequently associated with nodal involvement in the mediastinum. Proliferating cells consist of lymphoplasmacytoid cells associated with plasma cells and lymphoepithelial lesions. The so-called lymphomatoid granulomatosis is a large-cell lymphoma of B-cell phenotype with a rich component of T-cells having an angiocentric pattern of growth. Large cells often assume a Reed-Sternberg-like morphology.

Sarcomas developing primarily in the lung are exceptionally rare. Pleuropulmonary synovial sarcoma is increasingly recognized as a subtype of sarcoma, due to the recent identification of a distinctive chromosomal translocation specific to synovial sarcoma [63]. Figure 7.18 illustrates the cytological features of one such case in a 36-year-old woman who presented with a huge, sharply marginated tumor mass in the right lung. The cytological picture was prototypical of tumors with epithelioid or spindle cell morphology and illustrates the issue of the differential diagnosis of tumors arising within the chest. The harvest was very cellular, with large cohesive tissue clusters containing spindled to epithelioid cells; their nuclei were ovoid to elongated with a finely granular chromatin and small nucleoli. Immunohistochemistry performed on the cell-block sample demonstrated cellular positivity for EMA, bcl-2, CD56, and CD99, with negative expression of cytokeratins, CD34, S100 protein, and calretinin. The conclusive diagnosis of monophasic synovial sarcoma was based on the demonstration of the t(x;18) chromosomal

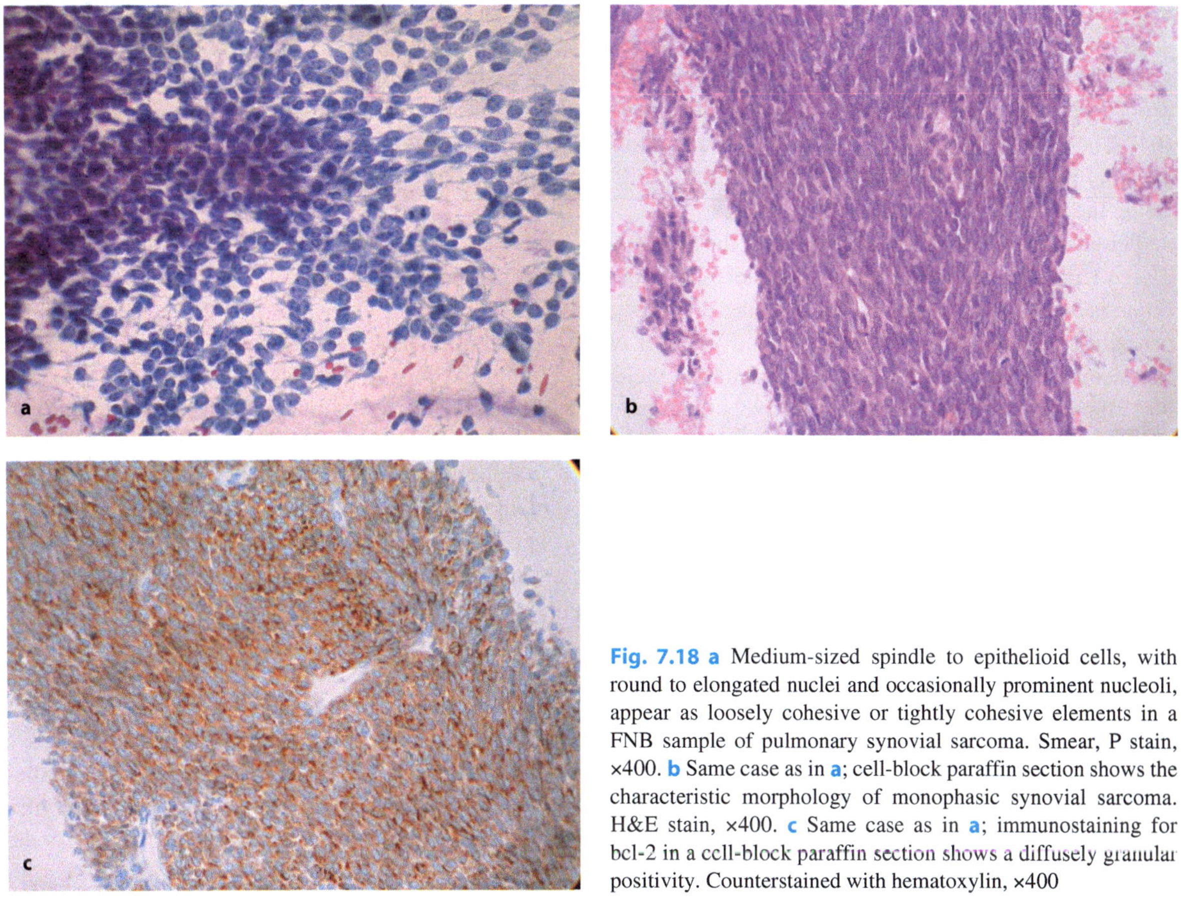

Fig. 7.18 a Medium-sized spindle to epithelioid cells, with round to elongated nuclei and occasionally prominent nucleoli, appear as loosely cohesive or tightly cohesive elements in a FNB sample of pulmonary synovial sarcoma. Smear, P stain, ×400. b Same case as in a; cell-block paraffin section shows the characteristic morphology of monophasic synovial sarcoma. H&E stain, ×400. c Same case as in a; immunostaining for bcl-2 in a cell-block paraffin section shows a diffusely granular positivity. Counterstained with hematoxylin, ×400

translocation by fluorescence in situ hybridization on cell-block material [63].

7.3 Mediastinum

Mediastinal lesions can be investigated by FNB, which in these cases is a safe, efficacious, and cost-effective technique. Patients tolerate the procedure well and there are no serious complications resulting from percutaneous tissue penetration of the needle when the procedure is carried out under CT scan or US guidance. A broad range of lesions can be detected within this anatomic compartment. Proper correlation with the patient's age and the location of the lesion within the mediastinal compartments are helpful in anticipating the possible diagnosis. In particular, lesions of the anterior mediastinum are likely to be thymoma, thymic cysts, lymphoma, thyroid lesions, or germ-cell tumors. Those in the middle mediastinum are frequently lymphoma or benign pericardial and bronchogenic cysts, while those in the posterior mediastinum are nerve sheath or neuronal tumors or bronchogenic or enteric cysts.

Metastatic disease is, however, the most frequent malignancy identified in the mediastinum. In particular settings, for example, in patients with non-small-cell lung cancers, the detection of mediastinal lymph node metastases is a crucial determinant of operability. CT-scan-assisted percutaneous fine-needle aspiration (FNA) is not the procedure of choice for such studies, and transbronchial needle aspiration is of poor accuracy due to its low sensitivity. Mediastinoscopy used to be the "gold standard" for determining the presence of nodal metastases in the mediastinum, until recently, when significant advances were made in alternative procedures based on the same principles as FNA but with different access. Lesions adjacent to the gastrointestinal tract are sampled by endoscopic ultrasound FNA biopsy while lesions along the more distal endobronchial wall are easily accessed and sampled by endobronchial US-guided FNA biopsy. The combination of the two procedures is a valid substitute for mediastinoscopy [64]. These procedures employ 22G needles and allow a highly representative sample to be obtained, facilitating the correct diagnosis.

Percutaneous FNB is well-accepted in the management of primary mediastinal malignancies. The technique is used after imaging as the first-line diagnostic procedure and, when possible, is coupled to CNB of the lesion in order to maximize the diagnostic yield. Not all primary tumors can be conclusively diagnosed using this approach, and mediastinoscopy or open thoracomy is still needed in a minority of cases. Powers et al., 1996 [65], carried out a large multi-institutional study on the diagnostic accuracy of percutaneous FNB of the mediastinum. They determined a sensitivity of 87% and a positive predictive value of 97% for the diagnosis of neoplasm.

7.3.1 *Tumors of the Thymus*

Thymic epithelial tumors have been traditionally classified into two main types: thymoma, which may be encapsulated or invasive and is histologically benign, and thymic carcinoma, which comprises a heterogeneous group of neoplasms that are histologically malignant. The prognosis of patients with thymomas varies considerably and several classifications have been proposed for these tumors. In 1999, the World Health Organization (WHO) proposed a consensus classification of thymic epithelial tumors [66]. This classification takes into account the morphology of the epithelial cells as well as the ratio of epithelial cells to lymphocytes. It was recently demonstrated that the WHO histological classification reflects the oncological behavior of thymoma, thus confirming the validity of this classification system for the assessment and treatment of patients with thymoma [67].

7.3.1.1 Thymoma

The WHO classification distinguishes six types: A, AB, B1, B2, B3, and C [66]. Types A, AB, and B1 have a less aggressive nature than types B2 and B3. Some variants are strongly associated with autoimmune disease but others are not. In our experience, FNB is not useful in the preoperative prediction of WHO histological types unless anaplasia is observed, but it is an invaluable method to confirm the diagnosis within the correct clinical-radiological context.

Cytomorphology

- Polymorphous population of non-cohesive lymphoid cells in the background (Fig. 7.19a).
- Cohesive tissue fragments consisting of oval to spindle epithelial cells intimately admixed with lymphoid cells (Fig. 7.19b).
- Epithelial cells possibly dominating the picture and appearing as aggregates of medium-sized oval to spindle-shaped elements (Fig. 7.19d).

Basically, the FNB appearance of thymoma is represented by a spectrum of lesions composed of a dual population of epithelial cells and lymphoid cells, which are variably admixed. At one end, there is a significant prevalence of lymphoid cells, with epithelial cells being barely perceptible (thymomas types AB, B1, B2 according to the WHO criteria). At the other end, lymphoid cells are poorly represented, with epithelial cells dominating the picture (thymoma type A) and possibly characterized by atypical features (thymoma type B3) [68,69]. Epithelial cells can be properly demonstrated by immunohistochemistry in cytological cell-block material based on their positivity for cytokeratins (Fig. 7.19c–e). Additional features are positivity for CD57 (thymoma B2 type), and CD5 and bcl-2 (thymoma type B3) [70]. The lymphoid cell component shows a B-cell phenotype and is CD20+.

7.3.1.2 Thymic Carcinoma

Thymic carcinoma (also known as type C thymoma) is a thymic epithelial tumor that exhibits a definite cytological atypia and a set of histological features non-specific to the thymus but rather similar to those observed in carcinomas of other organs. Variants include squamous cell, lymphoepithelioma, sarcomatoid, clear cell, mucoepidermoid, papillary, and undifferentiated tumors. Of note, the papillary adenocarcinoma variant can simulate mesothelioma

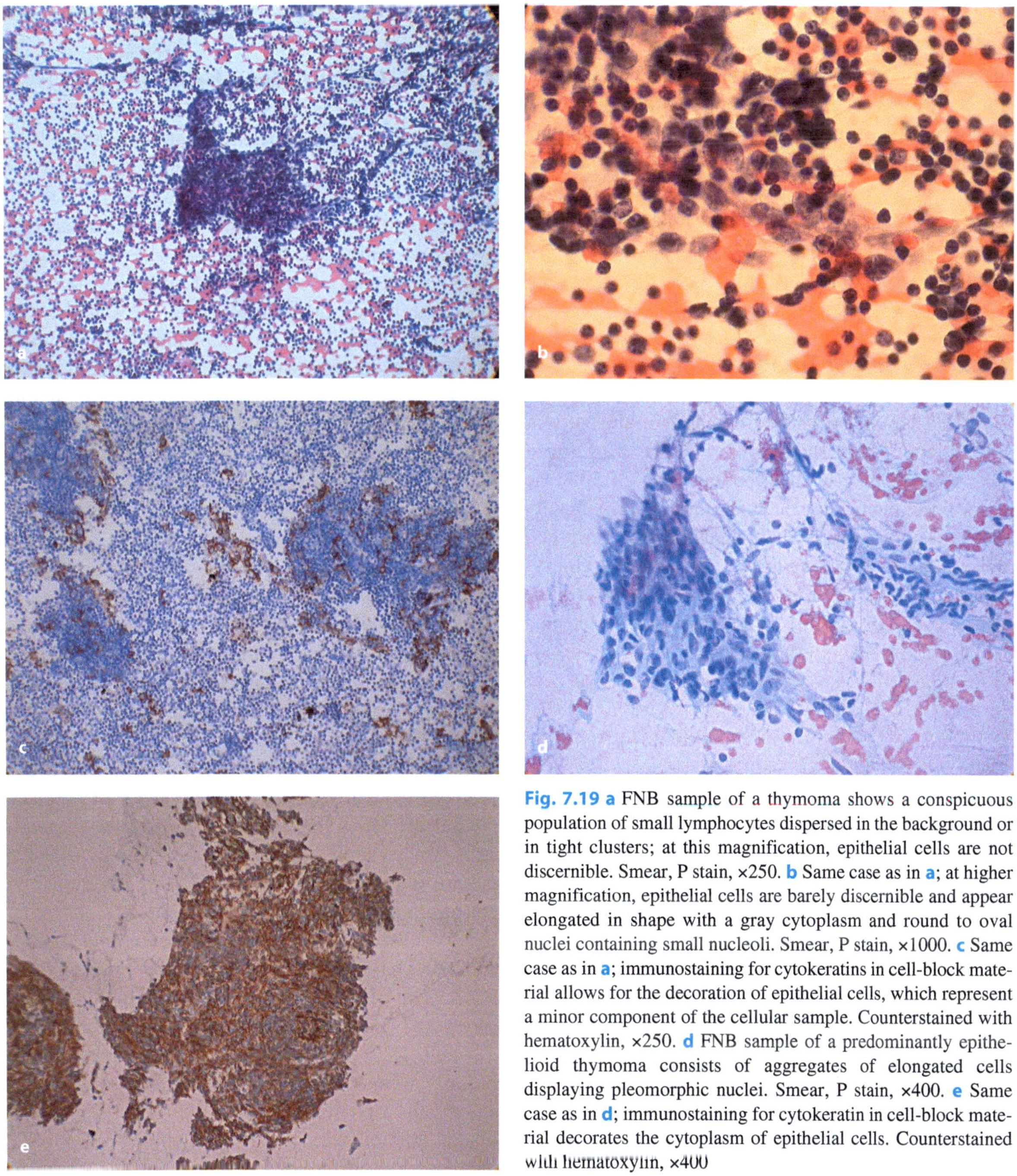

Fig. 7.19 a FNB sample of a thymoma shows a conspicuous population of small lymphocytes dispersed in the background or in tight clusters; at this magnification, epithelial cells are not discernible. Smear, P stain, ×250. b Same case as in a; at higher magnification, epithelial cells are barely discernible and appear elongated in shape with a gray cytoplasm and round to oval nuclei containing small nucleoli. Smear, P stain, ×1000. c Same case as in a; immunostaining for cytokeratins in cell-block material allows for the decoration of epithelial cells, which represent a minor component of the cellular sample. Counterstained with hematoxylin, ×250. d FNB sample of a predominantly epithelioid thymoma consists of aggregates of elongated cells displaying pleomorphic nuclei. Smear, P stain, ×400. e Same case as in d; immunostaining for cytokeratin in cell-block material decorates the cytoplasm of epithelial cells. Counterstained with hematoxylin, ×400

cytomorphologically. Indeed, in about 30% of patients the tumor cells show immunohistochemical expression of calretinin and other mesothelioma markers, which represents a potential trap in a correct differential diagnosis [71].

7.3.1.3 Neuroendocrine Tumors

The thymus can harbor typical and atypical carcinoid tumors as well as poorly differentiated small-cell carcinoma. These are very rare tumors. Upon FNB, carcinoid tumors display a uniform population of small round cells with central or slightly eccentric nucleoli. Nuclei dominate the cell and are conspicuous in their conformity of pattern or structure. Moderately and poorly differentiated neuroendocrine carcinoma primaries in the thymus are characterized by a more pleomorphic cellular population. In a series of three cases, we were able to demonstrate cytoplasmic button-like structures by May Grünwald-Giemsa staining (Fig. 7.20) [72].

7.3.2 Germ-Cell Tumors

Germ cell tumors occur predominantly in the anterior mediastinum and affect young adults, with most tumors developing in male patients. About 50% the tumors are mature cystic teratomas, approximately 18% are seminomas, 23% malignant mixed germ-cell tumors, and <10% immature teratoma or pure embryonal carcinoma [73]. The FNB diagnostic criteria are the same as those for the same tumors when detected in gonadal and extragonadal sites.

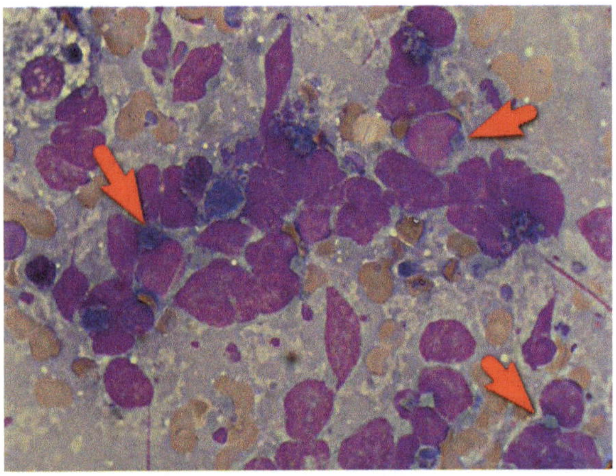

Fig. 7.20 FNB sample of a poorly differentiated neuroendocrine carcinoma growing primarily within the anterosuperior mediastinum; in May Grünwald Giemsa stained smears some characteristic button like inclusion bodies are seen within the cytoplasm of tumor cells (*arrows*). ×1000.

7.4 Pleura and Chest Wall

7.4.1 Malignant Mesothelioma

Mesothelioma is an aggressive malignancy that typically presents with pleural effusion due to diffuse involvement of the visceral and parietal surfaces of the pleura. Rarely, onset of the tumor is characterized by a concomitant solid nodule. The diagnosis is almost universally accomplished by cytopathological examination of the pleural fluid. In some cases, however, there is a mild pleural effusion and concomitant solid growth into the mediastinum and/or the chest wall, clinically and radiologically simulating a metastatic carcinoma. These nodular lesions are potential targets for FNB investigation [74,75]; often the likelihood of a solid-type malignant mesothelioma is underestimated in the differential diagnosis. In addition, FNB is recognized as a reliable method to diagnose recurrent malignant mesothelioma at the site of previous surgery, or metastatic mesothelioma in lymph nodes or the liver [76–78]. There are three main types of malignant mesothelioma cells: epithelioid, spindle/sarcomatoid, and mixed/biphasic. Epithelioid is the most common, accounting for 50–70% of cases. Figure 7.21 illustrates the FNB diagnostic yield of a solid and multinodular mediastinal tumor in a 59-year-old woman with a previous history of repeated pleural effusions that had been diagnosed cytologically as "mesothelial hyperplasia." The cytological picture is prototypical of tumors with an epithelioid cell morphology. Immunohistochemically, mesothelioma cells express CK7, calretinin, and CK5/6 and are characterized by membrane positivity for EMA. The distinction between pleural-based adenocarcinoma and mesothelioma may be an inordinately difficult decision when based on FNB material, especially when the harvest is dominated by papillary aggregates of small uniform polygonal cells with bland, monotonous nuclei containing prominent nucleoli. The differential diagnosis in this setting is based upon the results of the immunohistochemical survey, including the lack of calretinin positivity in adenocarcinoma cells and the detection of TTF-1 nuclear positivity, which demonstrates their derivation from the bronchial epithelium.

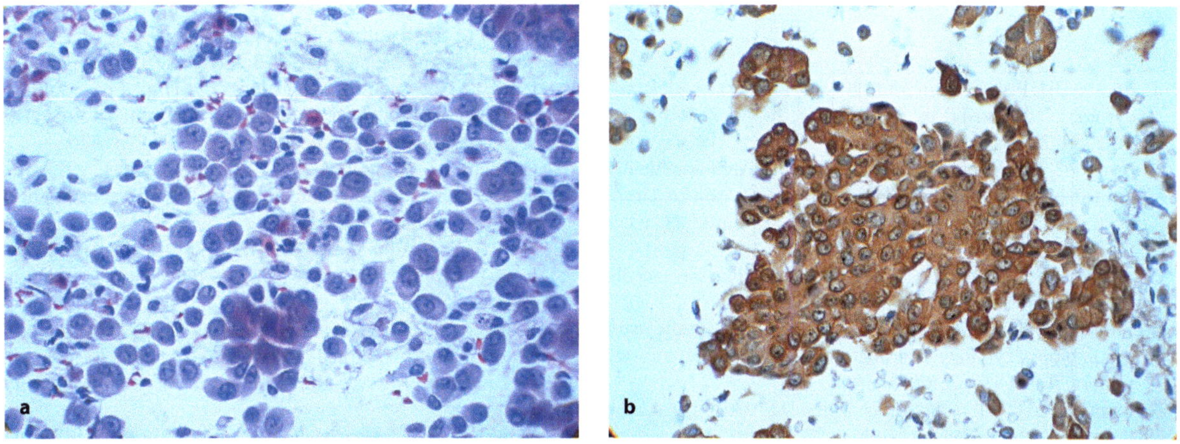

Fig. 7.21 a FNB sample collected from a solid multinodular mass growing into the anterior mediastinum and associated with pleural effusion. The smear consists of a population of large epithelioid cells with round nuclei and prominent nucleoli and seen in microacinar clusters or as non-cohesive elements. P stain, ×400. **b** Same case as in **a**; positive immunostaining for calretinin in cell-block material provides conclusive evidence of the mesothelial origin of the tumor cells. Counterstained with hematoxylin, ×400

7.4.2 Solitary Fibrous Tumor

Solitary fibrous tumor is the most common mesenchymal tumor of the pleura [79]. It is seen in adult patients, with a prevalence in the fifth and sixth decades of life. The patients are generally asymptomatic. On imaging, the tumor is usually well delimited, polypoid, and apparently encapsulated, and can appear to be attached to the pleura by means of a short pedicle. Histologically, solitary fibrous tumors are characterized by a variegated appearance due to the variable expression of a solid spindle cell component and a diffuse sclerosing component. The former can assume a fibrohistiocytic, hemangiopericytic, angiofibromatous, or neuroid appearance, often leading to misdiagnosis with other soft-tissue tumors. The cytological picture of this tumor in FNB samples has been studied in no more than 20 patients. In most cases, the diagnosis was reported as inconclusive [80]. In highly cellular tumors, smears show oval to spindle cells found in irregular three-dimensional aggregates (Fig. 7.22) or as loosely cohesive or isolated elements. Within the aggregates, numerous capillary vessels are seen. The definitive diagnosis is obtained by testing the immunohistochemical reactivity of these cells in cell-block material. They show the CD34+/bcl-2+/CD99+ profile and lack the expression of cytokeratin, EMA, S100P, and smooth muscle actin [81]. These features help differentiate solitary fibrous tumor from other spindle cell tumors, mainly malignant mesothelioma, spindle cell thymoma, and smooth muscle tumors. No more than 10% of the tumors behave aggressively. There is no chance of predicting malignancy by FNB cytological findings.

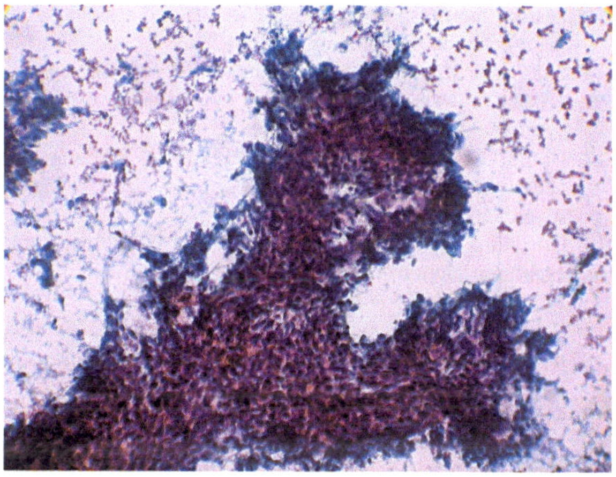

Fig. 7.22 FNB sample from a pleural-based soft-tissue tumor diagnosed as solitary fibrous tumor; the harvest consists of tight clusters of fibrocyte-like spindle cells arranged in a vorticoid pattern. Smear, P stain, ×400

References

1. Stanley JH, Fish GD, Andriole JG et al (1987) Lung lesions: cytologic diagnosis by fine-needle biopsy. Radiology 162:389–391.
2. Yang PC, Lee YC, Yu CJ, et al (1992) Ultrasonographically guided biopsy of thoracic tumors: a comparison of large-bore cutting biopsy with fine-needle aspiration. Cancer 69:2553–2560.
3. Allison DJ, Hemingway AP (1981) Percutaneous needle biopsy of the lung. BMJ 282:875–878.
4. Pilotti S, Rilke F, Gribaudi G et al (1982) Fine needle aspiration biopsy cytology of primary and metastatic pulmonary tumors. Acta Cytol 26:661–666.
5. Samuelsson L, Albrechtsson U, Tylen U (1982) Fine-needle biopsy of chest lesions. Radiologe 22:93–496.
6. Calhoun P, Feldman PS, Armstrong P et al (1986) The clinical outcome of needle aspirations of the lung when cancer is not diagnosed. Ann Thorac Surg 41:592–596.
7. Knudsen DU, Nielsen SM, Hariri J et al (1996) Ultrasonographically guided fine-needle aspiration biopsy of intrathoracic tumors. Acta Radiol 37:327–331.
8. Grode G, Faurschou P, Milman, N (1993) Percutaneous transthoracic fine-needle lung biopsy with 3 different needles: a retrospective study of results and complications in 224 patients. Respiration 60:284–288.
9. Zakowski MF, Gatscha RM, Zaman MB (1992) Negative predictive value of pulmonary fine needle aspiration cytology. Acta Cytol 36:283–286.
10. Collins CD, Breatnach E, Nath PH (1992) Percutaneous needle biopsy of lung nodules following failed bronchoscopic biopsy. Eur J Radiol 15:49–53.
11. Cristallini EG, Ascani S, Farabi R et al (1992) Fine needle aspiration biopsy in the diagnosis of intrathoracic masses. Acta Cytol 36:416–422.
12. Veale D, Gilmartin JJ, Sumerling MD et al (1988) Prospective evaluation of fine needle aspiration in the diagnosis of lung cancer. Thorax 43:540–544.
13. Milman N, Faurschou P, Grode G (1995) Diagnostic yield of transthoracic needle aspiration biopsy following negative fiberoptic bronchoscopy in 103 patients with peripheral circumscribed pulmonary lesions. Respiration 62:1–3.
14. Gasparini S, Ferretti M, Secchi EB et al (1995) Integration of transbronchial and percutaneous approach in the diagnosis of peripheral pulmonary nodules or masses: experience with 1,027 consecutive cases. Chest 108:131–137.
15, Böcking A, Klose KC, Kyll HJ et al (1995) Cytologic vs histologic evaluation of needle biopsy of the lung, hilum and mediastinum: sensitivity, specificity and typing accuracy. Acta Cytol 39:463–471.
16. Simpson RW, Johnson DA, Wold LE et al (1988) Transthoracic needle aspiration biopsy: review of 233 cases. Acta Cytol 32:101–104.
17. Klein JS, Salomon G, Stewart EA (1996) Transthoracic needle biopsy with a coaxially placed 20-gauge automated cutting needle: results in 122 patients. Radiology 198:715–720.
18. Yankelevitz DF, Henschke CI, Koizumi JH et al (1997) CT-guided transthoracic needle biopsy of small solitary pulmonary nodules. Clin Imaging 21:107–110.
19. Westcott JL, Rao N, Colley DP (1997) Transthoracic needle biopsy of small pulmonary nodules. Radiology 202:97–103.
20. Santambrogio L, Nosotti M, Bellaviti N et al (1997) CT-guided fine-needle aspiration cytology of solitary pulmonary nodules: a prospective, randomized study of immediate cytologic evaluation. Chest 112:423–425.
21. Cattelani L, Campodonico F, Rusca M et al (1997) CT-guided transthoracic needle biopsy in the diagnosis of chest tumours. J Cardiovasc Surg (Torino) 38:539–542.
22. Balslov S, Vestbo J, Viskum KA (1988) Value of Tru-cut lung biopsy in focal and diffuse lung disease. Thorax 43:147–150.
23. Weisbrod GL, Herman SJ, Tao LC (1987) Preliminary experience with a dual cutting edge needle in thoracic percutaneous fine-needle aspiration biopsy. Radiology 163:75–78.
24. Swischuk JL, Castaneda F, Patel JC et al (1998) Percutaneous transthoracic needle biopsy of the lung: review of 612 lesions. J Vasc Interv Radiol 9:347–352.
25. Winning AJ, McIvor J, Seed WA et al (1986) Interpretation of negative results in fine needle aspiration of discrete pulmonary lesions. Thorax 41:875–879.
26. Laurent F, Latrabe V, Vergier B et al (2000) CT-guided transthoracic needle biopsy of pulmonary nodules smaller than 20 mm: results with an automated 20-gauge coaxial cutting needle. Clin Radiol 55:281–287.
27. Nahman BJ, Van Aman ME, McLemore WE et al (1985) Use of the Rotex needle in percutaneous biopsy of pulmonary malignancy. AJR Am J Roentgenol 145:97–99.
28. Charig MJ, Phillips AJ (2000) CT-guided cutting needle biopsy of lung lesions: safety and efficacy of an out-patient service. Clin Radiol 55:964–969.
29. Greene R, Szyfelbein WM, Isler RJ et al (1985) Supplementary tissue-core histology from fine-needle transthoracic aspiration biopsy. AJR Am J Roentgenol 144:787–792.
30. Johnson RD, Gobien RP, Valicenti JF Jr (1983) Current status of radiologically directed pulmonary thin needle aspiration biopsy: an analysis of 200 consecutive biopsies and review of the literature. Ann Clin Lab Sci 13:225–239.
31. Geraghty PR, Kee ST, McFarlane G et al (2003) CT-guided transthoracic needle aspiration biopsy of pulmonary nodules: needle size and pneumothorax rate. Radiology 229:475–481.
32. Schreiber G, McCrory DC (2003) Performance characteristics of different modalities for diagnosis of suspected lung cancer: summary of published evidence. Chest 123: 115S–128S.
33. Rivera MP, Mehta AC (2007) American College of Chest Physicians. Initial diagnosis of lung cancer: ACCP evidence-based clinical practice guidelines (2nd edition). Chest 132:131S–148S.
34. Smolle-Juettner FM, Woltsche M, Roeger G et al (1996) Is preoperative percutaneous fine-needle aspiration cytology of intrathoracic lesions advisable in resectable patients? Eur J Cardiothorac Surg 10:1047–1050.
35. Libby DM, Smith JP, Altorki NK et al (2004) Managing the small pulmonary nodule discovered by CT. Chest 125:1522–1529.
36. Greif J, Marmur S, Schwarz Y, Man A, Staroselsky AN. Percutaneous core cutting needle biopsy compared with fine-needle aspiration in the diagnosis of peripheral lung

malignant lesions: results in 156 patients. Cancer 1998 84:144–147.

37. Travis WD, Brambilla E, Muller-Hermelink HK, Harris CC (eds) (2004) Pathology and Genetics of Tumours of the Lung, Pleura, Thymus and Heart. IARC Press, Lyon, p 10.
38. Aubry MC (2008) Pulmonary involvement by extrapulmonary neoplasms. In: Zander DS and Farver CF (eds) Pulmonary Pathology. Churchill Livingstone Elsevier, Philadelphia, pp 622–635.
39. Kobashi Y, Matsushima T, Irei T (2005) Clinicopathological analysis of lung cancer resembling malignant pleural mesothelioma. Respirology 10:660–665.
40. Travis WD, Brambilla E, Muller-Hermelink HK et al (eds) (2004) Pathology and Genetics of the Tumours of the Lung, Pleura, Thymus and Heart. World Health Organization Classification of tumours. IARC Press, Lyon.
41. Saleh HA, Haapaniemi J, Khatib G, Sakr W (1998) Bronchioloalveolar carcinoma: diagnostic pitfalls and immunocytochemical contribution. Diagn Cytopathol 18:301–306.
42. Silverman JF, Finley JL, Park HK et al (1985) Fine needle aspiration cytology of bronchioloalveolar-cell carcinoma of the lung. Acta Cytol 29:887–894.
43. Tao LC, Weisbrod GL, Pearson FG et al (1986) Cytologic diagnosis of bronchioloalveolar carcinoma by fine-needle aspiration biopsy. Cancer 57:1565–1570.
44. Chu P, Wu E, Weiss LM (2000) Cytokeratin 7 and cytokeratin 20 expression in epithelial neoplasms: a survey of 435 cases. Mod Pathol 13:962–972.
45. Tot T (2002) Cytokeratins 20 and 7 as biomarkers: usefulness in discriminating primary from metastatic adenocarcinoma. Eur J Cancer 38:758–763.
46. Alì G, Donati V, Loggini B et al (2008) Different estrogen receptor beta expression in distinct histologic subtypes of lung adenocarcinoma. Hum Pathol 39:1465–1473.
47. Maeshima AM, Omatsu M, Tsuta K et al (2008) Immunohistochemical expression of TTF-1 in various cytological subtypes of primary lung adenocarcinoma, with special reference to intratumoral heterogeneity. Pathol Int 58:31–37.
48. Kubba LA, McCluggage WG, Liu J et al (2008) Thyroid transcription factor-1 expression in ovarian epithelial neoplasms. Mod Pathol 21:485–490.
49. Siami K, McCluggage WG, Ordonez NG et al (2007) Thyroid transcription factor-1 expression in endometrial and endocervical adenocarcinomas. Am J Surg Pathol 31:1759–1763.
50. Kargi A, Gurel D, Tuna B (2007) The diagnostic value of TTF-1, CK 5/6, and p63 immunostaining in classification of lung carcinomas. Appl Immunohistochem Mol Morphol 15:415–420.
51. Mazziotta RM, Borczuk AC, Powell CA, Mansukhani M (2005) CDX2 immunostaining as a gastrointestinal marker: expression in lung carcinomas is a potential pitfall. Appl Immunohistochem Mol Morphol 13:55–60.
52. Johansson L (2004) Histopathologic classification of lung cancer: Relevance of cytokeratin and TTF-1 immunophenotyping. Ann Diagn Pathol 8:259–267.
53. Brambilla E, Lantuejoul S (2008) Neuroendocrine neoplasms. In: Zander DS and Farver CF (eds) Pulmonary Pathology. Churchill Livingstone Elsevier, Philadelphia, pp 563–577.
54. Collins BT, Cramer HM (1996) Fine needle aspiration cytology of carcinoid tumors. Acta Cytol 40:695–707.
55. Anderson C, Ludwig ME, O'Donnell M, Garcia N (1990) Fine needle aspiration cytology of pulmonary carcinoid tumors. Acta Cytol 34:505–510.
56. Szyfelbein WM, Ross JS (1988) Carcinoids, atypical carcinoids, and small-cell carcinomas of the lung: differential diagnosis of fine-needle aspiration biopsy specimens. Diagn Cytopathol 4:1–8.
57. Saqi A, Alexis D, Remotti F, Bhagat G.(2005) Usefulness of CDX2 and TTF-1 in differentiating gastrointestinal from pulmonary carcinoids. Am J Clin Pathol 123:394–404.
58. Delgado PI, Jorda M, Ganjei-Azar P (2000) Small cell carcinoma versus other lung malignancies: diagnosis by fine-needle aspiration cytology. Cancer 90:279–285.
59. Gherardi G, Marveggio C (1992) Immunocytochemistry in head and neck aspirates. Diagnostic application on direct smears in 16 problematic cases. Acta Cytol 36:687–696.
60. Cheuk W, Kwan MY, Suster S, Chan JK (2001) Immunostaining for thyroid transcription factor 1 and cytokeratin 20 aids the distinction of small cell carcinoma from Merkel cell carcinoma, but not pulmonary from extrapulmonary small cell carcinomas. Arch Pathol Lab Med 125:228–231.
61. Wiatrowska BA, Krol J, Zakowski MF (2001) Large-cell neuroendocrine carcinoma of the lung: proposed criteria for cytologic diagnosis. Diagn Cytopathol 24:58–64.
62. Hughes JH, Young NA, Wilbur DC et al (2005) Fine-needle aspiration of pulmonary hamartoma: a common source of false-positive diagnoses in the College of American Pathologists Interlaboratory Comparison Program in Nongynecologic Cytology. Arch Pathol Lab Med 129:19–22.
63. Mirzoyan M, Muslimani A, Setrakian S et al (2008) Primary pleuropulmonary synovial sarcoma. Clin Lung Cancer 9:257–261.
64. Wallace MB, Pascual JM, Raimondo M et al (2008) Minimally invasive endoscopic staging of suspected lung cancer. JAMA 299:540–546.
65. Powers CN, Silverman JF, Geisinger KR, Frable WJ (1996) Fine-needle aspiration biopsy of the mediastinum. A multi-institutional analysis. Am J Clin Pathol 105:168–173.
66. Rosai J (1999) Histological typing of tumors of the thymus. World Health Organization International Histological Classification of Tumors. 2nd Ed. Springer-Verlag, New York, Berlin.
67. Okumura M, Shiono H, Inoue M et al (2007) Outcome of surgical treatment for recurrent thymic epithelial tumors with reference to World Health Organization histologic classification system. J Surg Oncol 95:40–44.
68. Wakely PE Jr. (2008) Fine needle aspiration in the diagnosis of thymic epithelial neoplasms. Hematol Oncol Clin North Am 22:433–442.
69. Chieng DC, Rose D, Ludwig ME, Zakowski MF (2000) Cytology of thymomas: emphasis on morphology and correlation with histologic subtypes. Cancer 90:24–32.
70. Alexiev BA, Drachenberg CB, Burke AP (2007) Thymomas: a cytological and immunohistochemical study, with emphasis on lymphoid and neuroendocrine markers. Diagn Pathol 2:13.
71. Pan CC, Chen PC, Chou TY, Chiang H (2003) Expression of calretinin and other mesothelioma-related markers in thymic carcinoma and thymoma. Hum Pathol 4:1155–1162.

72. Gherardi G, Marveggio C, Placidi A (1995) Neuroendocrine carcinoma of the thymus: aspiration biopsy, immunocytochemistry, and clinicopathologic correlates. Diagn Cytopathol 12:158–164.
73. Rosai J (2004) Mediastinum. In: Rosai J (ed) Ackerman's surgical pathology, vol I, 9th edn. Mosby, New York.
74. Yu GH, Soma L, Hahn S, Friedberg JS (2001) Changing clinical course of patients with malignant mesothelioma: implications for FNA cytology and utility of immunocytochemical staining. Diagn Cytopathol 24:322–327.
75. Kapur U, Wojcik EM (2007) Fine-needle aspiration of malignant mesothelioma with unusual morphologic features: a case report. Diagn Cytopathol 35:174–178.
76. Pappa L, Machera M, Tsanou E et al (2006) Subcutaneous metastasis of peritoneal mesothelioma diagnosed by fine-needle aspiration. Pathol Oncol Res 12:247–250.
77. Cimbaluk D, Kasuganti D, Kluskens L (2006) Malignant biphasic pleural mesothelioma metastatic to the liver diagnosed by fine-needle aspiration. Diagn Cytopathol 34:33–36.
78. Tafazzoli A, Raza A, Martin SE (2005) Primary diagnosis of malignant mesothelioma by fine-needle aspiration of a supraclavicular lymph node. Diagn Cytopathol 33:122–125.
79. Ali SZ, Hoon V, Hoda S et al (1997). Solitary fibrous tumor. A cytologic-histologic study with clinical, radiologic, and immunohistochemical correlations. Cancer 81:116–121.
80. Cho EY, Han JJ, Han J, Oh YL (2007) Fine needle aspiration cytology of solitary fibrous tumours of the pleura. Cytopathology 18:20–27.
81. Liu CC, Wang HW, Li FY, Hsu PK et al (2008) Solitary fibrous tumors of the pleura: clinicopathological characteristics, immunohistochemical profiles, and surgical outcomes with long-term follow-up. Thorac Cardiovasc Surg 56:291–297.

Subject Index

A

B

C

D

E

F

G

H

I

S

T

U

V

W

Y

Z

Printed in July 2009

MIX
Papier aus verantwortungsvollen Quellen
Paper from responsible sources
FSC® C105338

If you have any concerns about our products,
you can contact us on
ProductSafety@springernature.com

In case Publisher is established outside the EU,
the EU authorized representative is:
Springer Nature Customer Service Center GmbH
Europaplatz 3, 69115 Heidelberg, Germany

Printed by Libri Plureos GmbH
in Hamburg, Germany